Pediatric Endocrinology

Guest Editor

ROBERT RAPAPORT, MD

PEDIATRIC CLINICS OF NORTH AMERICA

www.pediatric.theclinics.com

October 2011 • Volume 58 • Number 5

SAUNDERS an imprint of ELSEVIER, Inc.

W.B. SAUNDERS COMPANY
A Division of Elsevier Inc.

1600 John F. Kennedy Boulevard ● Suite 1800 ● Philadelphia, Pennsylvania 19103-2899

http://www.theclinics.com

THE PEDIATRIC CLINICS OF NORTH AMERICA Volume 58, Number 5
October 2011 ISSN 0031-3955, ISBN-13: 978-1-4557-1186-4

Editor: Kerry Holland

The Pediatric Clinics of North America (ISSN 0031-3955) is published bimonthly by Elsevier Inc., 360 Park Avenue South, New York, NY 10010-1710. Months of issue are February, April, June, August, October, and December. Periodicals postage paid at New York, NY and additional mailing offices. Subscription prices are $179.00 per year (US individuals), $423.00 per year (US institutions), $243.00 per year (Canadian individuals), $563.00 per year (Canadian institutions), $289.00 per year (international individuals), $563.00 per year (international institutions), $87.00 per year (US students and residents), and $149.00 per year (international and Canadian residents and students). To receive students/resident rare, orders must be accompanied by name of affiliated institution, date of term, and the signature of program/residency coordinator on institution letterhead. Orders will be billed at individual rate until proof of status is received. Foreign air speed delivery is included in all *Clinics* subscription prices. All prices are subject to change without notice. **POSTMASTER:** Send address changes to *The Pediatric Clinics of North America*, Elsevier Health Sciences Division, Subscription Customer Service, 3251 Riverport Lane, Maryland Heights, MO 63043. **Customer Service: 1-800-654-2452 (US and Canada). From outside of the US and Canada: 1-314-447-8871. Fax: 1-314-447-8029. For print support, E-mail: JournalsCustomerService-usa@elsevier.com. For online support, E-mail: JournalsOnlineSupport-usa@elsevier.com.**

Reprints. For copies of 100 or more, of articles in this publication, please contact the Commercial Reprints Department, Elsevier Inc., 360 Park Avenue South, New York, NY 10010-1710. Tel.: 212-633-3812; Fax: 212-462-1935; E-mail: reprints@elsevier.com.

The Pediatric Clinics of North America is also published in Spanish by McGraw-Hill Inter-americana Editores S.A., Mexico City, Mexico; in Portuguese by Riechmann and Affonso Editores, Rua Comandante Coelho 1085, CEP 21250, Rio de Janeiro, Brazil; and in Greek by Althayia SA, Athens, Greece.

The Pediatric Clinics of North America is covered in *MEDLINE/PubMed (Index Medicus), Excerpta Medica, Current Contents, Current Contents/Clinical Medicine, Science Citation Index, ASCA, ISI/BIOMED,* and *BIOSIS.*

Printed and bound by CPI Group (UK) Ltd, Croydon, CR0 4YY

Transferred to Digital Print 2011

GOAL STATEMENT

The goal of the *Pediatric Clinics of North America* is to keep practicing physicians and residents up to date with current clinical practice in pediatrics by providing timely articles reviewing the state-of-the-art in patient care.

ACCREDITATION

The *Pediatric Clinics of North America* is planned and implemented in accordance with the Essential Areas and Policies of the Accreditation Council for Continuing Medical Education (ACCME) through the joint sponsorship of the University Of Virginia School Of Medicine and Elsevier. The University Of Virginia School of Medicine is accredited by the ACCME to provide continuing medical education for physicians.

The University of Virginia School of Medicine designates this enduring material for a maximum of 15 *AMA PRA Category 1 Credit*(s)™ for each issue, 90 credits per year. Physicians should only claim credit commensurate with the extent of their participation in the activity.

The American Medical Association has determined that physicians not licensed in the US who participate in this CME activity are eligible for a maximum of 15 *AMA PRA Category 1 Credit*(s)™ for each issue, 90 credits per year.

Credit can be earned by reading the text material, taking the CME examination online at http://www.theclinics.com/home/cme, and completing the evaluation. After taking the test, you will be required to review any and all incorrect answers. Following completion of the test and evaluation, your credit will be awarded and you may print your certificate.

FACULTY DISCLOSURE/CONFLICT OF INTEREST

The University of Virginia School of Medicine, as an ACCME accredited provider, endorses and strives to comply with the Accreditation Council for Continuing Medical Education (ACCME) Standards of Commercial Support, Commonwealth of Virginia statutes, University of Virginia policies and procedures, and associated federal and private regulations and guidelines on the need for disclosure and monitoring of proprietary and financial interests that may affect the scientific integrity and balance of content delivered in continuing medical education activities under our auspices.

The University of Virginia School of Medicine requires that all CME activities accredited through this institution be developed independently and be scientifically rigorous, balanced and objective in the presentation/discussion of its content, theories and practices.

All authors/editors participating in an accredited CME activity are expected to disclose to the readers relevant financial relationships with commercial entities occurring within the past 12 months (such as grants or research support, employee, consultant, stock holder, member of speakers bureau, etc.). The University of Virginia School of Medicine will employ appropriate mechanisms to resolve potential conflicts of interest to maintain the standards of fair and balanced education to the reader. Questions about specific strategies can be directed to the Office of Continuing Medical Education, University of Virginia School of Medicine, Charlottesville, Virginia.

The faculty and staff of the University of Virginia Office of Continuing Medical Education have no financial affiliations to disclose.

The authors/editors listed below have identified no financial or professional relationships for themselves or their spouse/partner:

Ebe D'Adamo, MD; Denis Daneman, MBBCh, FRCPC; Daniela Driul, MD; Galia Gat-Yablonski, PhD; Carla Holloway, (Acquisitions Editor); Ian Holzman, MD; Christopher P. Houk, MD; Sharon J. Hyman, MD; Michelle Klein, MD; Peter A. Lee, MD, PhD; Karen Lin-Su, MD; Ágota Muzsnai, MD, PhD; Maria I. New, MD; Yeray Novoa, MD; Ferenc Péter, MD, PhD, DSc; Moshe Phillip, MD; Sayali A. Ranadive, MD; Karen Rheuban, MD (Test Author); Stephen M. Rosenthal, MD; Nicola Santoro, MD, PhD; Anpalakan Sathasivam, MD; Alfred Tenore, MD; Vidhya Viswanathan, MD; Diane K. Wherrett, MD, FRCPC; Michal Yackobovitch-Gavan, PhD.

The authors/editors listed below identified the following professional or financial affiliations for themselves or their spouse/partner:

Sonia Caprio, MD is an advisor for Daichi and Novo Nordisk.
Meilssa K. Crocker, MBA, MD is employed by the Children's Hospital Boston, and spouse owns stock in Agate Consulting.
Erica A. Eugster, MD is an industry funded research/investigator for Eli Lilly and Co.
Sherry L. Franklin, MD is on the Speakers' Bureau for Genentech, Pfizer, Inc., and Novo Nordisk, and is an industry funded research for Pfizer, Inc.
Mitchell E. Geffner, MD is an industry funded research/investigator for Eli Lilly, Inc., Genentech, Inc., Ipsen, Novo Nordisk, and Pfizer, Inc.; and is a consultant for Genentech, Inc., Ipsen, and Pfizer, Inc.
Derek LeRoith, MD, PhD is a consultant for Sanofi, BMS/AZ, and Merck.
Nelly Mauras, MD receives drug supply for research study for AstraZeneca, Genentech, and Novartis, and is an industry funded research/investigator for Genentech Center for Clinical Research in Endocrinology.
Saroj Nimkarn, MD is on the Speakers' Bureau for Pfizer, Inc. and Novo Nordisk.
Robert Rapaport, MD (Guest Editor) is a consultant and is on the Advisory Board for Novo Nordisk, is on the Speakers' Bureau for Lilly and Pfizer, Inc., and is an industry funded research/investigator for Pfizer, Inc.
Alan Rogol, MD is a consultant for Insmed, Inc., Ipsen, Inc., and Abbott; is on the Advisory Board for Dean/White Wave & Global and Stevia Inst.
Jack A. Yanovski, MD, PhD is an industry funded research/investigator for Roche.

Disclosure of Discussion of Non-FDA Approved Uses for Pharmaceutical Products and/or Medical Devices

The University of Virginia School of Medicine, as an ACCME provider, requires that all faculty presenters identify and disclose any off-label uses for pharmaceutical and medical device products. The University of Virginia School of Medicine recommends that each physician fully review all the available data on new products or procedures prior to clinical use.

TO ENROLL

To enroll in the Pediatric Clinics of North America Continuing Medical Education program, call customer service at 1-800-654-2452 or visit us online at www.theclinics.com/home/cme. The CME program is available to subscribers for an additional fee of $223.00.

Contributors

GUEST EDITOR

ROBERT RAPAPORT, MD
Professor of Pediatrics, Emma Elizabeth Sullivan Professor of Pediatric Endocrinology and Diabetes; Director, Division of Pediatric Endocrinology and Diabetes, Mount Sinai School of Medicine, New York, New York

AUTHORS

SONIA CAPRIO, MD
Department of Pediatrics, Yale University School of Medicine, New Haven, Connecticut

MELISSA K. CROCKER, MBA, MD
Pediatric Endocrine Fellow, Unit on Growth and Obesity, Program in Developmental Endocrinology and Genetics, Eunice Kennedy Shriver National Institute of Child Health and Human Development, National Institutes of Health, Department of Health and Human Services, Hatfield Clinical Research Center, Bethesda, Maryland

EBE D'ADAMO, MD
Department of Pediatrics, Yale University School of Medicine, New Haven, Connecticut; and Department of Pediatrics, University of Chieti, Chieti, Italy

DENIS DANEMAN, MBBCh, FRCPC
Division of Endocrinology, Department of Pediatrics, The Hospital for Sick Children and University of Toronto, Toronto, Ontario, Canada

DANIELA DRIUL, MD
Clinical Associate, Division of Pediatric Endocrinology, Department of Pediatrics DPMSC, University of Udine School of Medicine, Padiglione Petracco, Udine, Italy

ERICA A. EUGSTER, MD
Professor of Pediatrics and Director of Pediatric Endocrinology, Department of Pediatrics, Riley Hospital for Children, Indiana University School of Medicine, Indianapolis, Indiana

SHERRY L. FRANKLIN, MD
Assistant Clinical Professor, University of California San Diego School of Medicine, Rady Childrens Hospital of San Diego, California

GALIA GAT-YABLONSKI, PhD
The Jesse Z. and Sara Lea Shafer Institute for Endocrinology and Diabetes, National Center for Childhood Diabetes, Schneider Children's Medical Center of Israel; and Felsenstein Medical Research Center, Beilinson Campus, Petah Tikva, Israel

MITCHELL E. GEFFNER, MD
Professor of Pediatrics, Keck School of Medicine of the University of Southern California, Saban Research Institute of Children's Hospital of Los Angeles, Los Angeles, California

IAN HOLZMAN, MD
Professor of Pediatrics, Gynecology, and Reproductive Sciences; and Division
of Newborn Medicine, Mount Sinai School of Medicine, New York, New York

CHRISTOPHER P. HOUK, MD
Associate Professor of Pediatrics, Department of Pediatrics, Medical College of Georgia,
Augusta, Georgia

SHARON J. HYMAN, MD
Clinical Instructor, Division of Pediatric Endocrinology and Diabetes, Mount Sinai School
of Medicine, New York, New York

MICHELLE KLEIN, MD
Fellow, Division of Pediatric Endocrinology and Diabetes, Mount Sinai Hospital,
New York, New York

PETER A. LEE, MD, PhD
Professor of Pediatrics, Department of Pediatrics, Penn State College of Medicine,
Milton S. Hershey Medical Center, University Drive, Hershey, Pennsylvania; Department
of Pediatrics, Indiana University School of Medicine, Riley Hospital for Children,
Indianapolis, Indiana

KAREN LIN-SU, MD
Adrenal Steroid Disorders Program, Division of Pediatric Endocrinology, Mount Sinai
School of Medicine, New York, New York

NELLY MAURAS, MD
Division of Endocrinology and Metabolism, Nemours Children's Clinic; and Professor
of Pediatrics, Mayo College of Medicine, Jacksonville, Florida

ÁGOTA MUZSNAI, MD, PhD
Head Physician, Division of Endocrinology, St. Johns Hospital and United Hospitals
of North-Buda, Buda Children's Hospital, Bolyai-u., Budapest, Hungary

MARIA I. NEW, MD
Professor of Pediatrics, Professor of Genetics and Genomic Sciences and the Director
of Adrenal Steroid Disorders Program, Division of Pediatric Endocrinology, Mount Sinai
School of Medicine, New York, New York

SAROJ NIMKARN, MD
Adrenal Steroid Disorders Program, Division of Pediatric Endocrinology, Mount Sinai
School of Medicine, New York, New York

YERAY NOVOA, MD
Division of Pediatric Endocrinology and Diabetes, Mount Sinai Hospital, New York,
New York

FERENC PÉTER, MD, PhD, DSc
Professor, Department of Pediatrics, Division of Endocrinology, St. Johns Hospital and
United Hospitals of North-Buda, Buda Children's Hospital, Bolyai-u., Budapest, Hungary

MOSHE PHILLIP, MD
Professor, The Jesse Z. and Sara Lea Shafer Institute for Endocrinology and Diabetes,
National Center for Childhood Diabetes, Schneider Children's Medical Center of Israel;
Felsenstein Medical Research Center, Beilinson Campus, Petah Tikva, and Sackler
School of Medicine, Tel Aviv University, Tel Aviv, Israel

SAYALI A. RANADIVE, MD
Department of Endocrinology, Children's Hospital and Research Center Oakland, Oakland, California

ROBERT RAPAPORT, MD
Professor of Pediatrics, Emma Elizabeth Sullivan Professor of Pediatric Endocrinology and Diabetes; Director, Division of Pediatric Endocrinology and Diabetes, Mount Sinai School of Medicine, New York, New York

ALAN ROGOL, MD
Professor of Pediatrics, Department of Pediatrics, Indiana University School of Medicine, Riley Hospital for Children, Indianapolis, Indiana; Department of Pediatrics, University of Virginia, Charlottesville, Virginia

STEPHEN M. ROSENTHAL, MD
Professor of Pediatrics, Associate Program Director, Pediatric Endocrinology, and Director, Pediatric Endocrine Outpatient Services, University of California, San Francisco, San Francisco, California

NICOLA SANTORO, MD, PhD
Department of Pediatrics, Yale University School of Medicine, New Haven, Connecticut

ANPALAKAN SATHASIVAM, MD
Fellow, Division of Pediatric Endocrinology and Diabetes, Mount Sinai Hospital, New York, New York

ALFRED TENORE, MD
Professor and Chair of Pediatrics; and Director, Division of Pediatric Endocrinology, Department of Pediatrics DPMSC, University of Udine School of Medicine, Padiglione Petracco, Udine, Italy

VIDHYA VISWANATHAN, MD
Fellow in Pediatric Endocrinology, Section of Pediatric Endocrinology, Department of Pediatrics, Riley Hospital for Children, Indiana University School of Medicine, Indianapolis, Indiana

DIANE K. WHERRETT, MD, FRCPC
Division of Endocrinology, Department of Pediatrics, The Hospital for Sick Children and University of Toronto, Toronto, Ontario, Canada

MICHAL YACKOBOVITCH-GAVAN, PhD
The Jesse Z. and Sara Lea Shafer Institute for Endocrinology and Diabetes, National Center for Childhood Diabetes, Schneider Children's Medical Center of Israel, Petah Tikva, Israel

JACK A. YANOVSKI, MD, PhD
Head, Unit on Growth and Obesity, Program in Developmental Endocrinology and Genetics, Eunice Kennedy Shriver National Institute of Child Health and Human Development, National Institutes of Health, Department of Health and Human Services, Hatfield Clinical Research Center, Bethesda, Maryland

Contents

This article reviews factors that contribute to excessive weight gain in children and outlines current knowledge regarding approaches for treating pediatric obesity. Most of the known genetic causes of obesity primarily increase energy intake. Genes regulating the leptin signaling pathway are particularly important for human energy homeostasis. Obesity is a chronic disorder that requires long-term strategies for management. The foundation for all treatments for pediatric obesity remains restriction of energy intake with lifestyle modification. There are few long-term studies of pharmacotherapeutic interventions for pediatric obesity. Bariatric surgical approaches are the most efficacious treatment but, because of their potential risks, are reserved for those with the most significant complications of obesity.

The worldwide epidemic of childhood obesity in the last decades is responsible for the occurrence in pediatrics of disorders once mainly found in adults, such as the metabolic syndrome. A key factor in the pathogenesis of metabolic syndrome is insulin resistance, a phenomenon occurring mainly in obese subjects with a general resistance to the insulin effect only on carbohydrates metabolism. Given that the metabolic syndrome is driven by obesity, the prevalence of the latter will strongly influence the prevalence of metabolic syndrome. This article addresses the causes of metabolic syndrome and the relevance of obesity in the pediatric population.

Prevention of loss of b cells in type 1 diabetes is a major goal of current research. Knowledge of the genetic susceptibility, increasing ability to predict who may be at risk, recognition of the potential clinical impact of residual insulin secretion after diagnosis, and development of new immunomodulatory agents have supported an increasing number of clinical trials to prevent b-cell loss. Interventions can be targeted at 3 stages: before the development of autoimmunity (primary prevention), after autoimmunity is recognized (secondary prevention), or after diagnosis when significant numbers of b cells remain (tertiary prevention). Thus far, several agents show promise when given shortly after diagnosis, but no interventions before diagnosis have shown benefit. Knowledge in this area has grown quickly in recent years and will continue to grow rapidly with several international collaborative efforts underway.

Fluid homeostasis requires adequate water intake, regulated by an intact thirst mechanism and appropriate free water excretion by the kidneys, mediated by appropriate secretion of arginine vasopressin (AVP, also known as antidiuretic hormone). AVP exerts its antidiuretic action by binding to the X chromosome-encoded V2 vasopressin receptor (V2R), a G protein-coupled receptor on the basolateral membrane of renal collecting duct epithelial cells. After V2R activation, increased intracellular cyclic adenosine monophosphate mediates shuttling of the water channel aquaporin 2 to the apical membrane of collecting duct cells, resulting in increased water permeability and antidiuresis. Clinical disorders of water balance are common, and abnormalities in many steps involving AVP secretion and responsiveness have been described. This article focuses on the principal disorders of water balance, diabetes insipidus, and the syndrome of inappropriate antidiuretic hormone secretion.

Steroid 21 hydroxylase deficiency is the most common form of congenital adrenal hyperplasia (CAH). The severity of this disorder depends on the extent of impaired enzymatic activity, which is caused by various mutations of the 21 hydroxylase gene. This article reviews adrenal steroidogenesis and the pathophysiology of 21 hydroxylase deficiency. The three forms of CAH are then discussed in terms of clinical presentation, diagnosis and treatment, and genetic basis. Prenatal diagnosis and treatment are also reviewed. The goal of therapy is to correct the deficiency in cortisol secretion and suppress androgen overproduction. Glucocorticoid replacement has been the mainstay of treatment for CAH, but new treatment strategies continue to be developed and studied.

Clinical guidelines and consensus statements serve to summarize and organize current knowledge on diverse subjects and provide practical guidelines for proper clinical management. Recommendations should be based on research and evidence derived from appropriate sources. In 2008, more than 20 consensus statements were published in the pediatric literature alone. This article summarizes the salient points of the latest consensus statements jointly developed by multiple endocrine societies including the Lawson Wilkins Society for Pediatric Endocrinology and the European Society for Pediatric Endocrinology. As much as possible, the original intent and language of the statements was respected and paraphrased.

THE CLINICS ARE NOW AVAILABLE ONLINE!

Access your subscription at:
www.theclinics.com

FORTHCOMING ISSUES

December 2011
Pediatric Obesity
Miriam Vos, MD, and
Sarah E. Barlow, MD, MPH, Guest Editors

February 2012
Autism Spectrum Disorders (Practical Overview for Pediatricians)
Dilip R. Patel, MD, and
Donald E. Greydanus, MD, Guest Editors

April 2012
Pediatric Rheumatology
Khalid M. Ismail, MD, FAAP, FRCPC,
Guest Editor

RECENT ISSUES

August 2011
Interface Between Pediatric and Children's Mental Health
Sandra L. Friedrich, MD, and
Harsh K. Trivedi, MD
Guest Editors

June 2011
Pediatric Sleep Medicine Update
Judith A. Owens, MD, MPH
Jodi A. Mindell, PhD
Guest Editors

April 2011
Food Allergy in Children
Hemant P. Sharma, MD, MHS,
Robert A. Wood, MD, and
Max J. Cooper, MD, PhD, MBA
Guest Editors

ISSUE OF RELATED INTEREST

Endocrinology and Metabolism Clinics of North America, September 2010
Volume 39, Number 3
Type 1 Diabetes
Desmond A. Schatz, MD, Michael J. Haller, MD, and Mark A. Atkinson, PhD,
Guest Editors

Preface

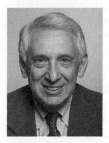

Robert Rapaport, MD
Guest Editor

The last issue of the *Pediatric Clinics of North America* devoted to pediatric endocrinology was published in 2005. That issue focused on pediatric diabetes. The past 6 years have been witness to tremendous advances in multiple areas in the field of pediatric endocrinology. I welcome this opportunity kindly provided by the editors and publishers of *Pediatric Clinics* to edit and coordinate the publication of an issue dedicated to pediatric endocrinology. This is an particularly opportune time in as much as I had recently had the pleasure of editing a two-volume issue of *Endocrinology and Metabolism Clinics of North America* devoted to Pediatric Endocrinology (Pediatric Endocrinology: Part I and II).[1,2] Therefore, with the assistance of the publishers and authors of the previous volumes, several of the articles appearing in those issues will be revised and/or reprinted in this volume.

In view of the huge strides made in genetics, genomics, proteomics, and personalized medicine, I thought it appropriate to start with an article devoted to genomics in pediatric endocrinology.

The number of smaller and younger infants who survive the neonatal period is ever increasing. It was important therefore to devote some attention to perinatal endocrinology and specifically to disorders of the thyroid gland in the newborn.

Growth disorders comprise the area that pediatric endocrinologists address perhaps more commonly than any other. Therefore it seemed important to devote articles to aspects of growth from basics on nutrition and bone growth to more generalized current indications regarding the use of growth hormone and ways of optimizing growth during puberty in children.

Significant new developments in etiology, recognition, and management in several areas of pediatric endocrinology have resulted in their inclusion within this compendium. They include hypogonadism and fertility preservation, disorders of water balance, and congenital adrenal hyperplasia.

Even though the last issue of *Pediatric Clinics* was devoted to pediatric diabetes, I felt that the worldwide increase in prevalence of both obesity as well as pediatric diabetes necessitated the inclusion of updates on pediatric obesity, metabolic syndrome, and the prevention of type 1 diabetes.

Pediatr Clin N Am 58 (2011) xv–xvi
doi:10.1016/j.pcl.2011.08.001
0031-3955/11/$ – see front matter © 2011 Elsevier Inc. All rights reserved.

pediatric.theclinics.com

Last, a review of a few selected consensus statements in pediatric endocrinology that deserves, I believe, a wide audience was included.

I would like to thank my colleagues worldwide who have graciously accepted to be contributors to this volume. This publication could not have been accomplished without the assistance and support of Kerry Holland, Senior Editor of Elsevier, and the hard work of my assistant, Yolanne Blake.

Thank you.

Robert Rapaport, MD
Division of Pediatric Endocrinology and Diabetes
Mount Sinai School of Medicine
One Gustave L. Levy Place
Box 1616
New York, NY 10029, USA

E-mail address:
robert.rapaport@mountsinai.org

REFERENCES

1. Rapaport R. Pediatric endocrinology: part I. Endocrinol Metab Clin North Am 2009; 38(3).
2. Rapaport R. Pediatric endocrinology: part II. Endocrinol Metab Clin North Am 2009;38(4).

Genomics in Pediatric Endocrinology— Genetic Disorders and New Techniques

Alfred Tenore, MD*, Daniela Driul, MD

KEYWORDS

- Genomics • Hormones • Pediatric endocrinology
- Positional cloning • DNA microarray

Recent advances in molecular biology, genetics, and clinical research are transforming the understanding of the molecular mechanisms of human diseases and in particular of endocrine disorders. It is now clear, more than ever, that disease is a function of genes, whether they are involved directly or indirectly through the environment. In the last 20 years, genetics has undergone a dramatic transformation. The significant advances that have occurred, through the completion of the sequencing of the human genome (Genomic Human Project)[1,2] and the development of new and powerful technology to study DNA, have moved molecular genetics from being a tool of the basic investigator to playing a mainstream role in medical practice, covering all aspects from diagnosis to treatment. Some of the implications of this change include:

Identification of genetic causal agents of some common endocrine disorders

Understanding the underlying molecular pathogenesis and pathophysiology of some common disorders

Development of new predictive tests for identifying carriers, allowing adequate genetic counseling and precocious prenatal diagnosis

Applications in the field of therapeutics with the development of new therapies stemming from an understanding of the molecular pathogenesis of endocrine disorders

Portions of this article were previously published in the *Endocrinology and Metabolism Clinics of North America*, 38:3.

Division of Pediatric Endocrinology, Department of Pediatrics DPMSC, University of Udine School of Medicine, Padiglione Petracco, Piazzale S.M. della Misericordia, 33100, Udine, Italy

* Corresponding author.

E-mail address: alfred.tenore@uniud.it

Pediatr Clin N Am 58 (2011) 1061–1081

doi:10.1016/j.pcl.2011.07.001

pediatric.theclinics.com

Functional or positional cloning technology and DNA recombinant technology have allowed the identification of genes that:

Encode for new hormones (eg, Leptin)
Are critical in the developmental process (ie, Involved in sexual differentiation or in the development of the pituitary gland[3])
Are responsible for multiple endocrine neoplasia (eg, menin protein in multiple endocrine neoplasia [MEN] 1[4] and rearranged during transfection [RET] in MEN 2[5]).

Furthermore, the molecular studies of hormone receptors and of the postreceptor signaling mechanisms have allowed understanding of the action of many hormones and the identification of new mutations that are capable of influencing hormone function, thus leading to different pathological situations (eg, insensitivity to growth hormone [GH],[6] insulin resistance[7]). At the present time, the molecular alterations of several monogenic endocrine disorders are known, and the diagnosis of such disorders may be established by means of mutational analysis.

The expansion of the Internet in the last years has allowed the storage, analysis, and rapid exchange of information worldwide concerning gene sequencing and has allowed the rapid completion of the sequencing of the human genome, making it easily and rapidly available for consultation to all scientists of the world. Several online databases are available containing information on genetic defects, allelic variants, modes of transmission, and clinical features. Web sites on genetic information include:

Genomics and its impact on Medicine and Society—http://www.ornl.gov/hmgs/publicat/primer
GeneMap—http://www.ncbi.nlm.nhi.gov/genemap99
GeneTests—http://www.geneclinics.org
National Organization for Rare Disorders—http://www.rarediseases.org
National Humane Genome Research Institute—http://www.genome.gov
Online Mendelian Inheritance in Man—http://www.ncbi.nlm.nhi.gov/Omim
Policy statements from the American College of Medical Genetics—http://www.faseb.org/genetics/acmg/polmenu.htm
Policy statements from American Academy of Pediatrics—http://www.aap.org/policy/pprgtoc.cfm.

Among these databases, the Online Mendelian Inheritance in Man (OMIM[8]) is probably the most complete and up-to-date. Other databases furnish information regarding the availability of the most accurate and recent genetic tests (www.genetests.org).

Molecular genetic studies also present important therapeutic implications. The first and most important therapeutic effect of recombinant DNA technology was the laboratory synthesis of hormones, which guaranteed greater availability and ease of use. The advantages of recombinant DNA technology are related to the fact that its use allows one to obtain large quantities of a specific peptide without risks of contamination that could be derived from human or animal extraction. Historically, insulin was the first hormone to be synthesized and approved for clinical use,[9] followed by recombinant human growth hormone (hGH)[10] in the early 1980s. At the present time, multiple peptide hormones (erythropoietin, thyrotropin, parathyroid hormone, follicle-stimulating hormone [FSH], and luteinizing hormone [LH]), growth factors (colony-stimulating factors), cytokines (interferons) and vaccines (hepatitis B virus) either are being used already or are in an advanced phase of study. Additional studies have made possible the synthesis of certain peptide hormones with genetically determined modifications leading to changes in their kinetics or metabolism and consequently to improved therapeutic results. A classic example is that of insulin analogues,[11] in which the modification of one amino acid has allowed one to obtain peptides with rapid or delayed actions.

In elucidating the molecular pathogenetic mechanisms of various disorders, genomics and proteomics also are allowing the creation of new therapeutic agents. The discovery that the mutation of the gene encoding for tyrosine kinase RET is responsible for the development of thyroid tumors is permitting the synthesis of kinase inhibitors to be used as possible chemotherapeutic agents.[5,12] Although still limited to the area of research, studies with gene therapy (ie, the transfer of genetic material in a specific patient) are a promise of the near future.[13]

Another application of the rapidly expanding field of molecular genetics is that of pharmacogenetics and pharmacogenomics. Although the terms tend to be used interchangeably, *pharmacogenetics* involves the clinical testing of genetic variation that gives rise to different responses to drugs. This discipline is enjoying much clinical interest; it is viewed as an outstanding opportunity to improve prescribing safety and efficacy, because it is known that there exist individual genetic variations in the metabolic handling of drugs. On the contrary, pharmacogenomics differs in that it refers to the influence of genetic variation on drug response in patients by correlating gene expression or single nucleotide polymorphisms with a drug's efficacy or toxicity and thereby attempts to develop rational means of optimizing drug therapy with respect to the patient's genotype in order to ensure maximum efficacy with minimal adverse effects. Such an approach promises the advent of personalized medicines, where drugs are optimized for each individual's unique genetic makeup.

If on the one hand it is true that the laboratory synthesis of hormones has reduced mortality caused by hormone deficiency states remarkably, it is also true that patients who require replacement therapy present with a suboptimal quality of life, which is manifested by an underlying imperfection related to replacement therapy.[14] The human genome project has disclosed the presence of polymorphisms, which are sequence variations of single nucleotides (SNPs) that may occur with variable frequency in the genome of the general population. Although many polymorphisms do not have any functional consequences, some may lead to subtle functional alterations in the gene product or gene expression and therefore may influence synthesis, secretion, or hormone sensitivity. For example, polymorphisms in exon 2 of the receptor for glucocorticoids are associated with a greater or lesser sensitivity to glucocorticoids.[15–17] Therefore, the aim of clinical endocrinology will be to apply this new genetic information on hormonal sensitivity in replacement therapy in order to optimize the dose and frequency of administrations. Such considerations assume greater importance if applied to the field of pediatric endocrinology, which is dedicated to treating growing individuals who are subject to prolonged hormone treatments.

The application of molecular genetic studies also may present the optimal therapeutic choice for a patient on the basis of the underlying genetic defect. Hong and colleagues give an example[18] when they describe the treatment of a child who had ambiguous genitalia caused by a mutation of the androgen receptor. The fact that this child was a carrier of a mutation of the receptor, which laboratory studies showed to consent binding to dihydrotestosterone, permitted the child to be treated with this hormone with favorable results and no need do undergo sex change.

The development of molecular genetic technology has allowed the identification of more than 1400 genes that are related directly to the development of pathological disorders. Among these, several endocrine disorders also are found (**Table 1**). Because it is not feasible to discuss all of the genetic/endocrinologic disorders within

Table 1
Principal genetic disorders in pediatric endocrinology

Disorder	Gene
Anterior pituitary	
Combined pituitary hormone deficiency	POUF1, PROP1, LHX3, HESX1
Isolated growth hormone deficiency	GH1, GHRHR, BTK
Hypogonadotropic Hypogonadism	GNRHR, KAL, LHB, FSHB
Isolated Thyrotropin Deficiency	TSHB
Adrenal gland	
Congenital adrenal hyperplasia	HSD3B2, CYP21, CYP11B1, CYP17
Congenital adrenal hypoplasia	DAX-1
Adrenoleukodystrophy x-linked	ABCD1
Familial glucocorticoid resistance	GCCR
Pheochromocytoma	RET, NF1, VHL
Thyroid gland	
Autosomal dominant hyperthyroidism	TSHR
Thyroid dysgenesis	PAX8
Impaired hormone synthesis	SLC5A5, DUOX2, TPO, TG
Pendred's syndrome	SLC26A4
Gonads	
5α-reductase deficiency	SRD5A2
Androgen insensitivity syndrome	AR
Estrogen resistance	ESR1
Gonadal dysgenesis	SRY
Male-limited precocious puberty	LHCGR
Persistent Müllerian duct syndrome type 1 and 2	AMH, AMHR2
Premature ovarian failure	FSHR
Pancreas	
Congenital hyperinsulinism	KCNJ11, GLUD1, ABCC8
Maturity-onset diabetes of the young types 1, 2, 3, 4, 5, 6	HNF4α, GCK, HNF1α, IPF1, HNF1β, Neurod1
Leprechaunism, Rabson-Mendenhall syndrome	INSR
Posterior pituitary	
Central diabetes insipidus	AVP
Nephrogenic diabetes insipidus	AVPR2, AQP2
Parathyroid gland	
Albright hereditary osteodystrophy	GNAS
Familial hypercalciuric/hypocalciuric hypercalcemia	CASR
Familial isolated hyper-/hypoparathyroidism	HRPT2, MEN1, CASR, PTH
Multiple endocrine systems	
Autoimmune polyendocrinopathy syndrome type 1	AIRE
Carney complex	PRKAR1A
Gardner syndrome	APC
McCune Albright syndrome	GNAS
MEN I	MEN 1
MEN IIA	RET
MEN IIB	RET

the constraints of this article, the reader is referred to the OMIM Web site for a more detailed discussion.

Gene alterations traditionally are classified according to:

The molecular nature of the DNA (ie, deletion, insertion, substitution of single nucleotide)

The consequences of transcription or translation (ie, null allele, nonsense, missense, and frameshift mutations)

The mutant protein produced (ie, partial or complete loss of function, acquisition of a new function, negative dominant effect).

In the field of endocrinology, disorders may be derived from mutations that structurally may be divided in alterations involving: the entire genome (ie, triploidy), the number of some chromosomes (eg, Turner or Klinefelter syndromes), or large parts of a chromosome (contiguous gene syndrome).

It is becoming more evident that diverse alterations of the same gene or of different genes could cause the same phenotype, because the function of the mutant protein also is involved. An example is represented by some forms of congenital hypothyroidism, where mutations of different genes involved in the various steps that lead to the synthesis of thyroid hormones all give the same phenotypic expression of thyroid hormone deficiency.[19] Mutations of a single gene, however, also may result in different clinical manifestations (eg, different point mutations of the CYP21 gene result in congenital adrenal hyperplasia in its various forms, with salt loss, virilization, or late onset[20]). It also must not be forgotten that because there may be additional mutations in the regulatory region or in the introns of a particular gene, the mutational analysis, which usually is limited to the encoding region of the gene, may result negative.

In the early 1960s, the field of endocrinology primarily was based on physiologic studies and on the determination of hormone levels. Based on this simplified concept, endocrine disorders traditionally were classified into four categories: (1) hormone deficiency disorders, (2) hormone excess disorders, (3) hormone resistance syndromes, and (4) tumors or disorders of endocrine glands without abnormal hormone secretion. Today, although the classification still holds, numerous conditions are explained by mutations in genes involved in the function or growth of endocrine tissues. From a functional point of view, the consequences of these mutations are variable and can be classified as either loss-of-function or gain-of-function; consequently, endocrine disorders may be divided into hypo- and hypersecretory disorders. A classical example of loss of function or gain of function is represented by disorders related to G protein coupled receptors. In fact, because of the advances in molecular biology techniques in the last 10 years, numerous peptide hormone receptors have been identified (parathyroid hormone [PTH], growth hormone-releasing hormone [GRH], thyrotropin [TSH], LH, FSH, and corticotropin [ACTH]) that are coupled to G protein. The G protein-coupled receptors are characterized by seven transmembrane-spanning domains. The G protein is a heterotrimeric protein made of three subunits (α, β, and γ) that behave as on–off switches in the transmission of the intracellular signal.

Numerous alterations of the G protein coupled receptor and the G protein have been identified. These mutations can be inhibitory or activating. In the former, the signal is not transmitted even in the presence of hormone, whereas in the latter, the signal is transmitted or even amplified in absence of hormone (constitutive activation).

GENETICALLY DETERMINED HYPOFUNCTIONAL ENDOCRINE DISORDERS

The various mechanisms that may be implicated in reduced hormone function include:

Defect of the gene for a particular hormone because of absence of the entire gene, deletion of part of the gene, or presence of single point mutations in the gene
Defects in the enzymes responsible for hormone synthesis
Production of a defective hormone
Absent transmission of the signal because of alterations in the receptor or in the intracellular mechanisms involved in signal transmission

Regardless of which of the four situations exist, the result is that there will be an inability to synthesize a functional peptide, and the patient will present with the clinical characteristics of a hormone deficiency state.

Short Stature

A typical example of a hyposecretion disorder in pediatric endocrinology is represented by familial isolated GH deficiency, of which four mendelian-transmitted forms are recognized: two autosomal-recessive (isolated growth-hormone deficiency [IGHD] types 1A and 1B), one autosomal-dominant type (IGHD type 2), and one x-linked type (IGHD type 3). In 1981, Phillips and colleagues[21] identified the absence of the GH1 gene that encodes for GH. Subsequently, other deletions have been identified of 6.7, 7.0, 7.6 and 45 kb, as well as single nucleotide mutations.[22–24] In all cases, the resultant effect is a complete inability to produce GH; therefore phenotypically, the subjects present a marked growth deficit from 6 months of age and develop anti-GH antibodies with the introduction of exogenous GH treatment (IGHD type 1A). In IGHD type 1B, which is characterized by a more variable and less severe phenotype, three mutations of the GH gene, responsible for producing an altered GH molecule and mutations of the GHRH gene[25] or of its receptor,[26,27] have been identified. IGHD Type 1B usually is not associated with the production of anti-GH antibodies once treatment begins. This probably is related to the fact there is a minimal production of GH. The autosomal-dominant IGHD type 2 is caused by changes in the splicing of GH mRNA, causing skipping or deletion of exon 3. IGHD type 3 has an x-linked mode of transmission and may be associated with hypogammaglobulinemia.

Deficiency of GH may caused not only by genetic alterations of the GH gene, but it may be secondary to gene mutations for PIT-1, PROP-1, HESX1, and LHX3[28] which are involved in the embryologic development of the adenohypophysis and therefore regulate the synthesis of GH. An additional possibility is the synthesis of a defective hormone often referred to as biologically inactive GH. This rare form of short stature is characterized by the presence of a GH molecule whose immunoreactive activity is normal but whose biological activity is reduced. In 1996, Takahashi and colleagues[29] reported the case of a patient who had a mutation in codon 77 in the GH1 gene that allowed GH to bind to the GHBP correctly but to bind erratically to the GH receptor, behaving in a dominant negative manner. This altered molecule inhibits tyrosine phosphorylation after its binding to the GHR, a step that is fundamental in signal transmission.

Genetic forms of short stature also may be caused by alterations affecting one of several steps that start with the binding of GH to its receptor (GH-R) and which therefore, include the disorders of insensitivity to GH. The most common of these is exemplified by Laron syndrome,[30] described for the first time in 1966, and caused by a defect of the GH receptor. Since that time, more than 30 different mutations of the GH-R have been identified that involve deletions, nonsense mutations, splice mutations, and frameshift mutations.[6] Most of these alterations are in the extracellular domain of the receptor and characteristically are associated with low serum levels of GHBP (transport protein for GH, which corresponds to the extracellular portion of the receptor). The alterations that deal with the transmembrane and the intracellular domain of the receptor are rare and characterized by having normal levels of GHBP.

In recent years, the complex mechanism of signal transmission of the GH receptor is becoming more clear, and rare cases of short stature have been identified with alterations of the signal transducer and activator of transcription 5 (STAT5),[31] a cytoplasmic protein, which, after being activated migrates to the nucleus, binds to DNA and activates transcription.[32]

Thyroid

Congenital hypothyroidism (CH) is the most frequent form of congenital endocrine disorder, resulting from either dysgenesis (hypoplasia, ectopia, or thyroid agenesis), representing approximately 80% to 85% of cases, or dyshormonogenesis, which results from altered synthesis of thyroid hormones and is responsible for the remaining 15% to 20% of cases. Even though the dysgenetic forms of CH generally tend to be sporadic in nature, rare mutations have been identified related to thyroid migration and differentiation. Approximately 3% of the cases of thyroid dysgenesis are related to mutations in the homeobox genes TTF1, TTF2 e, and PAX8.[33]

The forms of CH caused by dyshormonogenesis are related to defects in one of the steps necessary for thyroid hormone synthesis, secretion, and transport. The main mutations are related to the transport of iodine, to the thyroperoxidase enzyme, and to thyroglobulin synthesis/function. Hypothyroidism related to abnormal TSH synthesis is rare, but when present, it may be isolated or associated with other pituitary defects (as a result of mutations of pituitary transcription factors such as PIT1, PROP-1, LHX3 e, and HESX1). The isolated, familial deficit of TSH is rare. It has been described in Japanese families and is caused by a homozygous mutation of the β subunit of TSH, which is responsible for the synthesis of a β chain that is unable to bind the α subunit of TSH to produce the biologically active form of TSH.[34] The secretory deficiency of thyroid hormones also may result from alterations in the TSH receptor which belongs to the G protein coupled receptor family. This disorder is characterized by TSH insensitivity.[35] Aside from TSH resistance, other forms of resistance to thyroid hormones have been described, which in most cases have been caused by autosomal-dominant mutations of the β gene, which encodes for the thyroid hormone receptor (THR-β).[36]

Disorders of the Reproductive Axis

Various genes are involved in the development and function of the hypothalamic-pituitary-gonadal axis, whose defects may determine various phenotypic degrees of hypogonadism. Such mutations may involve the secretion of gonadotropin-releasing hormone (GnRH), the GnRH receptor, the gonadotropins LH and FSH or their receptors, and the synthesis of estrogens and androgens or their relative receptors.

During development, the normal migration of the GnRH-secreting neurons from the olfactory placode to the hypothalamus requires the presence of anosmin-1, an extracellular matrix glycoprotein whose gene, KAL, has been identified on the X chromosome (Xp22.3). Several mutations have been described, which include nonsense, missense, and frameshift mutations, and large deletions of the KAL gene[37] responsible for Kallmann's syndrome, the most frequent form of isolated deficiency of gonadotropins, characteristically associated with hyposmia or anosmia.

Gonadotropin deficiency may be associated with defects of the gene for the GnRH receptor (a G protein-coupled receptor), located on chromosome 4q13.1.[38,39] Alterations of the β-subunit of LH or FSH and inactivating mutations of their receptors have been described in recent years but found to be very rare.[39,40] The deficit of gonadotropins also may be associated with other hormone deficiencies caused by mutations of the PROP-1 and LHX3 genes, which are responsible for the embryonic development of the adenohypophysis.

Up to now, only a single case has been described of a mutation of the gene for the estrogen receptor. Smith and colleagues[41] reported the case of a man who was found to be homozygous for a mutation in exon 2, which determines the production of a truncated protein lacking both the portion that binds to DNA and the domain that binds the hormone. More than 300 different mutations have been described in the gene for the androgen receptor, however, responsible for androgen insensitivity syndrome.[42] In most cases, these are missense mutations that may determine an impaired response or complete absence of response to androgens.

Adrenals

Adrenal insufficiency may be caused by adrenal destruction, dysgenesis, or impaired steroidogenesis. Genetic alterations that are primarily responsible for the destruction of the adrenal gland are related either to the production of autoantibodies, as found in the autoimmune polyglandular syndromes (APS) because of mutations in the APS1 of the AIRE gene, or to adrenoleukodystrophy.

More than 60 mutations in the AIRE gene have been identified in people who have APS1.[43] Some of these genetic changes lead to the production of an abnormally short, nonfunctional version of the autoimmune regulator protein. Other mutations change single amino acids in critical regions of the protein.

Although there is an autosomal form of adrenoleukodystrophy, the most common cause (approximately 1 of 20,000 cases) is the x-linked form, where the location of the defective gene is Xq28. This disorder is characterized by excessive accumulation of very long-chain fatty acids (VLCFA with a 24–30 carbon skeleton). The gene (ABCD1 or ATP-binding cassette, subfamily D, member 1) encodes for a protein (ALDP) that transfers fatty acids into peroxisomes before they undergo β oxidation.[44] A dysfunctional gene leads to the accumulation of VLCFA with resultant myelin and adrenal gland degeneration, leading to progressive neurological disability and death.

The principal forms of adrenal dysgenesis are caused by mutation of the SF-1 gene, mutations of DAX1, which has been identified in approximately 200 individuals,[45] and familial glucocorticoid deficiency. In familial glucocorticoid deficiency (FGD), molecular defects of the ACTH receptor gene (MC2R), consisting of point mutations, are described in approximately 25% to 40% of patients.[46] Mutations in the MC2 receptor accessory protein (MRAP) are responsible for another estimated 15% to 20% of cases.[47] The remainder (approximately 50% to 60%) of patients with FGD have unknown mutations that may affect ACTH signal transduction, expression of the ACTH receptor, or differentiation of the adrenal cortex.

The causes of adrenal insufficiency caused by altered hormone synthesis are related to altered cholesterol metabolism (eg, Smith-Lemli-Opitz syndrome caused by mutation of the gene for 7-dehydrocholesterol reductase) and impaired steroidogenesis secondary to mutations of the StAR, CYP21, CYP11B1, CYP17, and HSD3B2 genes.

Neurohypophysis

Diabetes insipidus (DI) may be caused by an impaired synthesis of vasopressin or antidiuretic hormone (central DI) or peripheral resistance to the action of vasopressin (nephrogenic DI). More than 25 mutations have been identified in the encoding region of the gene for vasopressin. Vasopressin deficiency also may be associated with diabetes mellitus, deafness, and optic atrophy, characteristic findings in the DIDMOAD syndrome also known as Wolfram syndrome, whose gene, WFS1, was identified recently and found to encode for a transmembrane protein whose function is still not clear.[48,49]

Approximately 90% of cases of nephrogenic DI (congenital x-linked DI) are caused by inactivating mutations of the V2 receptor, which belongs to the G protein-coupled receptors. More than 180 mutations of the gene have been reported. In most of these cases, these involve mutations of single nucleotides that determine amino acid substitutions or translational frameshifts.[50] In the remaining 10%, there is an autosomal-recessive mode of transmission (congenital autosomal nephrogenic DI), and the gene for the V2 receptor is normal. These latter cases are caused by mutations of the gene for the Aquaporin-2 receptor, which is a molecule involved in the transmission of the signal after vasopressin binds to its V2 membrane receptor.[50] Approximately 20 different mutations have been reported of the gene, and in most cases, these involve missense mutations and more rarely nonsense of frameshift mutations.[50] Recently an autosomal-dominant mode of inheritance has been described caused by a mutation of the Aquaporin-2, which alters the capacity of the luminal membrane to increase the permeability of water in response to the V2 receptor-mediated signal.[51]

Maturity-Onset Diabetes of the Young

Various forms of diabetes caused by monogenic defects of the β cell function have been described.[52] These disorders are characterized by an onset usually before 20 to 30 years of age and an autosomal-dominant mode of transmission. Six specific genetic defects have been identified:

Maturity-onset diabetes of the young (MODY) 1 is caused by a loss-of-function mutation in the HNF4A gene on chromosome 20, which encodes for HNF4-α, a protein that controls the function of HNF1-α (MODY 3) and perhaps HNF1β (MODY 5) also.

MODY 2 is caused by any of several mutations in the GCK gene on chromosome 7 for glucokinase, which serves as the glucose sensor for the beta cell. This accounts for approximately 10% to 15% of the cases of MODY

MODY 3, the most common type of MODY (approximately 65%), is caused by mutations of the HNF1α gene, a homeobox gene on chromosome 12. HNF1α is a transcription factor thought to control a regulatory network important for differentiation of beta cells. Mutations of this gene lead to reduced beta cell mass or impaired function.

MODY 4 arises from mutations of the IPF1 homeobox gene on chromosome 13. IPF1 is a transcription factor vital to the development of the embryonic pancreas.

MODY 5 arises from mutations of the HNF1β gene located on chromosome 7. HNF1β is involved in early stages of embryonic development of several organs, including the pancreas.

MODY 6 arises from mutations of the gene for the transcription factor referred to as neurogenic differentiation 1 located on chromosome 2 in a region of the short arm known as IDDM7, because it includes genes affecting susceptibility to type 1 diabetes.[53]

Hypoparathyroidism

Pseudohypoparathyroidism (PHP) is the classical example of a hyposecretion disorder caused by alterations of the G protein. Two different forms of PHP are described, depending on whether the defect is localized above cyclic adenosine monophosphate (cAMP) production (PHP type 1) or below (PHP type 2). PHP type 1 can be subdivided further into types 1A, 1B, and 1C. Type 1A is related to alterations of the gene that encodes for the α subunit of the G protein (Gsα). Several mutations have been described that involve both missense and nonsense mutations and small deletions and insertions; however, the most common mutation involves deletion of four base pairs in exon 7. These mutations determine a reduced expression or function of the G protein and therefore also are associated with resistance to TSH, LH, and FSH, whose effects also are mediated by G protein coupled proteins. Characteristically, the clinical presentation also includes osteodystrophy. On the contrary, pseudo-pseudo-hypoparathyroidism (PPHP) differs in that it is characterized only by the presence of Albright's osteodystrophy, whereas the response to PTH is normal.[54] In both cases, one finds the same mutation of the α subunit; however, if the transmission of the genetic defect is of maternal origin, the result is PHP type 1A, if it is of paternal origin one develops pseudo-HPT. The signs of osteodystrophy are lacking in PHP type 1B, and genetically no alterations have been detected of either PTH or its receptor. PHP type 1C is characterized by the presence of multiple hormonal resistance and osteodystrophy, but the activity of the G protein complex is normal, possibly suggesting the presence of a defect involving a different mode of signal transmission.

GENETICALLY DETERMINED HYPERSECRETORY ENDOCRINE DISORDERS

The genetic causes of endocrine hypersecretion disorders are mutations that lead to either an increase in hormone synthesis or continued activation of the intracellular signaling mechanism in the absence of the normal stimulatory ligand (constitutive activation).

Gigantism

The excessive secretion of GH is often secondary to the presence of a pituitary tumor whose cause remains uncertain even if recent studies in acromegalic subjects suggest that many of these cases are secondary to mutations which causes constitutive activation of the α subunit of the G protein similarly to what happens in the McCune Albright syndrome. GH secreting pituitary tumors also have been described in association with neurofibromatosis, tuberous sclerosis, and the Carney complex.[55]

Precocious Puberty (McCune Albright Syndrome and Familial Male Precocious Puberty)

Hypersecretory disorders of the reproductive system are caused by activating mutations of the LH and FSH receptors. Activating mutations of the LH receptor have been described only in males and are responsible for familial male precocious puberty or testotoxicosis. Currently 15 mutations are known that involve the transmembrane domain of the receptor, the most frequent among these is the substitution Asp^{578}Gly.[40] The mutation has been identified only in patients from the United States. Kremer and colleagues[56] studied a cohort of European patients but were not able to find the mutation described in the United States; they, however, found the substitution Ile^{542}Leu in four German children, suggesting the hypothesis of a common ancestor responsible for this clustering. It appears that activating mutations of the LH receptor in females are not associated with any particular phenotype. In so far as the FSH receptor is concerned, only one case has been described thus far of an activating mutation (Asp^{567}Gly).[57,58]

Activating mutations of the α subunit of the G protein complex are responsible for incomplete precocious puberty in the McCune Albright syndrome. This syndrome, which is found more frequently in females, is characterized by a triad of findings consisting of: café-au-lait spots with irregular margins, polyostotic fibrous dysplasia, an endocrine disorder. The most common autonomous hyperfunctioning gland involved is the ovary, causing incomplete precocious puberty; however, other endocrine tissues may be involved such as the thyroid, the adrenal, the pituitary, or the parathyroids. The peculiarity of this syndrome is that the somatic mutations are expressed in mosaicism, implying that the portion of normal or mutated cells is variable in different tissues; this in turn is responsible for the phenotypic variability. Most cases described in the literature are caused by a single base substitution of arginine with histidine or cysteine in position 201 of the Gsα protein. Less frequent mutations involve the substitution of arginine with serine, glycine, or leucine.[59]

Hyperthyroidism

Graves disease (GD) brought about by the production of TSH receptor stimulating antibodies is the most common cause of hyperthyroidism and has a genetically related etiology. GD has been associated with certain HLA haplotypes (B8 and Dr3) and genetic determinants on chromosomes 14, 20, and X.[60] Certain families with hyperthyroidism have been described that have an autosomal-dominant mode of inheritance, with gain-of-function mutation of the TSH receptor.[35,61] Furthermore, it may represent the endocrine component of the McCune Albright syndrome through an activating mutation of the α subunit of the G protein in thyroid tissue.[62]

Congenital Hyperinsulinism

Marked advances in the last years also have been made in the understanding of the molecular basis of congenital hyperinsulinism. Although this disorder is rare (1 in 40,000 to 1 in 50,000), it is the most common cause of persistent neonatal hypoglycemia and is characterized by an inappropriately elevated insulin secretion in the presence of low blood glucose. The use of recently developed genetic techniques has permitted the elucidation of the complex mechanism involved in the regulation of insulin secretion and the identification of various mutations with an autosomal-dominant or -recessive mode of transmission responsible for this disorder. The principle role of the β cell in the secretion of insulin is played by the K$_{ATP}$-dependent ion-conducting channel, which is a complex of two proteins, the sulfonylurea receptor (SUR), and an inward rectifier potassium channel (KIR). An increase in the intracellular ATP/ADP ratio, following cellular glucose uptake by means of the Glut2 transporter and its phosphorylation by means of glucokinase (GK), determines the closure of the K$_{ATP}$ channel with consequent depolarization of the cellular membrane. This depolarization causes opening of the calcium channel with resultant calcium influx and the triggering of insulin exocytosis. It recently was shown that mitochondrial glutamate dehydrogenase induces insulin secretion in a K$_{ATP}$- and calcium-independent manner. Mutations that determine loss of function of the SUR1 and Kir 6.2, generally transmitted in an autosomal-recessive mode, or the increase in function of glucokinase and glutamate dehydrogenase, both transmitted in an autosomal-dominant mode, are responsible for persistent congenital hyperinsulinism. In most cases, the mutations are those of the components of the K$_{ATP}$-dependent channel. More than 100 mutations of ABCC8 (sulfonylurea receptor gene) and 20 mutations of KCNJ11 (inwardly rectifying potassium channel gene) have been reported. These mutations are responsible for the more severe diffuse form of hyperinsulinism not responsive to treatment with diazoxide. Recently other mutations of ABCC8[63–65] and one of Kir6.2[66] have been described that have an autosomal-dominant mode of transmission and are responsible for a less-severe form of congenital hyperinsulinism. The second most common cause of congenital hyperinsulinism is a mutation of glutamate dehydrogenase[67,68] that is associated with increased levels of ammonia, because the enzyme has a regulatory role in the metabolism of amino acids and urea. Much more rare is the hyperinsulinism caused by the five known mutations of glucokinase.[69]

NEW TECHNIQUES AND THEIR APPLICATION
Historical Background

Up to the 1980s, the only possible DNA analysis available for identifying genetic alterations was through the determination of the karyotype. The use of this type of study, however, only could identify aberrations in the number of chromosomes or gross structural abnormalities (translocation, deletions, or inversions greater than 2 Mb). In recent years, there have been marked advances in the analysis of the karyotype. Different and more effective means of isolating chromosomes have been developed using chemical agents that are more adapt at arresting the cell cycle in metaphase. Furthermore, the application of molecular techniques to cytogenetics has permitted an increase in the power of resolution. In the 1990s, the development of fluorescent in situ hybridization (FISH) made possible the identification of microscopic deletions or cryptic translocations[70] and thus paved the way for developing specific tests to diagnose different clinical presentations caused by such submicroscopic alterations (eg, Prader-Willi and Angelman syndromes[71]). The last 20 years not only have seen advances in the study of the karyotype, but also the development of numerous methods of manipulating DNA, so that diagnoses of single base pair mutations can be made easily. Such techniques are being applied to the study of DNA, RNA, and the protein encoded by a gene.

Polymerase Chain Reaction

The technique that has constituted a revolutionary advancement in the field of molecular genetics is the polymerase chain reaction (PCR), which became available in 1985.[72] Through the repetition of various cycles involving heat denaturation, primer annealing, and extension, the technique allows a rapid logarithmic amplification of targeted DNA or cDNA (DNA complementary to RNA) sequences, obtaining in a few hours up to a million copies of the sequence to study. The DNA obtained in this way may be subjected to other types of investigations such as restriction fragment length polymorphism (RFLP), allele-specific oligonucleotide hybridization, and DNA sequencing. An important application of PCR is in identifying a specific sequence of DNA in a biological sample. For example, this technique, through the amplification of the SRY gene, is utilized in the detection of parts of the Y chromosome in patients who have Turner syndrome.[73]

DNA Sequencing

Mutations may be identified by genetic tests either directly or indirectly. In the former, mutations are diagnosed because they change the size or sequence of a segment of DNA or because they alter a restriction site for endonuclease. The gold standard for the identification of a point mutation is DNA sequencing as described by Sanger and colleagues[74] in 1977. With this method, the sequence of each base pair is identified and compared with the sequence of the normal gene. Such a technique, however, is labor-intensive and expensive, and even if subsequent modifications such as automatic fluorescent sequencing[75,76] and pyrosequencing[77] technology have accelerated the technique, the major limitation is that it allows the analysis only of short DNA sequences.

Deletions even of a single base may determine different gel electrophoretic mobilities of the PCR-amplified DNA sequences. If mutations do not alter the size of the DNA fragment, they may alter the endonuclease restriction sites. These enzymes, derived from bacteria, are capable of splicing the DNA when they recognize a specific base sequence. Mutations of even a single nucleotide may remove one of these sequences or create a new one. Therefore, if these enzymes do not recognize the base sites to cut or if they recognize a new site, they alter the size of the resultant DNA fragments.[78] If the substitution of the base does not alter a restriction site, the mutation may be identified with the allele-specific oligonucleotide probe technique or its variant reverse line blot.[79] The disadvantage of these techniques is that the exact mutated sequence has to be known.

The completion of the sequencing of the human genome in 2001, 4 years ahead of the expected time, was the result of a worldwide collaborative endeavor of public and private institutions and facilitated immensely by the availability and rapid access of the gathered information through the Internet. The identification of the sequence of a genome, however, is only the first step towards understanding how an organism functions. In fact, knowing the exact sequence of the approximately 3,200,000,000 base pairs located in the 23 human chromosomes is not sufficient per se. Although it is important to know the gene sequences, it is of fundamental importance to know their organization in the context of the additional information contained in the surrounding DNA, which regulate gene expression.

It is known that two individuals may share at most 99.9% of DNA sequences but it is the remaining approximately 0.1% that are responsible for the genetically determined individual traits including disease susceptibility. Most of these variations in the 0.1% are caused by common variants of DNA (polymorphism) as a result of single nucleotide substitutions (SNP or single nucleotide polymorphism, approximately 1 per 1000 base pairs[80,81]), as insertions, deletions, or repeated polymorphism. Most of these variations usually have no functional significance in that they occur in 98% of the non-encoding genic sequences.

Positional Cloning and Linkage Analysis

Polymorphisms are identified easily, because they can cause the elimination or creation of new gene sequences that are recognized by restriction enzymes. The presence of an RFLP, even if it does not cause any clinical or biochemical change in an individual, may be used as a genetic marker, and therefore, as a marker for inheriting a specific allele for a particular disorder within a family. Such a discovery forms the basis for the technique referred to as positional cloning, which refers to a method of gene identification in which a gene for a specific phenotype is identified, with only its approximate chromosomal location known (candidate region). Initially, the candidate region can be defined using techniques such as linkage analysis, and positional cloning is used to narrow the candidate region until the gene and its mutations are found. Positional cloning typically involves the isolation of partially overlapping DNA segments from genomic libraries to progress along the chromosome toward a specific gene. During the course of positional cloning, the need arises to determine whether the DNA segment currently under consideration is part of the gene.

The study of such polymorphisms led to the identification of the gene responsible for MEN1. In fact, studying the genome of patients belonging to affected families, polymorphisms present in a small region of the long arm of chromosome 11 (11q13) were utilized as markers to see how they were coinherited with the disease (linkage analysis).[82,83] Among the genes identified in this region, one appeared to be mutated in patients affected with MEN1, and it encoded for a protein of 610 amino acids.[4] Only subsequently was it discovered that such a protein, which was named menin, is expressed at the nuclear level in many tissues and exhibits a tumor-suppressive function. In fact, experiments on mice that lacked a copy of MEN1 documented the development of tumors in the same tissues affected in MEN1.[84] Furthermore, in vitro studies of the reduction of expression of the gene have documented an increased cellular proliferation, whereas overexpression produced apoptosis.[85] Once the gene responsible for such a syndrome is identified, it is possible to diagnose the carrier state of mutations of the MEN gene, and thereby, in case of positive results, begin a periodic screening for the precocious identification of neoplasias as early as 5 years of age. This biochemical and radiologic monitoring would be needless if the subject were found to be genetically negative.[86]

Linkage analysis techniques are very useful in cases of disorders demonstrating a Mendelian mode of transmission and caused by alterations of a single gene, as opposed to multifactorial disorders in which the role of every single gene is minimal and in whose development also intervene environmental factors. In this era of genomics, however, one of the major challenges will be the elucidation of complex multifactorial disorders such as diabetes and hypertension. Linkage studies performed over the last 10 years have identified multiple loci more or less weakly associated with the development of type 1 diabetes mellitus (DM)[87–89] The HLA genes on the major histocompatibility complex and the gene for insulin are responsible for approximately 45% and 10%, respectively, for genetic susceptibility to type 1 DM. This information, however, is not sufficient to predict which individual will develop diabetes and therefore may benefit from possible preventive interventions.[90,91]

DNA Microarray and Functional Genomics

Another certain challenge of the genomic era goes far beyond the simple cataloguing of gene sequences. The capability to understand the function of each gene, its product, the regulation of its expression and tissue specificity will permit, in the future, one to understand in a comprehensive and integrated manner the structure and function of people. This part of genomics goes under the term functional genomics. The function of a protein often may be identified according to the sequence of its encoding gene. Examples of this are those products of transcription whose sequence shows homology with that of a family of proteins whose function already is known (ie, the family of G protein-coupled receptors characterized by their 7 transmembrane spanning domain). Based on this technique and with the information gathered from the sequencing of the genome, more than 400 members of this family have been identified, including hormone receptors and releasing factors of pituitary hormones, catecholamines, and parathormone.[92]

The concept of functional genomics also is based on a comparison of the genomes of other organisms that are structurally simpler and whose genes are therefore more easily identifiable. If the encoded sequences of people comprise less that 2% of the entire genome, this percent increases to 20% in the housefly, 70% in yeasts, and 85% in prokaryotes. Therefore, for example on the basis of similarities with the drosophila toll protein, it was possible to identify the family of more than 10 toll-like receptors with important immunologic functions.[93]

Recent progress in biotechnology is allowing enormous advances in the comprehension of gene function. DNA microarray and serial analysis of gene expression (SAGE) technology allow the simultaneous testing of the expression of thousands of genes and allow one to automatically identify the gene of interest. Two forms of microarray exist, which differ in the length of the DNA sequence bound to the matrix, either 20 to 25 base pairs (oligonucleotides) or several hundred base pairs (cDNA). Briefly, DNA microarray technology consists of an arrayed series of thousands of microscopic spots of specific DNA sequences, which can be a short section of a gene or other DNA element (probe) in order to hybridize a cDNA or cRNA sample (target). Probe–target hybridization usually is quantified by fluorescence-based detection to determine relative abundance of nucleic acid sequences in the target. This allows one to identify the transcriptome, which is a catalogue of all the genes expressed in a determined cell or tissue in a specific stage of development. In fact, Rainey and colleagues[94] studied the differences of gene expression between fetal and adult adrenal glands and identified 69 transcripts that presented a difference of expression greater than 2.5 times. The fetal adrenals were found to have higher transcription products in relation to steroid biosynthesis or growth (ie, insulin-like growth factor-2), whereas adult glands had greater transcripts that were related to cellular immunity and signal transduction.

DNA microarray technology has been revealed to be very useful for studies in the field of endocrinology, in particular for analyzing the cellular response to a specific stimulus. This has allowed the identification of 45 new genes expressed in the rat liver in response to TSH.[95] Microarray technology has had an enormous impact on scientific research with an explosion in the number of experiments on animal models (mice and monkeys) and people in the last few years. In the past, the analysis of the expression of a single gene required many days of hard work; today, with the use of this new technology, the analysis of thousands of gene expressions may be accomplished in just a few hours. Recent studies are elucidating further the complex regulatory system of the hypothalamic-pituitary-adrenal axis and on the mechanism that regulates the initiation of puberty.[96,97] The major impact of this technology, however, is in the gene analysis of tumors. Major advances have been made in recent years in the discovery of genes that are involved in the pathogenesis of various tumors, including those of the pituitary[98–100] and adrenals.[101]

This article cannot end without introducing the importance of bioinformatics, which is the application of information technology to the field of molecular biology. The rapid developments in genomic and other molecular research technologies have produced a tremendous amount of information, which, like pieces of a puzzle, need to be put together in order to form a comprehensive picture of the data accumulated. This need has led to the development of the extremely important field of computational biology, a branch of bioinformatics that refers to mathematical and computing approaches used to analyze and interpret the accumulated data so that they can make biological processes understandable.

SUMMARY

New discoveries in the field of genetics are occurring on a daily basis, leading to continuous changes in the way medicine has been practiced up to now. New molecular technologies and increasing information being acquired from the human genome are rapidly advancing knowledge of the cause of diseases and helping to elucidate the molecular and genetic pathways that regulate normal physiological endocrine processes. The sum of this information will allow accurate diagnosis of these disorders and provide novel molecular-oriented pharmacologic therapies to treat them.

Although all of these advances are scientifically directed to improve the modern way of life, the powerful nature of the continuously developing new molecular technologies in uncovering every aspect of past, present, and future health problems will raise important ethical implications that also need to be addressed.

REFERENCES

1. International Human Genome Sequencing Consortium. Initial sequencing and analysis of the humane genome. Nature 2001;409:860–921.
2. Venter J, Adams MD, Myers EW. The sequence of the humane genome. Science 2001;291:1304–51.
3. Rosenfeld M, Briata P, Dasen J, et al. Multistep signaling and transcriptional requirements for pituitary organogenesis in vivo. Recent Prog Horm Res 2000; 55:1–13.
4. Chandrasekharappa S, Guru S, Manickam P, et al. Positional cloning of the gene for multiple endocrine neoplasia type 1. Science 1997;276:404–7.
5. de Groot JW, Links TP, Plukker JT, et al. Ret as a diagnostic and therapeutic target in sporadic and ereditary endocrine tumors. Endocr Rev 2006;27:535–60.
6. Rosenbloom A. Growth hormone insensitivity: physiologic and genetic bases, phenotype, and treatment. J Pediatr Endocrinol Metab 1999;135:280–9.
7. Steiner D, Tager H, Chan S, et al. Lessons learned from molecular biology of insulin gene mutations. Diabetes Care 1990;13:600–9.
8. OMIM. Available at: http://www.ncbi.nlm.nih.gov/omim.
9. Riggs A. Bacterial production of human insulin. Diabetes Care 1981;4:64–8.
10. Rosenfeld RG, Aggarwal BB, Hintz RL, et al. Recombinant DNA-derived methionyl growth hormone is similar in membrane binding properties to humane pituitary growth hormone. Biochem Biophys Res Commun 1982;106(1):202–9.
11. Hirsch IB. Insulin analogues. N Engl J Med 2005;352:174–83.
12. Fagin JA. How thyroid tumors start and why it matters: kinase mutants as targets for solid pharmacotherapy. J Endocrinol 2004;183:249–56.
13. Pfeifer A, Verma IM. Gene therapy: promises and problems. Annu Rev Genomics Hum Genet 2001;2:177–211.
14. Romijn JA, Smit JWA, Lamberts SWJ. Intrinsic imperfections of endocrine replacement therapy. Eur J Endocrinol 2003;149:91–7.
15. Huizenga NA, Koper JW, De Lange P, et al. A polymorphism in the glucocorticoid receptor gene may be associated with an increased sensitivity to glucocorticoids in vivo. J Clin Endocrinol Metab 1998;83:144–51.
16. Van Rossum EF, Huizenga NA, Uitterlinden AG, et al. Identification of a restriction site polymorphism in the glucocorticoid receptor gene: association with increased sensitivity to glucocorticoids in vivo, corticosteroid-binding globulin and systolic blood pressure. Presented at the 84th Annual Meeting of the Endocrine Society. San Francisco, June 19–22, 2002.
17. Van Rossum EF, Koper JW, Uitterlinden AG, et al. A polymorphism in the glucocorticoid receptor gene with decreases sensitivity to glucocorticoids in vivo is associated with a healthier metabolic profile. Presented at the 84th Annual Meeting of the Endocrine Society. San Francisco, 2002.
18. Ong Y, Wong H, Adaikan G, et al. Directed pharmacological therapy of ambiguous genitalia due to androgen receptor gene mutation. Lancet 1999;354: 1444–5.
19. Kopp P. Perspective: genetic defects in the etiology of congenital hypothyroidism. Endocrinology 2002;143:2019–24.

20. White PC, New MI. Genetic basis of endocrine disease 2: congenital adrenal hyperplasia due to 21-hydroxylase deficiency. J Clin Endocrinol Metab 1992; 74(1):6–11.

21. Phillips JA III, Hjell BL, Seeburg PH. Molecular basis for familial isolated growth hormone deficiency. Proc Natl Acad Sci U S A 1981;78:6372–5.

22. Cogan JD, Phillips JA III. Growth disorders caused by genetic defects in the growth hormone pathway. Adv Pediatr 1998;45:337–61.

23. Wagner JK, Eble A, Hindmarsh PC, et al. Prevalence of human GH-1 alterations in patients with isolated familial growth hormone deficiency. Pediatr Res 1998; 43(1):105–10.

24. Mullis PE. Genetic control of growth. Eur J Endocrinol 2005;152:11–31.

25. Mullis PE, Patel M, Brickell PM. Isolated growth hormone deficiency: analysis of the growth hormone (GH) releasing hormone gene and the GH gene cluster. J Clin Endocrinol Metab 1990;70:187–91.

26. Cogan JD, Phillips JA III. Heterogeneous growth hormone gene mutations in familial GH deficiency. J Clin Endocrinol Metab 1993;76:1224–8.

27. Salvatori R, Fan X, Phillips JA III. Three new mutations in the gene for the growth hormone (GH)-releasing hormone receptor in familial isolated GH deficiency type Ib. J Clin Endocrinol Metab 2001;86:273–9.

28. Mullis PE. Genetics of growth hormone deficiency. Endocrinol Metab Clin North Am 2007;36:17–36.

29. Takahashi Y, Kaji H, Okimura Y, et al. Brief report: short stature caused by a mutant growth hormone. N Engl J Med 1996;334:432–6.

30. Laron Z, Pertzelen A, Mannheimer S. Genetic pituitary dwarfism with high serum concentration of growth hormone: a new inborn error of metabolism? Isr J Med Sci 1966;2:152–5.

31. Rosenfeld RG, Belgorosky A, Camacho-Hubner C, et al. Defects in growth hormone receptor signaling. Trends Endocrinol Metab 2007;18(4):134–41.

32. Schindler C, Darnell JE Jr. Transcriptional responses to polypeptide ligands. The JAK-STAT pathway. Annu Rev Biochem 1995;64:621–52.

33. De Felice M, Di Lauro R. Thyroid development and its disorders: genetics and molecular mechanisms. Endocr Rev 2004;25:722–46.

34. Medeiros-Neto GA, de Laserda L, Wondisford FE. Familial congenital hypothyroidism caused by abnormal and bioinactive TSH due to mutations in the β subunit gene. Trends Endocrinol Metab 1997;8(1):15–20.

35. Duprez L, Parma J, Van Sande J, et al. TSH receptor mutations and thyroid disease. Trends Endocrinol Metab 1998;9(4):133–40.

36. Gurnel M, Beck Peccoz P, Chaterjee VK. Resistance to the thyroid hormone. In: De Groot LJ, Jameson JL, editors. Endocrinology. 5th edition. Philadelphia: Elsevier-Saunders; 2006. p. 2227–38.

37. Hardelin JP. Kallmann syndrome: towards molecular pathogenesis. Mol Cell Endocrinol 2001;179:75–81.

38. Beranova M, Oliveira LM, Bedecarrats GY, et al. Prevalence, phenotypic spectrum, and modes of inheritance of gonadotropin-releasing hormone receptor mutations in idiopathic hypogonadotropic hypogonadism. J Clin Endocrinol Metab 2001;86:1580–8.

39. Kalantaridou S, Chrousos G. Monogenic disorders of puberty. J Clin Endocrinol Metab 2002;87(6):2481–94.

40. Themmen AP, Huhtaniemi IT. Mutations of gonadotropins and gonadotropin receptors: elucidating the physiology and pathophysiology of pituitary–gonadal function. Endocr Rev 2000;21(5):551–83.

41. Smith EP, Boyd J, Frank GR, et al. Estrogen resistance caused by a mutation in the estrogen receptor gene in a man. N Engl J Med 1994;331:1056–61.
42. Patterson MNH, Gottlieb P, Pinsky L. The androgen receptor gene mutations database. Nucleic Acids Res 1994;22:3560–2.
43. Peterson P, Peltonen L. Autoimmune polyendocrinopathy syndrome type 1 (APS1) and AIRE gene: new views of molecular basis of autoimmunity. J Autoimmun 2005;25:49–55.
44. Ligtenberg MJ, Kemp S, Sarde CO, et al. Spectrum of mutations in the gene encoding the adrenoleukodistrophy protein. Am J Hum Genet 1995;56: 44–50.
45. Phelan JK, McCabe ER. Mutations in NROB1 (DAX1) and NR5A (SF1) responsible for adrenal hypoplasia congenita. Hum Mutat 2001;18:472–87.
46. Flück CE, Martens JWM, Conte FA, et al. Clinical, genetic, and functional characterization of ACTH receptor mutations using a novel receptor assay. J Clin Endocrinol Metab 2002;87:4318–23.
47. Metherell LA, Chapple JP, Cooray S, et al. Mutations in MRAP, encoding a new interacting partner of the ACTH receptor, cause familial glucocorticoid deficiency type 2. Nat Genet 2005;37:166–70.
48. Inoue H, Tanizawa Y, Wasson J, et al. A gene encoding a transmembrane protein is mutated in patients with diabetes mellitus and optic atrophy (Wolfram syndrome). Nat Genet 1998;20(2):143–8.
49. Hardy C, Khanim F, Torres R, et al. Clinical and molecular genetic analysis of 19 Wolfram syndrome kindreds demonstrating a wide spectrum of mutations in WFS1. Am J Hum Genet 1999;65(5):1279–90.
50. Oksche A, Rosenthal W. The molecular basis of nephrogenic diabetes insipidus. J Mol Med 1998;76(5):326–37.
51. Mulders SM, Bichet DG, Rijss JP, et al. An aquaporin-2 water channel mutant which causes autosomal dominant nephrogenic diabetes insipidus is retained in the Golgi complex. J Clin Invest 1998;102:57–66.
52. Fajans SS, Bell GI, Polonsky KS. Molecular mechanisms and clinical pathophysiology of maturity-onset diabetes of the young. N Engl J Med 2001;345: 971–80.
53. Copeman JB, Cucca F, Hearne CM, et al. Linkage disequilibrium mapping of a type 1 diabetes susceptibility gene (IDDM7) to chromosome 2q31–q33. Nat Genet 1995;9(1):80–5.
54. Nakamoto JM, Sandstrom AT, Brickman AS, et al. Pseudohypoparathyroidism type Ia from maternal but not paternal transmission of a Gsα gene mutation. Am J Med Genet 1998;77(4):261–7.
55. Statakis CA, Carney JA, Lin JP, et al. Carney complex, a familial multiple neoplasia and lentiginosis syndrome: analysis of 11 kindreds and linkage to the short arm of chromosome 2. J Clin Invest 1996;97(3):699–705.
56. Kremer H, Martens JW, van Reen M, et al. A limited repertoire of mutations of the luteinizing hormone (LH) receptor gene in familial and sporadic patients with male LH-independent precocious puberty. J Clin Endocrinol Metab 1999;84: 1136–40.
57. Simoni M, Gromoll J, Nieschlag E. The follicle-stimulating hormone receptor: biochemistry, molecular biology, physiology and pathophysiology. Endocr Rev 1997;18:739–73.
58. Gromoll J, Simoni M, Nieschlag E. An activating mutation of the follicle-stimulating hormone receptor autonomously sustains spermatogenesis in a hypophysectomized man. J Clin Endocrinol Metab 1996;81:1367–70.

59. Lumbroso S, Paris F, Sultan C. Activating Gsα mutations: analysis of 113 patients with signs of McCune-Albright syndrome—a European collaborative study. J Clin Endocrinol Metab 2004;89:2107–13.

60. Pearce SHS, Kendall-Taylor P. Genetic factors in thyroid disease. In: Braverman LE, Utiger RD, editors. The thyroid: a fundamental and clinical text. 9th edition. Philadelphia: Lippincott Williams & Wilkins; 2005. p. 407–21.

61. Vassart G. Thyroid stimulating hormone receptor mutations. In: De Groot LJ, Jameson JL, editors. Endocrinolgy. 5th edition. Philadelphia: Elsevier-Saunders; 2006. p. 2191–200.

62. Weinstein LS, Shenker A, Gejman PV, et al. Activating mutations of the stimulating G protein in the McCune Albright syndrome. N Engl J Med 1991;325: 1688–95.

63. Huopio H, Reimann F, Ashfield R, et al. Dominantly inherited hyperinsulinism caused by a mutation in the sulfonylurea receptor type 1. J Clin Invest 2000; 106(7):897–906.

64. Thornton PS, MacMullen C, Ganguly A, et al. Clinical and molecular characterization of a dominant form of congenital hyperinsulinism caused by a mutation in the high-affinity sulfonylurea receptor. Diabetes 2003;52:2403–10.

65. Magge SN, Shyng SL, MacMullen C, et al. Familial leucine-sensitive hypoglycemia of infancy due to a dominant mutation of the beta cell–sulfonylurea receptor. J Clin Endocrinol Metab 2004;89:4450–6.

66. Lin YW, MacMullen C, Ganguly A, et al. A novel KCNJ11 mutation associated with congenital hyperinsulinism reduces the intrinsic open probability of beta cell ATP-sensitive potassium channels. J Biol Chem 2006;281:3006–12.

67. Miki Y, Taki T, Ohura T, et al. Novel missense mutations in the glutamate dehydrogenase gene in the congenital hyperinsulinism-hyperammonemia syndrome. J Pediatr 2000;136(1):69–72.

68. MacMullen C, Fang J, Hsu BY, et al. Hyperinsulinism/hyperammonemia syndrome in children with regulatory mutations in the inhibitory guanosine triphosphate-binding domain of glutamate dehydrogenase. J Clin Endocrinol Metab 2001;86: 1782–7.

69. de Lonlay P, Giurgea I, Sempoux C, et al. Dominantly inherited hyperinsulinaemic hypoglycaemia. J Inherit Metab Dis 2005;28(3):267–76.

70. Cremer T, Lichter P, Borden J, et al. Detection of chromosome aberrations in metaphase and interphase tumor cells by in situ hybridization using chromosome specific library probes. Hum Genet 1988;80:235–46.

71. Nativio DG. The genetics, diagnosis, and management of Prader-Willi syndrome. J Pediatr Health Care 2002;16:298–303.

72. Saiki RK, Scharf S, Faloona F, et al. Enzymatic amplification of β globin genomic sequences and restriction site analysis for diagnosis of sickle cell anemia. Science 1985;230:1350–4.

73. Kocova M, Siegel S, Wenger S, et al. Detection of Y chromosome sequence in Turner's syndrome by Southern blot analysis of amplified DNA. Lancet 1993; 342:140–3.

74. Sanger F, Nicklen S, Coulson A. DNA sequencing with chain-terminating inhibitors. Proc Natl Acad Sci U S A 1977;74:5463–7.

75. Prober JM, Trainor GL, Dam RJ. A system for rapid DNA sequencing with fluorescent chain-terminating dideoxynucleotides. Science 1987;238: 336–41.

76. Griffin HG, Griffin AM. DNA sequencing. Recent innovations and future trends. Appl Biochem Biotechnol 1993;38:147–59.

77. Ahmadian A, Ehn M, Hober S. Pyrosequencing: hystory, biochemistry and future. Clin Chim Acta 2006;363:83–94.
78. Rosenthal N. Molecular medicine: tools of the trade-recombinant DNA. N Engl J Med 1994;331:315–7.
79. Rudert W, Trucco M. Rapid detection of sequence variations using polymers of specific oligonucleotides. Nucleic Acids Res 1992;20:1146.
80. Wang DG, Fan JB, Siao JA, et al. Large-scale identification, mapping, and genotyping of single-nucleotide polymorphisms in the human genome. Science 1998;280:1077–82.
81. Sachidanandam R, Weissman D, Schmidt SC, et al. A map of human genome sequence variation containing 1.42 million single nucleotide polymorphisms. Nature 2001;409:928–33.
82. Nakamura Y. Localization of the genetic defect in multiple endocrine neoplasia type 1 within a small region of chromosome 11. Am J Hum Genet 1989;44:751–5.
83. Thakker RV. Linkage analysis of 7 polymorphic markers at chromosome 11p11.2-11q13 in 27 multiple endocrine neoplasia type 1 families. Ann Hum Genet 1993;57:17–25.
84. Bertolino P, Tong WM, Galendo D, et al. Heterozygous Men1 mutant mice develop a range of endocrine mimicking multiple endocrine neoplasia type1. Mol Endocrinol 2003;17:1880–92.
85. Yang Y, Hua X. In search of tumor-suppressing functions of menin. Mol Cell Endocrinol 2007;265:34–41.
86. Brandi ML. Guidelines for diagnosis and therapy of MEN type 1 and type 2. J Clin Endocrinol Metab 2001;86:5658–71.
87. Davies JL, Kawaguchi Y, Bennett ST, et al. A genome-wide scan search for human type 1 diabetes susceptibility genes. Nature 1994;371:130–6.
88. Cox NJ, Wapelhorst B, Morrison VA, et al. Seven regions of the genome show evidence of linkage to type 1 diabetes in a consensus analysis of 767 multiplex families. Am J Hum Genet 2001;69:820–30.
89. Mein CA, Esposito L, Dunn MG, et al. A search for type 1 diabetes susceptibility genes in families from the United Kingdom. Nat Genet 1998;19:297–300.
90. Polychronakos C. Impact of the human genome project on pediatric endocrinology. Horm Res 2003;59:55–65.
91. Anjos S, Polychronakos C. Mechanisms of genetic susceptibility to type I diabetes: beyond HLA. Mol Genet Metab 2004;81:187–95.
92. Howard AD, McAllister G, Freighner SD, et al. Orphan G protein-coupled receptors and natural ligand discovery. Trends Pharmacol Sci 2001;22:132–40.
93. Rock FL, Hardiman G, Timmans JC, et al. A family of human receptors structurally related to Drosophila toll. Proc Natl Acad Sci U S A 1998;95:588–93.
94. Rainey WE, Carr BR, Wang ZN, et al. Gene profiling of human fetal and adult adrenals. J Endocrinol 2001;171:209–15.
95. Feng X, Jiang Y, Meltzer P, et al. Thyroid hormone regulation of hepatic genes in vivo detected by complementary DNA microarray. Mol Endocrinol 2000;14:947–55.
96. Ojeda SR, Roth C, Mungenast A, et al. Neuroendocrine mechanisms controlling female puberty: new approaches, new concepts. Int J Androl 2006;29:256–63.
97. Ojeda SR, Lominiczi A, Mastronardi A, et al. Minireview: the neuroendocrine regulation of puberty. Is the time ripe for a systems biology approach? Endocrinology 2006;147(3):1166–74.
98. Qian X, Scheithauer BW, Kovacs K, et al. DNA microarrays: recent developments and application to the study of pituitary tissues. Endocrine 2005;28(1):49–56.

99. Minematsu T, Miyai S, Kajiya H, et al. Recent progress in studies of pituitary tumor pathogenesis. Endocrine 2005;28(1):37–41.
100. Morris DG, Musat M, Czirjak S, et al. Differential gene expression in pituitary adenomas by oligonucleotide array analysis. Eur J Endocrinol 2005;153: 143–51.
101. Igaz P, Wiener Z, Szabò P, et al. Functional genomics approaches for the study of sporadic adrenal tumor pathogenesis: clinical implications. J Steroid Biochem Mol Biol 2006;104:87–96.

Perinatal Endocrinology: Common Endocrine Disorders in the Sick and Premature Newborn

Sharon J. Hyman, MD[a],*, Yeray Novoa, MD[a], Ian Holzman, MD[b]

KEYWORDS

- Endocrine • Premature • Newborn • Ill • Low birth weight
- Small for gestational age

Endocrine disorders are common in infants in the neonatal ICU (NICU). They often are associated with prematurity, low birth weight (LBW) or very low birth weight (VLBW), and small size for gestational age. They also frequently occur in infants who are critically ill or stressed. The most common conditions encountered are thyroid disorders, adrenal insufficiency, calcium disorders (most commonly hypocalcemia), and disorders of glucose homeostasis (hypoglycemia and hyperglycemia).

THYROID DISORDERS

Among the most common endocrine disorders encountered in premature and ill newborns are disorders involving the thyroid gland. Specific to this population, the most frequent include transient hypothyroxinemia of prematurity, thyroid abnormalities related to nonthyroidal illness (sick euthyroid syndrome), and primary hypothyroidism, which is often transient and may manifest as a delayed rise of thyroid-stimulating hormone (TSH). Central (secondary or tertiary) hypothyroidism presents with a similar biochemical picture as hypothyroxinemia and should be excluded. The prevalence of central congenital hypothyroidism in the United States

Portions of this article were previously published in the *Endocrinology and Metabolism Clinics of North America*, 38:3.
[a] Division of Pediatric Endocrinology and Diabetes, Mount Sinai School of Medicine, One Gustave L. Levy Place, Box 1616, New York, NY 10029, USA
[b] Division of Newborn Medicine, Mount Sinai School of Medicine, One Gustave L. Levy Place, Box 1508, New York, NY 10029, USA
* Corresponding author.
E-mail address: sharon.hyman@mssm.edu

Pediatr Clin N Am 58 (2011) 1083–1098
doi:10.1016/j.pcl.2011.07.003
0031-3955/11/$ – see front matter © 2011 Elsevier Inc. All rights reserved.

pediatric.theclinics.com

previously had been reported as only 1 of 110,000 to 1 of 29,000 newborns; however the recent Dutch newborn screening program using measurements of thyroxine (T4), TSH, and T4-binding globulin (TBG) has been shown to detect a prevalence of 1 of 20,263 infants.[1] Van Tijn and colleagues showed central hypothyroidism to comprise 13.5% of all patients who had permanent congenital hypothyroidism. Neonatal hyper-thyroidism or thyrotoxicosis is rare, usually occurring in infants born to mothers who have autoimmune hyperthyroidism (Graves disease), and it is not specific to preterm and ill newborns.

This section reviews the physiology of thyroid function in the preterm infant and then focuses the discussion on the following conditions: transient hypothyroxinemia of prematurity, nonthyroidal illness, and primary hypothyroidism.

Thyroid Function in the Premature Newborn

In the preterm infant, the hypothalamic-pituitary-thyroid axis demonstrates decreased hypothalamic thyrotrophin-releasing hormone (TRH) production and secretion, a less robust response of the thyroid gland to TSH, reduced thyroid organification of iodine, and a reduction in the peripheral conversion of thyroxine (T4) to triiodothyronine (T3).[2,3] Concentrations of T4 and free T4 are therefore lower in the cord serum of preterm compared with term infants, and these concentrations correlate with gestational age and birth weight. Thyroid-binding globulin (TBG) concentrations are low also; TSH and T3 concentrations are normal to low.

After birth both, the normal neonatal surge of TSH and the rise in T4, free T4, and T3 concentrations are attenuated in the preterm infant.[2–4] In infants born at 30 to 37 weeks gestation, T4 and free T4 concentrations have been shown to increase after birth, peak between 12 and 72 hours, and then decline in a pattern similar to that of term infants.[5] In these infants, T4 and free T4 concentrations remain lower than those of term infants and then increase over 4 to 8 weeks to concentrations comparable with those of term infants.[2,4,5] Their TSH surge is similar to term infants in magnitude and timing (peak of approximately 70 µU/mL at 30 to 90 minutes).[5,6] In contrast, in the most premature or VLBW infants (less than 30 to 31 weeks gestation or less than 1500 g) T4 and free T4 concentrations decline progressively in the first 1 to 2 weeks after birth, after which there is progressive recovery.[2,4,6,7] Their TSH peak is significantly lower (approximately 8 µU/L) than that of full-term infants.[8] Transient hypothyroxinemia is therefore the most prevalent thyroid disorder of premature and LBW infants.

Transient Hypothyroxinemia of Prematurity

Transient hypothyroxinemia is characterized by temporary low concentrations of T4 and free T4 with normal or low concentrations of TSH.[3,8] It has been shown to occur with a frequency of 24% to 50% of premature and LBW/VLBW infants.[9] There has been no consensus regarding the concentrations considered to be low, partly because it is unclear as to what constitutes normal thyroxine concentrations in preterm infants.[8] Both absolute cut-off values and standard deviations below the mean have been used to define transient hypothyroxinemia.

The etiology of transient hypothyroxinemia is multifactorial and includes the loss of the maternal T4 transfer, a less responsive hypothalamic-pituitary-thyroid axis, low TBG concentrations, nonthyroidal illness, medications such as glucocorticoids and dopamine, which reduce pituitary secretion of TSH, and iodine deficiency and iodine exposure by means of antiseptics, drugs, and contrast media.[3,4,8]

Almost all reports document an association between hypothyroxinemia in preterm infants and adverse outcome.[2–4,6] Low thyroid hormone concentrations have been shown to be associated with increases in perinatal mortality and morbidities including intraventricular central nervous system hemorrhage and periventricular echolucencies, prolonged oxygen supplementation, and mechanical ventilation. In those infants who survive, an increased risk of neurodevelopmental complications, lower IQ, and cerebral palsy have been reported.

It is unclear, however, whether low thyroid hormone concentrations are causative of these acute and long-term complications or simply a reflection of severe illness in premature infants.[2,8] Consequently, numerous studies have been done with thyroid supplementation in preterm infants to determine whether treatment results in improvement in clinical outcome. Most of these studies showed that thyroxine supplementation did not improve complications, mortality, or neurodevelopmental outcomes.

A Cochrane review published in 2000[10] summarized four randomized or quasi-randomized controlled trials.[2] Chowdrey and colleagues[11] found no significant difference between preterm infants at 25 to 28 weeks gestation who received thyroxine treatment compared with placebo in terms of weight gain, linear growth, and head circumference at 10 months of age or psychomotor development at 12 and 24 months and found no difference in mortality. Vanhole and colleagues,[12] in a double-blind placebo controlled study in infants between 25 and 30 weeks gestation, found no effect on respiratory complications, intraventricular hemorrhage, growth, retinopathy of prematurity, and mortality between those receiving thyroxine treatment compared with placebo. Amato and colleagues,[13] in a study of infants less than 32 weeks gestation requiring more than 40% supplemental oxygen, found no significant difference in mortality and long-term respiratory complications between those receiving thyroxine and those who did not receive treatment. A double-blind, placebo-controlled study by Van Wassenaer and colleagues[14] of thyroxine supplementation in infants of 25 to 29 weeks gestation demonstrated no significant difference in respiratory disease, intraventricular hemorrhage, periventricular hemorrhage, or mortality. It also showed no significant difference in neurodevelopmental outcomes at 6, 12, and 24 months of age. Additional analysis by gestational age revealed a significant difference in the Bayley mental development index at 24 months in the thyroxine-treated infants of 25 to 26 weeks gestation at birth compared with placebo. A significantly lower mental development index, however, was shown in those infants treated with thyroxine compared with placebo in infants born at 27 to 29 weeks gestation. This raised the concern that thyroxine supplementation may be detrimental to preterm infants older than 26 weeks gestation.[2] In a Cochrane review of studies up to 2001,[15] a meta-analysis of five studies found no significant difference in mortality in infants given thyroid hormone supplementation compared with controls.[8] Another meta-analysis of two studies showed no significant difference in the incidence of cerebral palsy or the Bayley Mental Psychomotor Development indices.[15]

There is insufficient evidence to determine whether thyroxine supplementation in preterm infants who have transient hypothyroxinemia results in reductions in morbidity, mortality, or neurodevelopmental impairments.[16]

Nonthyroidal Illness (Sick Euthyroid Syndrome)

Preterm infants have an increased susceptibility to morbidities, including birth trauma, hypoxemia, acidosis, infection, hypoglycemia, and hypocalcemia.[3] These conditions, in addition to overall relative malnutrition, inhibit peripheral conversion of T4 to T3. Hence, a low concentration of T3, which is characteristic of preterm infants, is aggravated. Serum T3 concentrations may remain low for 1 to 2 months after birth. In addition to low T3 concentrations, these infants tend to have a variable but usually elevated reverse T3 concentration, normal or low total T4 concentration, and a free T4 concentration that is usually in the normal range for healthy preterm infants of matched weight and gestational age. Their TSH concentrations are low. Treatment of these thyroid abnormalities caused by nonthyroidal illness is not beneficial and therefore not recommended.

Primary Hypothyroidism

Primary hypothyroidism, characterized by low T4 and elevated TSH concentrations, occurs more commonly in preterm, VLBW, and ill infants than in term infants, and it is often transient.[4] Etiologies of primary hypothyroidism in this population of infants include iodine deficiency, increased susceptibility to the thyroid-suppressive effects of iodine in topical antiseptics,[17–21] and recovery from sick euthyroid syndrome.[21] Some infants have a delayed rise in the TSH concentration that is not detected until days to weeks after birth following initial newborn screens with normal TSH concentrations.[4,21] In addition to the etiologies already mentioned, other causes of this late rise of TSH include developmental delay in the maturation of the hypothalamic-pituitary-thyroid axis and exposure to medications frequently used in premature and ill newborns that can suppress initial TSH concentrations (eg, dopamine and glucocorticoids).[21] Studies of newborn screening databases have shown that this delayed rise of TSH occurs more frequently in VLBW infants.[22,23] In a retrospective study of infants in the NICU at the authors' institution, the authors determined the frequency of late rise of TSH to be 1.4%[21] Most of these infants were premature, and many had evidence of significant iodine exposure. In more than half of these infants, the elevation in TSH concentration persisted, continued to rise, or was severe enough to require treatment with thyroxine replacement.

Primary hypothyroidism, especially when detected as a delayed rise of TSH, is likely transient; in these infants, the long-term effects are not known but may include adverse developmental outcomes. Therefore, many investigators recommend retesting of VLBW infants and those in the NICU between 2 and 6 weeks of age to detect and treat this form of hypothyroidism in a timely manner.[4,21–23]

HYPOCALCEMIA

Hypocalcemia, defined as a serum total calcium concentration of less than 7.5 mg/dL or ionized calcium less than 1.2 mmol/L, is relatively common in infants in the NICU.[24,25] These infants may be asymptomatic, with hypocalcemia detected only on routine chemistries. They may present with specific symptoms of neuromuscular irritability including tremulousness, tetany, exaggerated startle response, seizures, and laryngospasm. Nonspecific symptoms such as apnea, cyanosis, tachycardia, tachypnea, vomiting, and feeding difficulties may be seen also.

The etiologies of neonatal hypocalcemia are considered in relation to the age at which it presents.[24] Early neonatal hypocalcemia occurs within the first 3 days of life and is common in the NICU, with an incidence in premature infants of 26% to 50%.[26] Late hypocalcemia develops afterwards, frequently between 5 and 10 days of life.[24–27]

Early Neonatal Hypocalcemia

Early hypocalcemia results from an exaggeration of the normal decline of serum calcium concentrations during the first 24 to 48 hours of life.[25] After birth, as the infant is withdrawn from the maternal supply of calcium through the placenta, the serum calcium concentration falls.[25] Parathormone (PTH) secretion is stimulated; however, the parathyroid gland's response is slow, resulting in a physiologic nadir in serum calcium concentrations within the first 48 hours of life. In some newborns, total and ionized calcium concentrations decline more rapidly and to lower nadir values.[24] This occurs most frequently in premature, small for gestational age, LBW, and asphyxiated infants, and in infants born to mothers with gestational or permanent diabetes mellitus.[24–27] In a study by Tsang and Oh,[26] 30% of LBW infants developed hypocalcemia at a mean age of 29 hours. The hypocalcemic infants were more ill and premature and had lower birth weights and lower calcium intake. Roberton and colleagues,[27] in a study of ill LBW infants, showed that 39% developed hypocalcemia within 96 hours of life. In addition to low birth weight, other factors associated with early hypocalcemia were low calcium intake and longer exposure to high inspired oxygen concentrations, reflecting the severity of their illnesses.

In premature infants, early hypocalcemia has been attributed to an attenuated physiologic postnatal rise in PTH secretion, a relative resistance of the renal tubules to PTH, and prolonged elevation of calcitonin concentrations.[24,25] In LBW infants hypocalcemia also may be caused by the rapid skeletal accretion of calcium and relative resistance of the intestinal tract and bone to calcitriol.[24] Asphyxiated and perinatally stressed newborns often have a reduced calcium intake, an increased phosphate load caused by cellular injury, and elevated calcitonin resulting in hypocalcemia.

The frequency of hypocalcemia in infants of mothers who have diabetes is approximately 50%.[24] The etiology is multifactorial and hypothesized to be caused by significant maternal urinary excretion of calcium and magnesium, resulting in reduced placental transfer of calcium and magnesium, decreased neonatal secretion of PTH, elevated neonatal calcitonin, and deficient intake and impaired absorption of calcium by the infant.

Common treatments in the NICU have been associated with early hypocalcemia.[24] Aminoglycoside antibiotics increase urinary excretion of calcium and magnesium. Compounds that complex with and sequester calcium, such as phosphates, citrate, and fatty acids, can lower ionized calcium concentrations. Ionized calcium also can be reduced in infants given bicarbonate, which increases calcium binding to albumin.

Late Neonatal Hypocalcemia

Hypocalcemia also can occur in infants in the NICU after 3 days of age. One of the most frequent causes is excessive intake of phosphate, usually through the diet.[24,25] Other etiologies include chronic renal insufficiency caused by renal hypoplasia or obstructive nephropathies, hypomagnesemia, and vitamin D deficiency associated with maternal vitamin D insufficiency.[24,25]

Hypoparathyroidism in infancy usually is caused by delayed maturation of parathyroid gland function.[24] It also may be caused by parathyroid gland dysembryogenesis, however.[24,25] The most common forms of dysgenesis are the DiGeorge and velocardiofacial syndromes, in which there is maldevelopment of the third and fourth branchial pouches. These syndromes usually are associated with microdeletions of chromosome 22q11.2.[24,25,28–30] The clinical phenotype and severity of infants who have this chromosomal anomaly are variable. They often have characteristic facial and aortocardiac anomalies. Infants who have classic DiGeorge syndrome have the triad of hypocalcemia caused by parathyroid gland hypoplasia, defective T-lymphocyte function and impaired cell-mediated immunity caused by impaired thymic differentiation, and conotruncal defects of the heart or aortic arch. Syndromes associated with 22q11.2 deletions have been grouped as the CATCH-22 syndromes (cardiac anomalies, abnormal facies, thymic hypoplasia or aplasia, cleft palate, and hypocalcemia with deletion at 22q). Some infants who have deletions of 22q11.2 may have neonatal hypoparathyroidism as the only manifestation. Hypoparathyroidism may be permanent but is often transient, with resolution during infancy and possible recurrence during times of stress or severe illness.[30]

Evaluation and Management of Neonatal Hypocalcemia

In infants who have persistent or recurrent hypocalcemia, the following should be obtained before initiating treatment: serum total and ionized calcium, magnesium, phosphate, creatinine, calcidiol, calcitriol, intact PTH, and spot urinary calcium and creatinine concentrations.[24] Decreased PTH concentrations are common in early hypocalcemia, but persistently low concentrations suggest impaired PTH secretion. Elevated PTH concentrations occur in infants who have PTH resistance, renal insufficiency, or vitamin D deficiency. Low calcidiol concentrations usually occur in vitamin D deficiency associated with maternal vitamin D insufficiency. Low calcitriol concentrations can be caused by severe renal insufficiency, hypoparathyroidism, or 1 alpha hydroxylase deficiency. Elevated calcitriol implies vitamin D resistance. Serum total and ionized calcium, phosphate, and intact PTH should be measured in mothers of infants who have unexplained hypocalcemia. In infants who have suspected DiGeorge syndrome, evaluation should include a complete blood cell count and T (CD4) lymphocyte counts. A chest radiogram may be useful to look for a thymic shadow. The diagnosis is confirmed by a microdeletion of chromosome 22q11.2 by fluorescent in situ hybridization (FISH).

Treatment of newborns who have acute or symptomatic hypocalcemia is accomplished best by the intravenous infusion of calcium salts; 10% calcium gluconate (9.3 mg/mL of elemental calcium) is used most commonly.[24,25] In asymptomatic newborns, treatment generally is indicated when the total serum calcium concentration is less than 6 mg/dL in the preterm infant and less than 7 mg/dL in the term infant. Calcium supplementation can be given either by the intravenous or oral route, depending on the clinical status of the infant. Effective oral therapy involves adding calcium glubionate or calcium carbonate to a low phosphate formula such as Similac PM 60/40 (calcium to phosphate ratio of 1.6:1) to establish an overall ratio of calcium to phosphate intake of 4:1. Additional therapy depends on the cause of hypocalcemia. Infants who have hypoparathyroidism require calcitriol in addition to calcium supplementation to restore and maintain eucalcemia. Infants who have vitamin D deficiency will benefit from vitamin D supplementation. If magnesium concentrations are low, treatment with intravenous or intramuscular magnesium sulfate is essential for correction of the hypocalcemia.

ADRENAL INSUFFICIENCY

The maturation of the hypothalamic-pituitary-adrenal (HPA) axis is a complex process that starts in utero and involves interaction between maternal, placental, and fetal factors.[31] The intrauterine environment shields the fetus from significant maternal cortisol exposure until late in gestation, and stimulates the activation of the axis toward the latter part of the pregnancy.

There are two placental actions crucial to the normal development of the axis. The first one is the oxidation of cortisol to cortisone (biologically inactive) by 11B hydroxysteroid hydrogenase type 2 (11B-HSD2), thus limiting fetal exposure to maternal cortisol. During the first part of gestation, maternal cortisol crosses the placenta, exerting negative feedback on the fetal HPA axis and suppressing fetal cortisol production. Placental 11B-HSD2s activity is low during the first half of gestation and increases during the last trimester, thereby decreasing the negative feedback to the fetal HPA axis and stimulating production of fetal corticotropin (ACTH). This results in the necessary stimuli for developing the adrenal neocortex. The second factor is placental corticotropin-releasing factor (CRH). In contrast to hypothalamic CRH, its production is stimulated by cortisol, and increases toward term, also stimulating fetal adrenal steroid production.[32]

In response to the above signals, the fetal adrenal gland undergoes massive hypertrophy during the latter part of gestation,[33] primarily in the fetal zone. Its main products are dehydroepiandrosterone and dehydroepiandrosterone-sulfate, because through most of gestation, the fetal adrenal gland is deficient in 3BHSD activity. As a consequence, the fetus cannot produce cortisol de novo before 23 weeks of gestation, and normally does not do so until as late as 30 weeks, when the higher levels of ACTH stimulate the development of the cortex. Instead, cortisol is synthesized from placental progesterone, thus bypassing the need for 3BHSD. However, the circumstances that lead to premature delivery can accelerate the maturation of the adrenal cortex, and 3BHSD activity may appear earlier.[34]

In preterm infants, there is an incomplete response to stress. This diminished response seems to mainly occur at the level of the adrenal gland, and it also seems to be limited to the first 2 weeks of life[35] (temporary adrenocortical insufficiency of the premature [TAP]). Normal cortisol values for infancy remain a topic of disagreement. Even though some authors have provided data for preterm infants after birth and during the first weeks of life,[36–39] along with results of ACTH[40] and CRH[35] stimulation tests, there is no consensus regarding normality.[41] Normal values may be as low as 1 to 2 μg/dL.[42] To further complicate the issue, antenatal circumstances, such as maternal glucocorticoid administration, can have an effect on the infant's adrenal response.[35]

A diminished neonatal adrenal response may place the infant at an increased risk for morbidity and mortality. Cortisol has several actions:

Regulates protein, carbohydrate, lipid, and nucleic acid metabolism
Maintains vascular responsiveness to circulating vasoconstrictors
Opposes the increase in capillary permeability during acute inflammation
Regulates extracellular water by reducing movement of water into cells and by promoting free water excretion
Suppresses the inflammatory response
Modulates central nervous system processing and behavior[31]

In the preterm infant, inadequate adrenal function has been associated with hypotension[41] and the development of bronchopulmonary dysplasia (BPD).[43] Standard- and low-dose ACTH stimulation tests have been used to diagnose adrenal insufficiency in preterm and critically ill infants.[44–46]

Hypotension

TAP might play a role in the appearance of refractive hypotension in VLBW infants. Low cortisol concentrations have been related to low blood pressure and poor response to inotrope treatment.[41] Also, increased effectiveness and faster response to inotrope treatment have been shown when treating premature infants who have refractory hypotension with low-dose hydrocortisone,[47] but this finding has been disputed.[39]

Bronchopulmonary Dysplasia

Infants who developed bronchopulmonary dysplasia (BPD) have been shown to have a significantly lower response to ACTH stimulation tests when compared with controls,[48] and lower basal cortisol values,[49,50] although not by all authors.[51] Also, these infants have shown early increases in markers of lung inflammation,[52] and thus it has been hypothesized that inadequate cortisol activity leads to amplified inflammatory responses, resulting in chronic lung disease.

The use of low-dose hydrocortisone (1 mg/kg/d) to prevent early adrenal insufficiency in preterm infants has shown a significant increase in survival without oxygen dependence at 36 weeks postmenstrual age[53] when compared with controls. Larger studies have not confirmed these results, although they have shown an increased risk of spontaneous gastrointestinal perforation[54] in the hydrocortisone-treated infants.

Before one can understand fully the role cortisol plays in the extrauterine development of the preterm infant, normality ranges have to be defined, taking into account factors such as gestational age, postconceptional age, use of antenatal corticosteroids, and the degree of stress affecting the premature infant.[41]

HYPOGLYCEMIA

The definition of hypoglycemia has been debated for decades. Currently there is no consistent definition of hypoglycemia in terms of either diagnostic or therapeutic concentrations.[55–57] Koh and colleagues[58,59] in 1986 and 1992 performed a review of multiple pediatric textbooks and surveys of neonatal pediatricians to determine threshold concentrations used to define hypoglycemia.[57] In the first study, they identified definitions of hypoglycemia in term neonates ranging from 18 to 45 mg/dL from textbooks and 18 to 70 mg/dL from surveys.[59] A comparison of both studies showed that the median threshold concentration had increased significantly between 1986 and 1992.[57] In 1992, most pediatricians considered a safe blood glucose concentration to be greater than 36 mg/dL.[58]

Many pediatric endocrinologists currently define hypoglycemia as a plasma glucose concentration of less than 50 mg/dL for diagnostic purposes.[55] They consider a plasma glucose concentration of 70 mg/dL as the lowest concentration acceptable during hypoglycemia treatment. It is important to keep in mind that bedside glucometers are screening instruments and may not be entirely accurate for measuring hypoglycemia.

The goal of neonatal glucose homeostasis is to provide the brain and other vital organs with sufficient glucose for energy. Newborn infants have high glucose turnover rates of approximately 4 to 6 mg/kg/min. At birth, when the transplacental glucose supply is interrupted, most healthy term newborns are able to quickly initiate glucose production to meet their high glucose demands.[57,60] This occurs by means of increases in plasma catecholamines, glucagon, and cortisol, in combination with a decrease in plasma insulin concentrations that promote glycogenolysis, gluconeogenesis, lipolysis, fatty acid oxidation, and muscle protein breakdown. Hepatic glucose production by glycogenolysis and gluconeogenesis, which is estimated to be 4 to 6 mg/kg/min in term newborns, is the only source of glucose until feeding is established. In term newborns, liver glycogen stores are depleted within approximately 12 hours of birth. Glucose production by gluconeogenesis begins about 2 hours after birth and peaks after 12 hours. Lipolysis generates free fatty acids that are used for oxidative metabolism and the production of ketones. Both free fatty acids and ketones can be used by tissues as an energy source, thereby decreasing the demands of these tissues for glucose.

Certain groups of newborns are at risk of developing transient hypoglycemia. These include premature infants and those who have intrauterine growth retardation (IUGR) and low metabolic reserves.[57,60,61] Preterm infants have limited glycogen stores, because glycogen storage takes place primarily during the third trimester. In addition to low glycogen stores, preterm infants and those who have IUGR also have decreased accumulation of protein and fat. As a result, their ability to maintain glucose production by glycogenolysis and gluconeogenesis for more than short periods of fasting is limited. It also has been shown that the activity of glucose-6-phosphatase, a key enzyme for gluconeogenesis and glycogenolysis, is low in preterm infants. In addition, lipolysis and ketogenesis are limited because of a lack of fat-stores in adipose tissue, resulting in lower free fatty acid and ketone body concentrations. These infants are therefore at higher risk of the harmful effects of hypoglycemia.[62]

Infants who have high expenditure of energy, such as those with perinatal asphyxia, sepsis, hypoxia, and hypothermia, are also at risk for hypoglycemia. Infants who have asphyxia or stress at the time of delivery can have hypoglycemia caused by hyperinsulinism.[62,63] This also can be seen in infants who have intrauterine growth retardation and in those born to mothers who have diabetes. This type of hyperinsulinism is usually transient, resolving within days to weeks after birth. The glucose requirement of these infants is high, however, and they frequently require dextrose infusion rates of 20 mg/kg/min or greater to control blood glucose concentrations. Sometimes these infants have more prolonged hypoglycemia lasting several months, requiring treatment with diazoxide.

Infants without obvious risk factors for transient hypoglycemia, those requiring high glucose infusion rates to maintain euglycemia, or those who have persistent or recurrent hypoglycemia warrant an evaluation to determine the etiology to optimally treat. Etiologies to consider include congenital hyperinsulinism, hormone deficiencies, and metabolic disorders.[57]

Infants who have congenital hyperinsulinism typically present within the first few days of life with symptomatic hypoglycemia that is persistent.[57,64,65] Some infants, but not all, are macrosomic because of exposure to perinatal hyperinsulinemia. Their glucose infusion rates to maintain euglycemia are elevated, usually greater than 8 mg/kg/min[64] and sometimes exceed 15 to 20 mg/kg/min.[63,65] Biochemically, they have an inappropriately normal or elevated serum insulin concentration at the time of hypoglycemia with low serum fatty acid and ketone body concentrations.[63,64] The serum lactate and ammonia concentrations may be elevated in some forms of congenital hyperinsulinism. These infants also demonstrate an inappropriately good glycemic response (an increase of more than 30 mg/dL) to glucagon at the time of hypoglycemia.[63,65] The most common genetic causes are autosomal recessive mutations in the genes (on chromosome 11p15.1) encoding the two subunits SUR1 and KIR6.2 of the pancreatic KATP channels, which result in unregulated insulin secretion.[57,63,64,66] The second most common form of congenital hyperinsulinism is the hyperinsulinism/hyperammonemia syndrome, which is associated with sporadic or dominantly inherited mutations of glutamate dehydrogenase. These infants typically demonstrate protein-induced (leucine sensitive) hypoglycemia.[64] A rare cause of hyperinsulinism involves a mutation of the glucokinase gene. The histopathological lesions associated with congenital hyperinsulinism are described as diffuse or focal,[57,63-65,67] and recently 18-fluoro-DOPA positron emission tomography (PET) scanning has been shown to be effective in distinguishing focal from diffuse forms.[65] Medical management of hyperinsulinism includes diazoxide, somatostatin analogs, calcium channel blockers, and a protein (leucine)-restricted diet. If medical therapy fails to control hypoglycemia, surgery is necessary with selective resection of focal lesions or subtotal pancreatectomy for the diffuse form.

Deficiencies of the counter-regulatory hormones cortisol and growth hormone can present with severe hypoglycemia, which may be the first sign of multiple pituitary hormone deficiencies. Midline defects (eg, cleft palate) and micropenis may be seen on physical examination. The biochemical profile is similar to hyperinsulinism. If cortisol or growth hormone deficiencies are suspected, other pituitary hormone concentrations should be evaluated, particularly thyroid hormone concentrations, to determine which hormone replacement is necessary.[57,67]

Metabolic disorders that can present with hypoglycemia include glycogen storage disorders, defects in gluconeogenesis, defects in amino acid metabolism, and fatty acid oxidation disorders.[57] Newborn screening evaluates for many of these conditions; however, in the setting of persistent or recurrent hypoglycemia, these disorders need to be excluded.

Any newborn who has risk factors for hypoglycemia (eg, maternal diabetes, intrauterine growth retardation, preterm birth, perinatal stress), physical examination findings associated with known causes of hypoglycemia (eg, midline defects, hepatomegaly), or any symptom that might be consistent with hypoglycemia should be evaluated.[56] The initial blood glucose measurement usually is performed by glucometer to obtain a rapid result; however, a sample also should be sent to the laboratory for confirmation. Management of the infant's hypoglycemia should be based on clinical signs, the blood glucose concentration and trend over time, and response to enteral feedings.

Multiple diagnostic algorithms have been suggested to assist with determining the specific etiology of hypoglycemia.[55,65,67] These may be helpful when an infant has hypoglycemia that is persistent, recurrent, or difficult to manage, or if the infant does not have any obvious risk factors for hypoglycemia. Regardless of the specific approach, the evaluation should involve obtaining a critical sample at the time of hypoglycemia. This sample includes a preserved glucose concentration to confirm hypoglycemia along with a blood gas to determine if acidosis is present, urinalysis for measurement of ketones, lactate concentration, free fatty acid concentration, insulin concentration, and growth hormone and cortisol concentrations. The absence of acidosis, along with absent or low concentrations of free fatty acids and ketones, is strongly suggestive of hyperinsulinism (either transient or congenital). This pattern, however, also can be seen with hormone deficiencies.[55] Diagnosis will depend on the insulin, cortisol, and growth hormone concentrations. If free fatty acid concentrations are elevated, fatty acid oxidation disorders should be suspected.

The presence of acidosis with an elevated lactate concentration and absent ketones suggests disorders of gluconeogenesis and glycogenolysis.[55] Ketoacidosis occurs in certain glycogen storage disorders and may be seen with deficiencies of growth hormone and cortisol.

In addition to the biochemical profile, other clues to the diagnosis of hypoglycemia include the relation to meals and the presence or absence of hepatomegaly.[65] Determining the specific etiology of hypoglycemia is imperative to determining the appropriate treatment for the infant.

HYPERGLYCEMIA

Hyperglycemia is a common occurrence in the VLBW infant, especially in the first week of life. Estimates of as many as greater than 80% of all infants weighing less 1500 g may be affected, with the highest numbers seen in the infants who are also growth-restricted.[66] There is no consensus as to what glucose concentration should be defined as hyperglycemia, but recent publications have used a blood glucose concentration greater than 150 to 180 mg/dL (8.3 to 10 mmol/L),[68] because this is concentration at which many premature infants begin to have glycosuria. It is known that hyperglycemia correlates with gestational age, birth weight, illness and stress, neonatal corticosteroid therapy, and intravenous glucose administration.[69] The incidence of hyperglycemia may be increasing because of the recent emphasis on early intravenous alimentation.

Not unexpectedly, there are significant complications from untreated hyperglycemia, including hyperosmolality, an osmotic diuresis, dehydration and, possibly, intracranial bleeding and additive effects on ischemic brain injury. It also has been suggested that hyperglycemia is a risk factor for retinopathy of prematurity[70] and early death and overall morbidity.[71]

The etiology of significant hyperglycemia for most premature infants receiving intravenous glucose at infusion rates exceeding the normal glucose turnover of approximately 6 mg/kg/min[72] is thought to be caused by multiple factors related to prematurity. These include an inability to inhibit gluconeogenesis, relative insulin resistance (possibly related to elevated growth hormone, cortisol, and catecholamine concentrations), defective proinsulin processing, and delayed secretion.[69] The use of early intravenous lipid infusions also may increase glucose by serving as a preferential oxidative substrate and inhibiting insulin's hepatic effects.[73] Because many small and ill premature infants are unable to receive adequate oral/gastric feedings, several enteroinsular hormones (gastrointestinal peptide, pancreatic polypeptide) are not secreted.[74]

The management of hyperglycemia is rather straightforward; either the rate of glucose infusion is decreased, or exogenous insulin is infused. There continues to be controversy, however, about the use of insulin because of the concerns of inadvertently causing hypoglycemia or hypokalemia. There is a risk of accidentally increasing the infusion rate and also the unknown dosage effect caused by insulin binding to the intravenous tubing and infusion bag. Because the addition of an exogenous insulin infusion not only treats hyperglycemia but also allows for the provision of adequate calories, it is common in some neonatal units to routinely infuse insulin in the smallest babies. Because neonates appear to have a maximal oxidative capacity of 12 mg/kg/min,[74] management requires carefully titrating both glucose and insulin infusions. A reasonable intravenous insulin infusion rate is 0.01 to 0.1 U/kg/h with the lowest dose preferred for the initial infusion. To prevent insulin absorption to intravenous tubing, a solution of insulin (5 U/mL) should be used as a priming solution in the tubing and left for 20 minutes, then replaced by the actual infusate.[75]

Although hyperglycemia related to prematurity is a common occurrence, transient and permanent neonatal diabetes (developing from birth through the first 3 to 4 months) is extremely rare, estimated to occur in 1 of 400,000 to 500,000 live births.[76] Neonatal diabetes may occur as an isolated defect or as part of a multisystem syndrome, with overlap in the putative defects in both of these and those cases that appear to be transient. For the most part, neonatal diabetes does not seem to have an autoimmune etiology. Transient diabetes is known to predispose the individual to type 2 diabetes later in life.[77] Both transient and permanent diabetes often are associated with intrauterine growth restriction.[78]

Transient diabetes has been reported with uniparental isodisomy of chromosome 6 and an unbalanced duplication of paternal chromosome 6. Pancreatic β-cell ATP-sensitive K+ channels are hetero-octamers assembled from Kir6.2 and the high-affinity sulfonylurea receptor 1 (SUR1) encoded by the ABCC8 gene. Mutations in the gene have been associated with transient and permanent diabetes. These mutations also have given rise to type 2 diabetes[79] and with associated neurologic symptoms.[80] Ketoacidosis has been a common occurrence at presentation.

Permanent diabetes has been reported to be caused by mutations in the insulin promoter factor-1 implicated in pancreatic development[80] and with complete deficiency of glucokinase activity.[81] Patients who have glucokinase deficiency are growth-restricted at birth, require insulin shortly after birth, and have parents who have hypergly-cemia.[81] Mutations in the insulin gene can cause disruption of the beta cells and the early onset of diabetes (although they may be diagnosed later than the traditional infants who have diabetes).[82] Neonatal diabetes also has been mapped to chromosome 10p12.1-p13 in a family in which affected individuals were severely growth-restricted, microcephalic, and had agenesis of the cerebellum. The hyperglycemia in these affected individuals was severe and unresponsive to insulin infusion.[83] Heterozygous activation mutations in the gene encoding for Kir6.2 (the ATP-sensitive potassium channel subunit) is a common cause of permanent neonatal diabetes. It is also seen as part of the neuro-logic syndrome DEND (developmental delay, epilepsy and neonatal diabetes).[84] Muta-tions in the potassium channel conceivably may be amenable to therapy with sulfonylureas, but this remains to be shown. Other causes of transient and permanent neonatal diabetes are managed, if possible, with insulin.

REFERENCES

1. van Tijn DA, de Vijlder JJM, Verbeeten B Jr, et al. Neonatal detection of congenital hypothyroidism of central origin. J Clin Endocrinol Metab 2005;90(6):3350–9.
2. Ogilvy-Stuart AL. Neonatal thyroid disorders. Arch Dis Child Fetal Neonatal Ed 2002;87(3):F165–71.
3. Kratzsch J. Thyroid gland development and defects. Best Pract Res Clin Endo-crinol Metab 2008;22(1):57–75.
4. Rapaport R, Rose SR, Freemark M. Hypothyroxinemia in the preterm infants: the benefits and risks of thyroxine treatment. J Pediatr 2001;139:182–8.
5. Cuestas RA. Thyroid function in healthy premature infants. J Pediatr 1978;92(6): 963–7.
6. van Wassenaer AG, Kok JH. Hypothyroxinaemia and thyroid function after preterm birth. Semin Neonatol 2004;9:3–11.
7. Mercado M, Yu VYH, Francis I, et al. Thyroid function in very preterm infants. Early Hum Dev 1988;16:131–41.
8. Williams FLR, Visser TJ, Hume R. Transient hypothyroxinaemia in preterm infants. Early Hum Dev 2006;82(12):797–802.
9. Uhrmann S, Marks KH, Maisels MJ, et al. Frequency of transient hypothyroxinae-mia in low birthweight infants. Arch Dis Child 1981;56:214–7.
10. Osborn DA. Thyroid hormone for preventing of neurodevelopmental impairment in preterm infants. Cochrane Database Syst Rev 2000;(2):CD001070.
11. Chowdhry P, Scanlon JW, Auerbach R, et al. Results of controlled double-blind study of thyroid replacement in very low birth weight premature infants with hypo-thyroxinaemia. Pediatrics 1984;73:301–5.
12. Vanhole C, Aerssens P, Naulaers G, et al. L-thyroxine treatment of preterm newborns: clinical and endocrine effects. Pediatr Res 1997;42:87–92.
13. Amato M, Pasquier S, Carasso A, et al. Postnatal thyroxine administration for idio-pathic respiratory distress syndrome in preterm infants. Horm Res 1988;29:301–5.
14. van Wassenaer AG, Kok JH, de Vijlder JJ, et al. Effects of thyroxine supplemen-tation on neurologic development in infants born at less than 30 weeks' gestation. N Engl J Med 1997;42:87–92.
15. Osborn DA. Thyroid hormones for preventing neurodevelopmental impairment in preterm infants. Cochrane Database Syst Rev 2001;(4):CD001070.
16. Osborn DA, Hunt RW. Postnatal thyroid hormones for preterm infants with tran-sient hypothyroxinaemia. Cochrane Database Syst Rev 2007;(1):CD005945.

17. Weber G, Vigone MC, Rapa A, et al. Neonatal transient hypothyroidism: aetiological study. Italian collaborative study on transient hypothyroidism. Arch Dis Child Fetal Neonatal Ed 1998;79(1):F70–2.
18. l'Allemand D, Gruters A, Beyer P, et al. Iodine in contrast agents and skin disinfectants is the major cause for hypothyroidism in premature infants during intensive care. Horm Res 1987;28(1):42–9.
19. Smerdely P, Boyages SC, Wu D, et al. Topical iodine-containing antiseptics and neonatal hypothyroidism in very low birth weight infants. Lancet 1989;2(8664): 661–4.
20. Gordon CM, Rowitch DH, Mitchell ML, et al. Topical iodine and neonatal hypothyroidism. Arch Pediatr Adolesc Med 1995;149:1336–9.
21. Hyman SJ, Greig F, Holzman I, et al. Late rise of thyroid stimulating hormone in ill newborns. J Pediatr Endocrinol Metab 2007;20(4):501–10.
22. Mandel SJ, Hermos RJ, Larson CA, et al. Atypical hypothyroidism and the very low birth weight infant. Thyroid 2000;10:693–5.
23. Larson C, Hermos R, Delaney A, et al. Risk factors associated with delayed thyrotropin elevations in congenital hypothyroidism. J Pediatr 2003;143:587–91.
24. Root AW, Diamond FB Jr. Disorders of mineral homeostasis in the neonate and infant. In: Sperling MA, editor. Pediatric endocrinology. 3rd edition. Philadelphia: Saunders Elsevier; 2008. p. 691–706.
25. Hsu SC, Levine MA. Perinatal calcium metabolism: physiology and pathophysiology. Semin Neonatol 2004;9:23–36.
26. Tsang RC, Oh W. Neonatal hypocalcemia in low birth weight infants. Pediatrics 1970;45:773–81.
27. Roberton NR, Smith MA. Early neonatal hypocalcemia. Arch Dis Child 1975;50: 604–9.
28. Driscoll DA, Budarf ML, Emanuel BS. A genetic etiology for DiGeorge syndrome: consistent deletions and microdeletions of 22q11. Am J Hum Genet 1992;50: 924–33.
29. De la Chapelle A, Herva R, Koivisto M, et al. A deletion in chromosome 22 can cause DiGeorge syndrome. Hum Genet 1981;57:253–6.
30. Greig F, Paul E, DiMartino-Nardi J, et al. Transient congenital hypoparathyroidism: resolution and recurrence in chromosome 22q11 deletion. J Pediatr 1996;128:563–7.
31. Watterberg KL. Adrenocortical function and dysfunction in the fetos and neonate. Semin Neonatol 2004;9:13–21.
32. Pepe GJ, Albrecht ED. Actions of placental and fetal adrenal steroid hormones in primate pregnancy. Endocr Rev 1995;16:608–48.
33. Mediano S, Jaffe RB. Developmental and functional biology of the primate fetal adrenal cortex. Endocr Rev 1997;18:378–403.
34. Parker CR Jr, Faye-Peterson O, Stankovic AK, et al. Immunohistochemical evaluation of the cellular localization and ontogeny of 3B-hydroxysteroid dehydrogenase/delta 5-4 isomerase in the human fetal adrenal gland. Endocr Res 1995; 21:69–80.
35. Ng PC, Lam WK, Lee CH, et al. Reference ranges and factors affecting the human corticotropin-releasing hormone test in preterm, very low birth weight infants. J Clin Endocrinol Metab 2002;87(10):4621–8.
36. Wittekind CA, Arnold JD, Leslie GI, et al. Longitudinal study of plasma ACTH and cortisol in very low birth weight infants in the first 8 weeks of life. Early Hum Dev 1993;33:191–200.
37. Al Saedi S, Dean H, Dent W, et al. Reference ranges for serum cortisol and 17-OH-progesterone levels in preterm infants. J Pediatr 1995;126:985–7.

38. Heckmann M, Wudy SA, Haack D, et al. Reference range for serum cortisol in well preterm infants. Arch Dis Child Fetal Neonatal Ed 1999;81:F171–4.
39. Aucott SW, Watterberg KL, Shaffer ML, et al. Do cortisol concentrations predict short-term outcomes in extremely low birth weight infants? PROPHET study group. Pediatrics 2008;122:775–81.
40. Hingre RV, Gross SJ, Hingre KS, et al. Adrenal steroidogenesis in very low birth weight preterm infants. J Clin Endocrinol Metab 1994;78(2):266–70.
41. Ng PC. Is there a normal range of serum cortisol concentration for preterm infants? Pediatrics 2008;122:873–5.
42. Arnold J, Leslie G, Bowen J, et al. Longitudinal study of plasma cortisol and 17-hydroxyprogesterone in very low birth weight infants during the first 16 weeks of life. Biol Neonate 1997;72(3):148–55.
43. Ng PC, Lee HC, Lam CWK, et al. Transient adrenocortical insufficiency of prematurity and systemic hypotension in very low birthweight infants. Arch Dis Child Fetal Neonatal Ed 2004;89:F119–26.
44. Karlsson R, Kallio J, Toppari J, et al. Timing of peak serum cortisol values in preterm infants in low-dose and the standard ACTH tests. Pediatr Res 1999; 45(3):367–9.
45. Bolt RJ, Van Weissenbruch MM, Popp-Snijders C, et al. Maturity of the adrenal cortex in very preterm infants is related to gestational age. Pediatr Res 2002; 52(3):405–10.
46. Bolt RJ, Van Weissenbruch MM, Popp-Snijders, et al. Fetal growth and the function of the adrenal cortex in preterm infants. J Clin Endocrinol Metab 2002;87(3): 1194–9.
47. Ng PC, Lee CH, Bnur FL, et al. A double-blind, randomized, controlled study of a stress dose of hydrocortisone for rescue treatment of refractory hypotension in infants. Pediatrics 2006;117:367–75.
48. Watterberg KL, Scott SM. Evidence of early adrenal insufficiency in babies who develop bronchopulmonary dysplasia. Pediatrics 1995;85:120–5.
49. Banks BA, Stouffer N, Cnaan A, et al. Association of plasma cortisol and chronic lung disease in preterm infants. Pediatrics 2001;107:494–8.
50. Nykanen P, Antila E, Heinonen K, et al. Early hypoadrenalism in premature infants at risk for bronchopulmonary dysplasia or death. Acta Paediatr 2007; 96:1600–5.
51. Merz U, Pfaffle R, Peschgens T, et al. The hypothalamic-pituitary-adrenal axis in preterm infants weighting ≤1250 g: association with perinatal data and chronic lung disease. Acta Paediatr 1998;87:313–7.
52. Watterberg KL, Demmers LM, Scott SM, et al. Chorioamnionitis and early lung inflammation in babies who develop bronchopulmonary dysplasia. Pediatrics 1996;97:210–5.
53. Watterberg KL, Verdes JS, Gifford KL, et al. Prophylaxis against early adrenal insufficiency to prevent chronic lung disease in premature infants. Pediatrics 1999;104:1258–63.
54. Watterberg KL, Gerdes JS, Cole CH, et al. Prophylaxis of early adrenal insufficiency to prevent bronchopulmonary dysplasia: a multicenter trial. Pediatrics 2004;114:1649–57.
55. Langdon DR, Stanley CA, Sperling MA. Hypoglycemia in the infant and child. In: Sperling MA, editor. Pediatric endocrinology. 3rd edition. Philadelphia: Saunders Elsevier; 2008. p. 422–43.
56. Rozance PJ, Hay WW. Hypoglycemia in newborn infants: features associated with adverse outcomes. Biol Neonate 2006;90:74–86.

57. Sunehag AL, Haymond MW. Glucose extremes in newborn infants. Clin Perinatol 2002;29:245–60.
58. Koh TH, Vong SK. Definition of neonatal hypoglycemia: is there a change? J Paediatr Child Health 1996;32(4):302–5.
59. Koh TH, Eyre JA, Aynsley-Green A. Neonatal hypoglycaemia: the controversy regarding definition. Arch Dis Child 1988;63:1386–8.
60. Mitanchez D. Glucose regulation in preterm newborn infants. Horm Res 2007;68:265–71.
61. Hume R, Burchell A, Williams FLR, et al. Glucose homeostasis in the newborn. Early Hum Dev 2005;81:95–101.
62. Hawdon JM. Hypoglycaemia and the neonatal brain. Eur J Pediatr 1999;158(Suppl 1):S9–12.
63. Stanley CA. Hyperinsulinism in infants and children. Pediatr Clin North Am 1997;44(2):363–74.
64. Hussain K. Diagnosis and management of hyperinsulinaemic hypoglycaemia of infancy. Horm Res 2008;69:2–13.
65. Valayannopoulos V, Romano S, Mention K, et al. What's new in metabolic and genetic hypoglycaemias: diagnosis and management. Eur J Pediatr 2008;167:257–65.
66. Hays SP, Smith EO, Sunehag AL. Hyperglycemia is a risk factor for early death and morbidity in extremely low birth-weight infants. Pediatrics 2006;118:1811–8.
67. Palladino A, Bennett MJ, Stanley CA. Hyperinsulinism in infancy and childhood: when an insulin level is not always enough. Clin Chem 2008;54(2):256–63.
68. Beardsall K, Vanhaesebrouck S, Ogilvy-Stuart AL, et al. A randomized controlled trial of early insulin therapy in very low birth weight infants, NIRTURE (neonatal insulin replacement therapy in Europe). BMC Pediatr 2007;7:29–39.
69. Kairamknonda VR, Khashu M. Controversies in the management of hyperglycemia in the ELBW infant. Indian Pediatr 2008;45:29–38.
70. Garg R, Agthe AG, Donohue PK, et al. Hyperglycemia and retinopathy of prematurity in very low birth weight infants. J Perinatol 2003;23:186–94.
71. Bochicchio GV, Sung J, Joshi M, et al. Persistent hyperglycemia is predictive of outcome in critically ill trauma patients. J Trauma 2005;58:921–4.
72. Thureen PJ. Early aggressive nutrition in the neonate. Pediatr Rev 1999;44:e45–55.
73. van Kempen AAMW, van der Crabben SN, Ackermans MT, et al. Stimulation of gluconeogenesis by intravenous lipids in preterm infants: response depends on fatty acid profile. Am J Physiol Endocrinol Metab 2006;290:e723–30.
74. Berseth CL. Effect of early feeding on maturation of the preterm infant's small intestine. J Pediatr 1992;120:947–53.
75. Mena P, Llanos A, Uauy R. Insulin homeostasis n the extremely low birth weight infant. Semin Perinatol 2001;25:436–46.
76. Shield JP, Gardner RJ, Wadsworth EJ, et al. Aetiopathology and genetic basis of neonatal diabetes. Arch Dis Child Fetal Neonatal Ed 1997;76:F39–42.
77. Shield JP, Baum JD. Is transient neonatal diabetes a risk factor for diabetes later in life? Lancet 1993;341:693.
78. Shield JP. Neonatal diabetes: new insights into etiology and implications. Hormone Res 2000;53(Suppl S1):7–11.
79. Vaxillaire M, Dechaume A, Busiah K, et al. New ABCC8 mutations in relapsing neonatal diabetes and clinical features. Diabetes 2007;56:1737–41.
80. Stoffers DA, Zinken NT, Stanojevic V, et al. Pancreatic agenesis attributable to a single nucleotide deletion in the human IPF-1 gene coding sequence. Nat Genet 1997;15:106–10.

81. Njolstad PR, Sagen JV, Bjorkhaug L, et al. Permanent neonatal diabetes caused by glucokinase deficiency. Diabetes 2003;52:2854–60.
82. Stoy J, Edghill EL, Flanagan SE, et al. Insulin gene mutations as a cause of permanent neonatal diabetes. Proc Natl Acad Sci U S A 2007;104:15040–4.
83. Sellick GS, Garrett C, Houlston RS. A novel gene for neonatal diabetes maps to chromosome 10p12.1-p13. Diabetes 2003;52:2636–8.
84. Gloyn AL, Diatloff-Zito C, Edghill EL, et al. KCNJ11 activating mutations are associated with developmental delay, epilepsy and neonatal diabetes syndrome and other neurological features. Eur J Hum Genet 2006;14:824–30.

Congenital Disorders of the Thyroid: Hypo/Hyper

Ferenc Péter, MD, PhD, DSc[a],*, Ágota Muzsnai, MD, PhD[b]

KEYWORDS

- Hypothyroidism • Hyperthyroidism • Congenital
- Disorders of thyroid • Goiter

This article summarizes the ontogenesis and genetics of the thyroid with regards to its possible congenital dysfunction and briefly refers to the roles of the mother-placenta-fetal unit, iodine effect, and organic and functional changes of the negative feedback mechanism, as well as maturity and illness, in some forms of congenital hypo- and hyperthyroidism. This article also describes the published literature and the authors' data on the clinical aspects of congenital hypothyroidism, on the alternating hypo- and hyperthyroidism in the neonatal period, and on neonatal hyperthyroidism.

ONTOGENESIS OF THYROID FUNCTION AND GENETIC BACKGROUND OF ALTERED THYROID FUNCTION

The ontogenesis of thyroid function involves the development of the fetal thyroid gland and its maturation, as well as the evolution of the hypothalamic-pituitary-thyroid axis. The developing thyroid is first visible in the floor of the primitive pharynx by embryonic day E20 to E22. Endodermal epithelium cells form the thyroid anlage, distinguishing themselves from their neighbors in a process defined as *specification*. A defect in this process should result in thyroid agenesis. During the second stage of early thyroid morphogenesis, the thyroid anlage invades the surrounding mesenchyme, forming a bud that proliferates and migrates from the pharyngeal floor through the anterior midline of the neck. The thyroid primordium becomes a bilobed structure by day E24 to E32 and reaches its final position around day E48 to E50. At the same time, small rudimentary follicles become evident and migrating C cells, derived from the ultimobranchial bodies, disseminate into the thyroid. Around day E51, the process of

Portions of this article were previously published in the *Endocrinology and Metabolism Clinics of North America*, 38:3.

[a] Department of Pediatrics, Division of Endocrinology, St Johns Hospital and United Hospitals of North-Buda, Buda Children's Hospital, 1023 Bolyai-u. 5-9, Budapest, Hungary
[b] Division of Endocrinology, St Johns Hospital and United Hospitals of North-Buda, Buda Children's Hospital, 1023 Bolyai-u. 5-9, Budapest, Hungary
* Corresponding author.
E-mail address: peter_f@budaigyk.hu

lobulation is complete, resulting in the definitive external form of the gland. An error during lobulation results in hemiagenesis, and an impaired descent results in ectopic thyroid tissue. Usually, the terminal differentiation of the thyroid follicular cells occurs when migration is complete (by 10–12 weeks). Specific proteins essential for thyroid hormone biosynthesis and secretion appear progressively: thyroglobulin (10–11 weeks), thyroid peroxidase, sodium/iodine symporter (12–13 weeks), thyrotropin receptor, thyroid oxidases, and pendrin. Defected, decreased, or absent production of these proteins results in dyshormonogenesis. All inborn errors of thyroid hormono-genesis are associated with a normally placed gland. In the last stages of embryonic life, the thyroid increases in size and continues to grow until term.

The hypothalamic-pituitary-thyroid axis is functional at midgestation. Thyrotropin is detectable in fetal serum as early as the 12th week and increases from the 18th week until term. The maturation of the hypothalamic-pituitary-thyroid feedback control is demon-strated by a fetal thyrotropin response to exogenously administered thyrotropin-releasing hormone at around 25 weeks' gestation and also by the observation in the third trimester of a progressive rise in the ratio of free thyroxine (FT_4) to thyrotropin.

Congenital hypothyroidism is a heterogeneous condition resulting from a decreased or absent action of thyroid hormone. It is usually a sporadic disorder with 85% of cases caused by abnormal thyroid gland development (dysgenesis) and the remaining 15% due to inborn error of thyroid hormonogenesis. Less common causes are thyroid hormone resistance, decreased thyroxine (T_4) cellular transport, thyrotropin resis-tance, and decreased thyrotropin synthesis or secretion. Growing evidence[1–3] confirms that almost every thyroidal and nonthyroidal disorder has a molecular genetic component (**Table 1**).

SOME OTHER AETIOPATHOGENETIC FACTORS

In addition to developmental and genetically determined damage to the thyroid, tran-sient or permanent congenital hypo- or hyperthyroidism may also be affected by factors related to the mother-placenta-fetal unit, the iodine effect (deficiency or excess), organic and functional changes of the negative feedback mechanism, and the status of maturation and health/illness at birth and in the first period of life. These factors are discussed below.

Mother-Placenta-Fetal Unit

It is well established that in iodine-deficient areas, the maternal thyroid hormone level can be too low to provide an adequate fetal hormone level, especially in the first trimester. However, convincing data suggest that maternal thyroid disorders (eg, overt or subclinical hypothyroidism, hypothyroxinemia) during pregnancy in iodine-sufficient areas can also result in neurointellectual impairment of children.[4,5]

Maternal hyperthyroidism can also cause significant risk for the offspring (see below). One of the reasons for such a close connection is the importance of the mother-placenta-fetus unit[6] with regards to the hypothalamic-pituitary-thyroid axis and influencing factors. Other maternal autoimmune thyroid diseases can be risk factors of primary dysfunction in the offspring as well.[7] **Fig. 1** shows the potential role of the mother-placenta-fetus unit in some congenital thyroid dysfunctions.

Iodine Deficiency or Excess

Iodine deficiency can cause transient hypothyroidism or even impaired neurocognitive development. The deficiency is more common in known mild or moderate iodine-deficient areas in Europe.[8] However, recent data suggest that women of reproductive age remain the most likely group to have low iodine excretion in the United States,[9] which is a risk to their offspring. Urinary iodine excretion is a good indicator of the status of iodine supplementation at the population level.[10,11] Neonatal thyrotropin screening results can also reflect the prevalence of iodine deficiency in a population.[12]

Iodine excess also can cause thyroid suppression. This excess can be caused by drugs, contrast agents, antiseptic solutions, or nutrition (eg, seaweed in Japan).[13] Premature infants are especially sensitive to both iodine deficiency and excess.[14]

Organic and Functional Changes of the Negative Feedback Mechanism (Central Resistance; Change of "Set Point")

The normal range for serum thyrotropin versus FT_4 in healthy infants (depicted between the first and 90th percentiles) were published by Fisher and colleagues.[15] The elevation of serum thyrotropin relative to FT_4 (values to the right of the line marking the 99th percentile) indicates pituitary resistance to the negative feedback of T_4 on thyrotropin secretion. There are organic (mainly genetic) and functional (mainly environmental) forms of these changes[7]: In permanent thyroid hormone resistance or in central congenital hypothyroidism with hypothalamic-pituitary organic damage, both parameters (thyrotropin and FT_4) are low. Recently, evidence has confirmed central congenital hypothyroidism in the offspring of insufficiently treated pregnant Graves patients (both parameters are low, mostly transiently; see below). In cases where maturity of the negative feedback is delayed (serum thyrotropin remains elevated in the presence of high or high-normal FT_4 concentration) mostly transient and functional (both parameters are high). Researchers have found similar, but more permanent changes in children with Down syndrome: Thyrotropin may be elevated with normal T_4/FT_4.[16,17]

Role of Maturation and Illness

Despite the birth rates have decreased in developed countries, the proportion of premature, very low birth weight and ill newborns needing intensive care for weeks or months has increased. Parallel to this trend have been improved effectiveness of medical treatment and higher survival rates. Thyroid function in premature, very low birth weight, and seriously ill infants is characterized by either slightly decreased or markedly low thyrotropin and T_4 levels after birth and during the first weeks of life. This transient hypothyroidism may occur because of delay in maturation of the hypothalamic-pituitary-thyroid axis, the effect of medications used on the intensive care unit (eg, dopamine, glucocorticoid), or recovery from the sick euthyroid syndrome. In some cases, the iodine content of antiseptics can cause suppression of thyroid function.

Several trials on T_4 supplementation have been published and are in progress in this group of infants, but the results so far have been controversial. Further studies are needed to determine the indications, protocols, and duration of such a supplementation. Recently, Fisher reviewed this topic.[18]

Cases of primary congenital hypothyroidism have been identified amongst these infants. Thyroid function of these neonates should also be monitored by serial serum thyrotropin measurements to detect its late rise and to start early T_4 replacement in proven cases of primary hypothyroidism.[19,20]

CONGENITAL HYPOTHYROIDISM
Screening

Congenital hypothyroidism is the most common congenital endocrine disorder and treatable cause of mental retardation. The published incidence of primary

Table 1
Molecular basis of disturbances in thyroid development, thyroid hormone synthesis, transport and action, and hypothalamic-pituitary-thyroid axis

Phenotype (by Morphology or Function)	Gene	Role of Gene in Organogenesis/Protein Function	Associated Disorders
Dysgenesis			
Aplasia or hemiagenesis or hypoplasia (ectopic or eutopic)	TITF1/NKX2.1	Development of both follicular and C-cells	Choreoathetosis, respiratory distress syndrome, pulmonary disease
	PAX8	Thyroid follicular cell development	Renal agenesis
	TITF2/FOXE1	Migration of thyroid precursor cells	Cleft palate, choanal atresia, bifid epiglottis, spiky hair (Bamforth syndrome)
Resistance to thyrotropin	GNAS1	Signaling protein	Osteodystrophy (hereditary Albright syndrome)
Hypoplasia (eutopic); resistance to thyrotropin	TSHR	Thyroid differentiation, thyrotropin receptor	-
Inborn error of thyroid hormonogenesis			
Enlarged thyroid	TITF1, PAX8, TITF2/FOXE1	During later stages, regulation of thyroid-specific gene expression	-
	TPO	Thyroid differentiation; iodide organification	-
	TG	Thyroid differentiation; structural prohormone	-
	NIS	Iodide transport from the blood into thyroid cell (basal membrane)	-
	PDS	Iodide transport from thyroid cell to follicular lumen (apical membrane)	Sensorineural deafness (Pendred syndrome)
	DUOX1/THOX1 DUOX2/THOX2	Thyroidal hydrogen peroxide generation	-
	DEHAL1	Deiodination for iodide recycling	-

	Gene	Function	Associated features
Thyroid hormone transporter defect			
Thyroid hormone resistance	MCT8	Transmembrane T$_4$, triiodothyronine, reverse triiodothyronine, diiodothyronine transport	Severe neurologic abnormalities
	THRB	Nuclear thyroid hormone receptor	Hyperactivity, learning disability
Abnormal thyroid function test	SBP2	Synthesis of selenoproteins	Delayed puberty (suspected)
Impaired hypothalamic-pituitary-thyroid axis			
Secondary/tertiary hypothyroidism	LHX3	Early pituitary development	CPHD, pituitary mass, rigid cervical spine
	LHX4		CPHD, sella turcica defect
	PROP1	Expression of all pituitary cell lineage	CPHD, pituitary mass
	POU1F1	Generation and cell-type specification	Growth hormone, prolactine deficiency
	HESX1, PHF6	Forebrain, midline, and pituitary development	Septo-optic dysplasia, Chronic pulmonary heart disease, epilepsy
	TRHR	Thyrotropin-releasing hormone receptor	-
	TSHB	Thyrotropin β subunit	-
Other			
Transient congenital hypothyroidism	DUOX2/THOX2	Partial defect in hydrogen peroxide production	-
Permanent hyperthyroidism	TSHR	Gain-of-function of thyrotropin receptor	-

Abbreviation: CPHD, combined pituitary hormone deficiency.

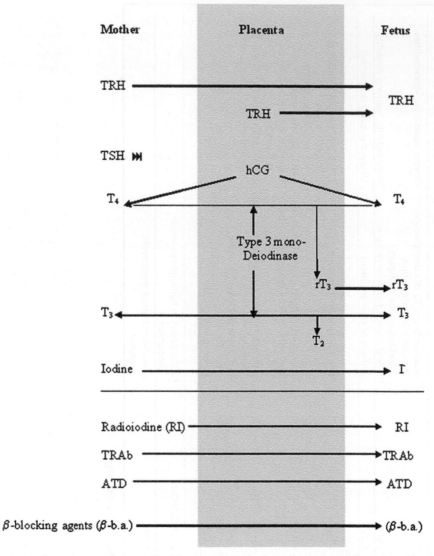

Fig. 1. Mother-placenta-fetus unit with regards to the hypothalamic-pituitary-thyroid axis. ATD, antithyroid drugs; hCG, human choriogonin; I, iodine; rT3, reverse triiodothyronine; T_2, diiodothyronine; T_3, triiodothyronine; TRAb, thyrotropin receptor antibodies; TRH, thyrotropin-releasing hormone; TSH, thyrotropin.

hypothyroidism increases: at present it varies from 1 in 1000 to 1 in 3500 live births depending on the iodine sufficiency, laboratory methods, screening practice (changes in test cutoffs), demographic and other unknown factors.[20] Depending on the iodine sufficiency, the incidence of primary hypothyroidism varies from 1 in 2500 to 1 in 4000 live births. Permanent secondary (thyrotropin deficient) and tertiary (thyro-tropin-releasing hormone deficient) hypothyroidism is rare, with an incidence of 1:50,000 and 1:100,000 respectively. Prevention of cretinism and optimal neurologic development can be achieved in affected infants by early introduction of hormonal replacement. Screening, based on measurement of hormone levels, aims to pick up hypothyroid children soon after birth because clinical features are not specific during the perinatal period.

The cost/benefit ratio determines the method and ultimately the strategies of the screening program. A full drop of whole blood is obtained by skin puncture on day 1 to 4 of life and is dried on filter paper. Samples are sent to screening laboratories via mail. Measurement of T_4, thyrotropin, or both is performed after an eluation process and a two-tiered approach is used. In Europe, Japan, and Australia, a primary thyrotropin determination was introduced as its sensitivity and specificity is greater than T_4 measurement. In North America the primary T_4 test is followed by backup thyrotropin determination in cases with a low T_4 level (usually the lowest 10th–20th percentile). Nowadays Canada and some states in the United States have switched to a primary thyrotropin program. Recently in the Netherlands, a primary T_4/backup-thyrotropin program was supplemented by a thyroxin-binding globulin measurement. Using the three-arm method, the incidence of congenital hypothyroidism increased up to 1:1800 in the Netherlands.[21] A second TSH determination in newborns with border-line TSH results also elevates the incidence mostly with milder forms, in which cases thyroid in situ is present.[22]

Despite the technical development in laboratory methods, some false-negative results still occur with both the commonly used screening programs. A primary thyrotropin strategy will miss the rare secondary and tertiary hypothyroidism, thyroxin-binding globulin deficiency, and hyperthyroxinemia, while a primary T_4/backup-thyrotropin program will miss compensated hypothyroidism. Apart from those infants missed depending on the exact strategy employed, infants with atypical congenital hypothyroidism (delayed thyrotropin rise) will be missed because their thyrotropin and T_4 levels are normal on initial screening.

Clinical Manifestation

Classic features of congenital hypothyroidism (lethargy, hypotonia, large tongue, hoarse cry, umbilical hernia, mottled dry skin, poor feeding, constipation) develop in the first 3 months of life and cannot be seen practically in countries where screening programs have been introduced. Babies identified by an abnormal laboratory result typically present with only some vague clinical symptoms during the first few postnatal weeks. After the 10 years of screening for congenital hypothyroidism, we evaluated the clinical signs of 87 recalled newborns suspected for thyroid hypofunction and developed a scoring system, which was subsequently evaluated.

Thyrotropin measurement was used from the blood spot taken from newborns aged 4 to 5 days. All newborns with elevated thyrotropin level were admitted to our hospital for further investigation and treatment. They were assessed by history and complete physical examination. More than 10 unspecific signs and history data were analyzed from their records to identify any factors that could predict congenital hypothyroidism: thyroid disorder in the family, concomitant congenital defect, large posterior fontanel, exuberant hair, enlarged tongue, constipation, umbilical hernia, hypoactivity, lethargic cry, wide nasal bridge, dry skin, and icterus.

The congenital hypothyroidism group (true positive, n = 67) and the reference group (false positive, n = 20) did not differ significantly in regard to the length of gestation (40 vs 39 weeks), birth weight (3330 vs 3240 g) and age at investigation (20 vs 22 days). By linear discriminant analysis, there were some significant differences ($P \leq .05$) and some nonsignificant differences ($P > .05$) between the two groups (**Table 2**).

Eight parameters that appeared significant in the hypothyroid group were ranked by screening thyrotropin value and weighted for further analysis: large posterior fontanel,

Table 2
Occurrence and significance of findings in newborns with elevated thyrotropin level at screening

Findings	Positive[a]	Negative[b]	P
Thyroid disorders in father's family	0	1	.51
Thyroid disorders in mother's family	14	3	.79
Concomitant congenital defect	9	0	.18
Large posterior fontanel	52	4	.00
Exuberant hair	11	0	.12
Enlarged tongue	22	0	.00
Constipation	16	0	.04
Umbilical hernia	23	2	.02
Hypoactivity	45	8	.03
Lethargic, hoarse cry	6	0	.38
Wide nasal bridge	15	0	.05
Dry skin	48	7	.00
Icterus	37	4	.02

[a] Hypothyroidism proved (n = 67).
[b] Hypothyroidism not proved (n = 20).

umbilical hernia, and dry skin were scored as 2, while enlarged tongue, constipation, hypoactivity, wide nasal bridge and icterus were scored as 1. Blood-spot thyrotropin was scored by numbers derived from the ratio of measured thyrotropin to the cutoff limit for normal thyrotropin. The classification system based on a score greater than 6 was correct for congenital hypothyroidism in 99% of cases. Signs summarized in **Table 3** are characteristic for congenital hypothyroidism at around 3 weeks of life.[22]

The scoring system delineates the manifestation of primary hypothyroidism in newborns and helps to differentiate hypothyroid infants from infants with a false-positive screening result. The extent of these nonspecific signs depends on the cause, severity, and duration of the hypothyroid status.

Fig. 2 summarizes the recommended diagnostic and therapeutic algorithm in congenital hypothyroidism.[23]

Prognosis

If T_4 replacement is adequate, somatic development in children with congenital hypothyroidism is similar to that in normal children. That is, height and weight are normal.

Table 3
Clinical signs and scoring for congenital hypothyroidism screened by thyrotropin measurement

Clinical Sign	Score	Clinical Sign	Score
Large posterior fontanel	2	Constipation	1
Umbilical hernia	2	Hypoactivity	1
Dry skin	2	Wide nasal bridge	1
Enlarged tongue	1	Icterus	1
Blood-spot thyrotropin: multiply by digit derived from measured/cutoff ratio			1
Cutoff value			>6

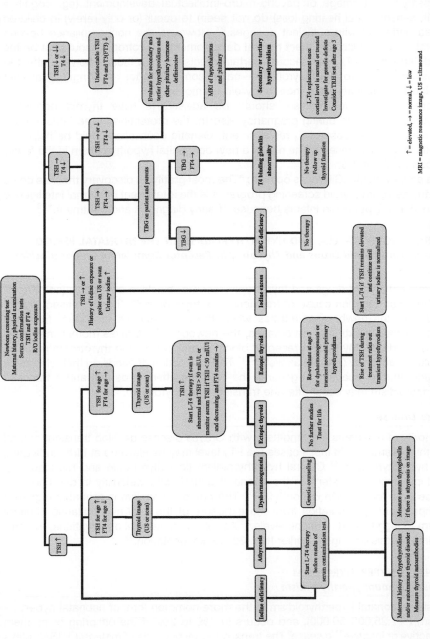

Fig. 2. Recommended diagnostic and therapeutic algorithm in congenital hypothyroidism. TSH, thyrotropin; R/O, rule out; TBG, thyroxin-binding globulin; T3(FT3), triiodothyronine (free triiodothyronine); TRH, thyrotropin-releasing hormone.

Also, retardation of bone maturation is also reversible in children with congenital hypo-thyroidism if T_4 replacement is adequate. Early (onset of replacement before 2 weeks of age) and high-dosage (initial dose of 10–15 µg/kg/d) treatment (**Table 4**) appears necessary.[24–26] Damage of psycho-neuro-intellectual development (eg, cognitive deficit, sensorineural hearing loss) do not seem to occur (or only rarely) in children treated early and with sufficient dosages.[27] However, the noncompliance beyond the first 3 years of life can affect mental development. Thyrotropin should not be the only determinant of T_4 dose because certain infants—mostly those who were affected by severe in utero hypothyroidism—have some (shorter or longer) transient hypothalamic-pituitary resistance to thyroid hormones.

Women with hypothyroidism should be advised to have thyroid hormones measured before and during pregnancy also for the protection of the fetus; mostly they need a higher dose of T_4 replacement. Genetic counseling could be helpful in genetic thyroid dysgenesis: The risk of a new congenital hypothyroidism in the family is probably about 2%.

We agree with MacGillivray's opinion: "The most gratifying discovery that has come from the newborn thyroid screening programs is the attainment of normal intelligence in congenital hypothyroid infants because of early diagnosis and treatment."[28]

ALTERNATING HYPO-, EU-, AND HYPERTHYROIDISM IN THE NEONATAL PERIOD
Maternal Antithyroid Drugs and Thyrotropin Receptor Stimulating and/or Blocking Antibodies

Maternal antithyroid drugs and thyrotropin receptor blocking antibodies (see **Fig. 1**) are the most common cause of transient hypothyroidism.[29] The decreased thyroid function of the newborn normalizes when these substances disappear from the infant's blood. In extremely rare cases, the newborn of a Graves mother may have antithyroid drugs, thyrotropin receptor blocking antibodies, and thyrotropin receptor stimulating antibody (TRSAb) as well.[30,31] The elimination depends on their clearance rate and starting quantity. In general, the blocking effect ends first and a transient hyperthyroidism may occur after the transient hypothyroidism.

Graves Disease

A minority of newborns from mothers with Graves disease develop transient central hypothyroidism.[32–35] In these cases the FT_4 level may be elevated at birth, indicating fetal hyperthyroidism.[33] Central hypothyroidism (low thyrotropin and reduced FT_4) develops earlier[33] or later[34] in the neonatal period, with variability in duration, and can be even longer than 6 months.[32,34] The pathomechanism is probably triggered by impairment of maturation from the exposure of the fetal hypothalamic-pituitary system to high thyroid hormone levels.[35] According to several observations, the critical time for this damage is earlier than 32 weeks' gestation.[32]

NEONATAL HYPERTHYROIDISM
Neonatal Immunhyperthyroidism

Transient neonatal hyperthyroidism is the more common form of neonatal hyperthyroidism (~1:25,000–50,000), and occurs in 1% to 2% of the offspring of mothers with active or inactive[31] disease. The transplacental passage of maternal TRSAb plays a key role in the pathogenesis of this disease. The elevated TRSAb level results in hyperthyroidism in utero from the second trimester as the fetal thyrotropin receptors respond to fetal thyrotropin or maternal TRSAb. Consequently, this form of hyperthyroidism begins in the fetal period and the short- and long-term outcome of the disease

Table 4
Relationship between IQ and important parameters of congenital hypothyroidism patients

| Start of L-T₄ | Dose µg/kg/day | Serum Thyroxin-Level Before Replacement | | | | | |
| | | <3 µg/dl | | >3 µg/dl | | Total | |
		n	IQ	n	IQ	Total	IQ
Day 7-13	>10	3	108.7 ± 26.5	5	113.6 ± 13.6	8	
	<10	3	106.3 ± 8.0	6	115.0 ± 6.7	9	
Total				11	114.4 ± 9.8ᵃ	17	111.9 ± 12.9ᵇ
Day 14-26	>10	8	101.4 ± 11.4	4	103.8 ± 12.8	12	
	<10	15	101.4 ± 12.2	14	103.6 ± 8.4	29	
Day >26		6		5		11	
Total				23	104.2 ± 9.2ᵃ	52	103.0 ± 10.0ᵇ
Total number		35	104.6 ± 10.5ᶜ	34	109.7 ± 7.9ᶜ	69	

ᵃ $p = 0.005$.
ᵇ $p = 0.004$.
ᶜ $p = 0.049$.

depends on the activity and duration of fetal and neonatal hyperthyroidism. Therefore, the treatment of Graves disease during pregnancy is very important and the correct management can act as a preventive method for the development of neonatal disease.

In a recent study, fetuses of 72 mothers were monitored monthly from 22 weeks' gestation by the fetal heart rate, the sonography of the fetal thyroid and bone (distal femoral ossification center), and, in some cases, the fetal T_4 and thyrotropin levels.[36] These results influenced the antithyroid drug treatment of the mothers. In this controlled trial, there was one death (with fetal thyrotoxicosis) and five newborns needed antithyroid drug therapy. According to this prospective and systematic study at 32 weeks' gestation, the sensitivity of fetal thyroid sonography was 92% and the specificity was 100% for the diagnosis of fetal neonatal dysfunction.[36]

Hyperthyroidism may manifest in the newborn immediately after birth or after a few days or months (see above).

Diagnosis
Early diagnosis and commencement of therapy is essential for good prognosis. The list of possible findings include tachycardia (heart rate >160/min), arrhythmias, cardiac failure, hyperactivity, irritability, restlessness, hyperreflexia, sleep disturbance, sweating, goiter, prominent eyes, narrow sutures, craniosynostosis, advanced bone age, vomiting, hyperphagia, icterus, diarrhea, poor weight-gain, hepatosplenomegaly, lymphadenopathia, and thrombocytopenia.

Serum T_4/FT_4, T_3/FT_3, are higher and serum thyrotropin level is lower than the normal range of the same gestational age.[37] The measurement of serum thyrotropin receptor antibodies (TRAb; or TRAK [TSH-Rezeptor-Autoantikörper (German)]) can be important for the early differential diagnosis.

Treatment
The development of intrauterine hyperthyroidism can be prevented by the administration of antithyroid drugs to the mother (see above). However, an overdose of antithyroid drugs may cause iatrogenic fetal hypothyroidism and goiter. The prolonged use (several months) of β-adrenergic blocking agent therapy by the mother may result in retarded fetal growth or postnatal bradycardia and hypoglycemia of the newborn.[38]

The optimal treatment of this condition would involve the neutralization or elimination of TRSAbs immediately in the newborn's blood. The Rees Smith group has recently described the characterization of a blocking-type human monoclonal autoantibody to the thyrotropin receptor (5C9), which could be used as a specific inhibitor of thyroid stimulation by thyrotropin receptor autoantibodies in patients with Graves disease.[39] However other groups have suggested that the widespread use of this therapy is not imminent, and more research is needed in this field.[40]

The following medical modalities are used to decrease the thyroid hormone synthesis and release: antithyroid drug therapy, high-dose iodine treatment, and intravenous human immunoglobulin therapy.

The basic treatment in neonates is antithyroid drug administration (methimazole 0.5–1.0 mg/kg/d or propylthiouracil 5–10 mg/kg/d in divided doses), but this is effective only after 1 to 2 weeks.

In severe thyrotoxicosis (with high TRSAb titer) inorganic iodine or iodinated contrast agents can block the release of thyroid hormones faster by iodine (eg, Lugol drops: one every 8 hours for a few days), but this also can take up to 7 to 10 days to normalize thyroid hormone levels.[41] Subsequently, in many serious cases the phenomenon of "iodine escape" occurs with worsening of symptoms. This risk exists in the newborns with extremely high TRSAb titer, when there is no chance to decrease the T_4 level in a few weeks. Early reports suggested that oral iodinated radiographic contrast agents (eg, iopanoic acid or sodium ipodate 0.1–0.2 g/d or 0.5 g every 3 days) might be useful to treat the thyrotoxicosis. Their value is also limited in long-term therapy because of escape from its inhibitory effect on the thyroid hormone synthesis.[41] Both preparations are no longer available in North America.

Therefore, as an alternative treatment—by analogy with human immunoglobulin therapy of neonatal autoimmune diseases (eg, immune thrombocytopenic purpura, Rh hemolytic disease)[42]—human immunoglobulin was given intravenously (1-1 g on the first and fourth day after admission) to an 8-day-old seriously thyrotoxic (T_4: 23.3 µg/dl; triiodothyronine: 6 ng/mL; thyrotropin: 0.0 mIU/L; TRAb: 78.0%) newborn.[43] Her symptoms and hormone levels normalized in 5 days (**Fig. 3**) and

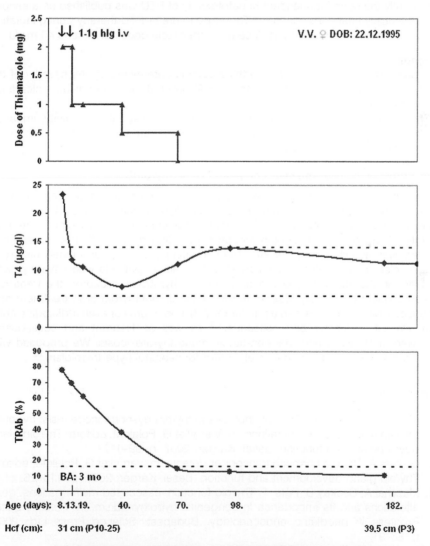

hIg = human immunoglobulin, TRAb = TSH Receptor Antibodies, BA = bone age,
Hcf = head circumference, P = percentile

Fig. 3. Some clinical and laboratory data of patient with neonatal thyrotoxicosis.

she is now a normal teenager.[43] After this successful treatment, an animal experiment was published by the Volpe group[44] confirming our result: The thyroid function was inhibited with human immunoglobulin in severe combined immunodeficient mice xenografted with Graves tissues probably because of antiidiotypic suppression.[44]

Tachycardia can be treated with β-blockers (propranolol 2 mg/kg/d in divided doses) or digoxin if cardiac failure is present. Extremely severe cases can also be treated with glucocorticoids.

Due to the pathogenesis of transient neonatal thyrotoxicosis (the "pathogen factor" is the maternal TRSAb), the most important parameter for follow-up of patients is the TRAb. Treatment should be stopped after the normalization of TRAb to reduce the risk of relapse.

Recently the dose-independent hepatotoxicity of PTU was published as a serious and potentially fatal complication.[45] Therefore to prefer PTU therapy during lactation is no more recommended.[46] The dose of methimazole does not exceed 40 mg/d.

Prognosis

The prognosis of the neonatal hyperthyroidism is determined by the severity of the fetal hyperthyroidism, the height of the TRSAb level at birth, and also its clearance rate in the newborn.[47]

The possible long-term morbidities include brain damage (hyperactivity, impaired intellect) and skeletal damage (advance of bone age, craniosynostosis), which start most frequently in the fetal period.

Non-Autoimmune or Permanent Congenital Hyperthyroidism

Non-autoimmune or permanent congenital hyperthyroidism, a form of neonatal thyrotoxicosis, is a very rare, but potentially serious disease. It can be nonfamilial or familial (autosomal-dominant inheritance). The nonfamilial variation may be either a de novo germline[48] or somatic thyrotropin receptor–activating mutation.[49] The disease can present with neonatal onset, or after the neonatal period without a family history of Graves disease and without elevated TRSAb levels. In patients who have a proven mutation in the stimulating G protein or in the thyrotropin receptor, the treatment option should be more aggressive. In milder forms, antithyroid drug treatment may be successful, but there is also a role for total thyroidectomy or even radioiodine ablation. Recently, Chester and colleagues[50] as well as Hébrant and colleagues[51] reviewed the topic of neonatal non-autoimmune thyrotoxicosis. We proposed with Foley a diagnostic and therapeutic algorithm for neonatal hyperthyroidism.[52]

REFERENCES

1. Moreno JC, Visser TJ. New phenotypes in thyroid dyshormonogenesis: hypothyroidism due to DUOX2 mutations. In: Van Vliet G, Polak M, editors. Thyroid gland development and function. Basel: Karger; 2007. p. 99–117.
2. Grüters A. Thyroid hormone transporter defects. In: Van Vliet G, Polak M, editors. Thyroid gland development and function. Basel: Karger; 2007. p. 118–26.
3. Muzsnai A, Csókay B, Péter F. Thyroid function, associated malformations, gene alterations and its importance in congenital hypothyroidism. In: Péter F, editor. Progress in paediatric endocrinology. Budapest: Science Press Ltd; 2008. p. 88–91.
4. Haddow JE, Palomaki GR, Allan WC, et al. Maternal thyroid deficiency during pregnancy and subsequent neuro-psychological development of the child. N Engl J Med 1999;341:549–55.

5. Pop VJ, Brouwers EP, Vadert HL, et al. Maternal hypothyroxinaemia during early pregnancy and subsequent child development: a 3-year follow-up study. Clin Endocrinol 2003;59:282–8.
6. Spiliotis BE. Thyroid function in the newborn and infant. In: Krassas GE, Rivkees SA, Kiess W, editors, Diseases of the thyroid in childhood and adolescence. Pediatr Adolesc Med. Basel: Karger; 2007. 11: p.44–55.
7. Péter F. Thyroid dysfunction in the offspring of mothers with autoimmune thyroid diseases [commentary]. Acta Paediatr 2005;94:1008–10.
8. Delange FM, Dunn JT. Iodine deficiency. In: Braverman LE, Utiger RD, editors. The thyroid. 9th edition. Philadelphia: Lippincott Williams & Wilkins; 2005. p. 264–88.
9. Caldwell KL, Miller GA, Wang RY, et al. Iodine status of the U.S. population, National Health and Nutrition Examination Survey 2003–2004. Thyroid 2008;18:1207–14.
10. Péter F, Muzsnai Á, Bourdoux P. Changes of urinary iodine excretion of newborns over a period of twenty years. J Endocrinol Invest 2003;26(Suppl 2):39–42.
11. Dorey CM, Zimmermann MB. Reference values for spot urinary iodine concentrations in iodine-sufficient newborns using a new pad collection method. Thyroid 2008;18:347–52.
12. Burns R, Mayne PD, O'Herlihy C, et al. Can neonatal TSH screening reflect trends in population iodine intake? Thyroid 2008;18:883–8.
13. Nagataki S. The average of dietary iodine intake due to the ingestion of seaweeds is 1.2 mg/day in Japan. Thyroid 2008;18:667–8.
14. Delange FM, Dalhem A, Bourdoux P, et al. Increased risk of primary hypothyroidism in premature infants. J Pediatr 1984;105:462–9.
15. Fisher DA, Nelson JC, Carlton EI, et al. Maturation of human hypothalamic-pituitary-thyroid function and control. Thyroid 2000;10:229–34.
16. Péter F, Halász G, Kirilina S, et al. Hypothyroid type FT4/TSH ratio in mongolism [Abstr] Proc 22nd Ann Meet ESPE. Budapest, August 29–31, 1983. p. 17.
17. Meyerovitch J, Sterl M, Antebi F, et al. Loss of TSH set points in Down syndrome [abstr]. Horm Res 2007;68(Suppl 1):23.
18. Fisher DA. Thyroid function and dysfunction in premature infants. Pediatr Endocrinol Rev 2007;4:317–28.
19. Rapaport R. Thyroid function in the very low birth weight newborn: rescreen or reevaluate? [editorials]. J Pediatr 1995;128:287–9.
20. LaFranchi SH. Increasing incidence of congenital hypothyroidism: some answers, more questions. J Clin Endocrinol Metab 2011;96:2395–7.
21. Kempers MJE, Lanting CI, van Heijst AFJ, et al. Neonatal screening for congenital hypothyroidism based on thyroxin, thyrotropin, and thyroxin-binding globulin measurement: potentials and pitfalls. J Clin Endocrinol Metab 2006;9:3370–6.
22. Deladoëy J, Ruel J, Giguére Y, et al. Is the incidence of congenital hypothyroidism increasing? A 20-year retrospective population-based study in Quebec. J Clin Endocrinol Metab 2011;96:2422–9.
23. Muzsnai A. Some aspects for optimization of hormone substitution in congenital hypothyroidism, (Hungarian) PhD Thesis, Budapest, 1991.
24. Péter F, Muzsnai Á, Szigetvári A. Intellectual assessment of hypothyroid children detected by screening. Acta Med Austriaca 1992;19:60–1.
25. Bongers-Schokking JJ, Koot HM, Wiersma D, et al. Influence of timing and dose of thyroid hormone replacement on development in infants with congenital hypothyroidism. J Pediatr 2000;136:292–7.
26. Péter F, Gráf R, Blatniczky L, et al. Neuropsychological development of children with congenital hypothyroidism recognized by neonatal screening. Pediatr Res 2001;49(Suppl 2):158A.

27. Rovet JF. In search of the optimal therapy for congenital hypothyroidism. J Pediatr 2004;144:698–700.
28. MacGillivray MH. Congenital hypothyroidism. In: Pescovitz OH, Eugster EA, editors. Pediatric endocrinology. Philadelphia: Lippincott Williams & Wilkins; 2004. p. 490–507.
29. Brown RS, Bellisario RL, Botero D, et al. Incidence of transient congenital hypothyroidism due to maternal thyrotropin receptor-blocking antibodies in over one million babies. J Clin Endocrinol Metab 1996;81:1147–51.
30. Zakarija M, McKenzie JM. Pregnancy associated changes in the thyroid-stimulating antibody of Graves' disease and the relationship to neonatal hyperthyroidism. J Clin Endocrinol Metab 1983;57:1036–41.
31. McKenzie JM, Zakarija M. The clinical use of thyrotropin receptor antibody measurements. J Clin Endocrinol Metab 1989;69:1093–6.
32. Higuchi R, Miyawaki M, Kumagai T, et al. Central hypothyroidism in infants who were born to mothers with thyrotoxicosis before 32 weeks' gestation: 3 cases. Pediatrics 2005;115:e623–5.
33. Matsura N, Konishi J, Fujieda K, et al. TSH receptor antibodies in mothers with Graves' disease and outcome in their offspring. Lancet 1988;1:14–7.
34. Mandel SH, Hanna CE, LaFranchi SH. Diminished thyroid-stimulating hormone secretion associated with neonatal thyrotoxicosis. J Pediatr 1986;109:662–5.
35. Kempers MJ, van Tijin DA, van Trotsenburg AS, et al. Central congenital hypothyroidism due to gestational hyperthyroidism: detection where prevention failed. J Clin Endocrinol Metab 2003;88:5851–7.
36. Luton D, Le Gac I, Vuillard E, et al. Management of Graves' disease during pregnancy: the key role of fetal thyroid gland monitoring. J Clin Endocrinol Metab 2005;90:6093–8.
37. Péter F, Foley TP Jr. Hyperthyroxinemia. In: Hochberg Z, editor. Practical algorithms in pediatric endocrinology. 2nd edition. Basel: Karger; 2007. p. 92–3.
38. Lazarus JH. Thyroid disease during pregnancy. In: Krassas GE, Rivkees SA, Kiess W, editors, Diseases of the thyroid in childhood and adolescence. Pediatric and Adolescent Medicine, vol. 11. Basel: Karger; 2007;11:25–43.
39. Sanders J, Evans M, Betterle C, et al. A human monoclonal autoantibody to the thyrotropin receptor with thyroid-stimulating blocking activity. Thyroid 2008;18:735–46.
40. Rapoport B, McLachlan SM. Whiter TSH receptor blocking antibodies in the treatment of Graves' disease? Thyroid 2008;18:695–6.
41. Cooper DS. Treatment of thyrotoxicosis. In: Braverman LE, Utiger RD, editors. The thyroid. Ninth edition. Philadelphia: Lippincott Williams & Wilkins; 2005. p. 665–94.
42. Berkowitz RL, Bussel JB, McFarland JG. Alloimmune thrombocytopenia: state of the art 2006. Am J Obstet Gynecol 2006;195:907–13.
43. Péter F, Kalmár Á, Kucsera R, et al. Human immunoglobulin therapy in serious neonatal Graves' disease. Long term (9 yrs) follow up [abstract]. Horm Res 2005;64(Suppl 1):249–50.
44. Resetkova E, Kawai K, Volpe R. Administration of normal human immunoglobulins (hIgs) inhibited thyroid function and humoral responses from Graves' tissues xenografted into severe combined immunodeficient (SCID) mice [abstr]. Thyroid 1996;6(Suppl 1):S2.
45. Rivkees SA, Mattison DR. Propylthiouracil (PTU)-induced liver failure and recommendations for the discontinuation of PTU use in children. Int J Pediatr Endocrinol 2009;2009:132–41.

46. Karras S, Tzotzas T, Krassas GE. Toxicological considerations for antithyroid drugs in children. Expert Opin Drug Metab Toxicol 2011;7:399–410.
47. Hung W, Sarlis NJ. Autoimmune and non-autoimmune hyperthyroidism in pediatric patients: a review and personal commentary on management. Pediatr Endocrinol Rev 2004;2:21–38.
48. Kopp P, Van Sande J, Parma J, et al. Brief report: congenital hyperthyroidism caused by a mutation in the thyrotropin receptor gene. N Engl J Med 1995; 332:150–4.
49. Hung W, Sarlis NJ. Molecular genetics of thyroid disorders in the neonate: a review. J Endocrinol Genet 2001;2:193–213.
50. Chester J, Rotenstein D, Ringkananout U, et al. Congenital neonatal hyperthyroidism caused by germline mutations in the TSH receptor gene. J Pediatr Endocrinol Metab 2008;21:479–86.
51. Hébrant A, van Staveren WCG, Maenhaut C, et al. Genetic hyperthyroidism: hyperthyroidism due to activating TSHR mutations. Eur J Endocrinol 2011;164: 1–9.
52. Foley TP Jr, Péter F. Neonatal hyperthyroidism. In: Hochberg Z, editor. Practical algorithms in pediatric endocrinology. 2nd edition. Basel: Karger; 2007. p. 82–3.

Nutrition and Bone Growth in Pediatrics

Galia Gat-Yablonski, PhD[a,b], Michal Yackobovitch-Gavan, PhD[a], Moshe Phillip, MD[a,b,c],*

KEYWORDS

• Nutrition • Growth • Children • Ghrelin • Leptin • Growth plate

Longitudinal growth in humans is generally divided into four major periods that differ in both the rate of linear gain as well as the major hormones that control it: prenatal period, infancy, childhood, and pubertal period.

The process begins the moment a zygote is created from sperm and oocyte and starts to divide. The zygote becomes embedded in the endometrium to receive essential nutrients through the uterus wall. The most rapid growth during the lifetime takes place in utero, when a complete fetus of about 50 cm in length is produced from a single cell in just 9 months. After birth, the baby continues to grow at a reduced speed during infancy and childhood, followed by a growth spurt during puberty. Thereafter, the growth rate slows, until final height is achieved. This article focuses on the role of nutrition in linear growth in children, without attending to the specific nutritional demands of each period. A detailed description of diseases that lead to insufficient food consumption is beyond the scope of this article.

Growth and development are specific hallmarks of childhood. In most children, they occur spontaneously, with no interruption. A complex system controls the initiation, rate, and cessation of growth. The association between nutrition and linear growth in children is well accepted. The growth of the human skeleton requires an adequate supply of many different nutritional factors. Some, such as proteins, lipids, and carbohydrates, form the "building materials"; others play regulatory roles. Classical nutrient deficiencies lead to stunting (energy, protein, and zinc), rickets (vitamin D), and other bone abnormalities (copper, zinc, vitamin C). However, the exact mechanism whereby nutrition modulates cellular activity during bone elongation is still not known.

Portions of this article were previously published in the *Endocrinology and Metabolism Clinics of North America*, 38:3.

[a] The Jesse Z. and Sara Lea Shafer Institute for Endocrinology and Diabetes, National Center for Childhood Diabetes, Schneider Children's Medical Center of Israel, 14 Kaplan Street, Petah Tikva 49202, Israel

[b] Felsenstein Medical Research Center, Beilinson Campus, Petah Tikva 49100, Israel

[c] Sackler School of Medicine, Tel Aviv University, Tel Aviv 69978, Israel

* Corresponding author. Institute of Endocrinology and Diabetes, National Center for Childhood Diabetes, Schneider Children's Medical Center of Israel, 14 Kaplan Street, Petah Tikva 49202, Israel.

E-mail address: mosheph@post.tau.ac.il

Pediatr Clin N Am 58 (2011) 1117–1140
doi:10.1016/j.pcl.2011.07.008
0031-3955/11/$ – see front matter © 2011 Elsevier Inc. All rights reserved.

pediatric.theclinics.com

Most of the studies that explored the role of specific nutrients in linear growth focused on malnourished children in developing countries. They found that in populations with marginal or poor nutritional status, increased intake of high-protein foods from animal and other sources stimulated weight gain and linear growth. Only a few studies were performed in developed countries, where food is not limited and the daily intake of dietary protein is sufficient to cover physiologic requirements.[1] Moreover, most of the latter focused on children with idiopathic short stature, who are often characterized as poor eaters and lean,[2,3] or on patients with eating disorders. Thus, their data need to be interpreted accordingly.

Linear growth is the product of an elaborate cascade of events that takes place in the cartilaginous growth center of the long bones, the epiphyseal growth plate (EGP). It involves the sequential replacement of chondrocytes of the EGP by osteoblasts, a process regulated by complex interactions among hormones, local growth factors, and components of the extracellular matrix, namely collagens and proteoglycans.[4] Endochondral ossification begins with the proliferation of early chondrocytes, followed by their alignment in columns, and finally, their maturation into hypertrophic chondrocytes. The hypertrophic cells then cease dividing and increase in volume by 5- to 10-fold by the ingress of water (**Fig. 1**). They begin to secrete extracellular matrix (ECM) consisting of collagen type X, as well as matrix vesicles (small particles that serve as centers of mineralization). Thereafter, the chondrocytes undergo programmed cell death, with calcification of the ECM, enabling the invasion of blood vessels and osteoblasts. The cartilage scaffold is thus replaced with bone tissue. This reorganization of the ECM is essential for proper maturation of the EGP.[5] The hormones and local factors that control these events may be directly or indirectly affected by the nutritional status.

In this article, we describe the evidence-based knowledge gained to date on the effect of food on specific growth-stimulating hormones (**Fig. 2**). In addition, we describe the effects of nutrition on the growth plate, with a focus on growth-related genes and suggest the involvement of novel factors such as sirtuins and microRNAs. We also describe the current knowledge on the effect of energy, vitamins, and micronutrients on growth, as shown in epidemiologic studies in humans.

HORMONES
Growth Hormone: Insulin-like Growth Factor-I

During childhood, linear growth is predominantly regulated by Growth Hormone (GH), a 191-amino acid polypeptide synthesized and secreted by somatotrophs of the

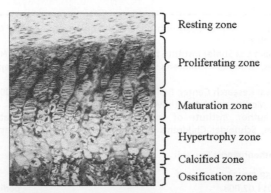

Resting zone

Proliferating zone

Maturation zone

Hypertrophy zone

Calcified zone

Ossification zone

Fig. 1. Organization of the EGP.

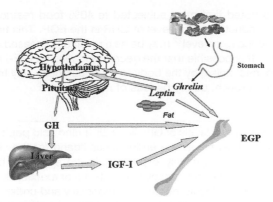

Fig. 2. The effect of nutrition on growth.

anterior pituitary gland. Besides promoting linear growth, GH also exerts metabolic effects on numerous tissues and organs. Its release from the pituitary is regulated by a complex interplay of hypothalamic, pituitary, and circulating factors. In the hypothalamus, GH secretion is stimulated by GH-releasing hormone (GHRH) and inhibited by somatostatin.

GH affects growth directly, by binding to its receptors in the growth plate, and also indirectly, via insulin-like growth factor (IGF)-I, a 70-amino acid peptide. GH stimulates many body tissues to produce IGF-I, especially the liver, thereby increasing circulating IGF-I levels and the local production of IGF-I in the EGP.

IGF-I serves as both the main mediator of GH action and as a GH-independent growth factor. Its direct effect on growth is best exemplified in utero: fetuses with deficient IGF-I production or a defect in the IGF-I receptor show significant growth delay, whereas fetuses with GH deficiency do not.[6] Mice studies of targeted mutagenesis of the genes encoding IGF-I and its receptor, IGF-IR, found that IGF-I −/−mice had a birth weight of 60% of their wild-type littermates, and IGF-IR −/−mice had a birth weight of 45% of normal. The IGF-IR −/−mice all died immediately postpartum from respiratory failure.[7] Human inactivation mutations in the IGF-I gene are also associated with growth retardation.[8,9] All the human mutations in the IGF-IR gene identified so far are associated with severe intrauterine growth retardation (IUGR) (length deficit of −0.3 to −5.8 SDS depending on the specific mutation).[6,9–14]

The mediatory effect of IGF-I on GH activity comes into play postnatally. IGF-I acts through its receptor, IGF-IR, which is expressed on all tissues except the liver, including cells of the EGP. It stimulates cell proliferation and differentiation and protects cells from apoptosis. In the EGP, IGF-I stimulates growth and differentiation in a spatial-dependent fashion.[15,16]

Multiple studies have shown that GH and IGF-I concentrations are responsive to changing nutritional status[17,18] and intake of amino acids and free fatty acids. Fasting induces a GH-resistant state, although its exact effect on the GH/IGF-I axis remains unclear. Whereas fasting increased serum GH levels in humans, rabbits, sheep, cows and pigs, it reduced serum GH levels in mice and rats; nevertheless, in all animals examined, IGF-I levels were reduced. The effect was more pronounced with protein restriction.[19] Down-regulation of either systemic or local IGF-I production was assumed to play a role.

Accordingly, fasting was found to lead to a decrease in the rate of longitudinal bone growth and reduced length of the EGP.[20–23] Heinrichs and colleagues[20] reported an increase in GH receptor (GHR) and IGF-I mRNA levels in rabbits after short fast, whereas our group noted that mice subjected to 40% food restriction for 10 days showed a dramatic reduction in the level of GHR in the EGP. This finding suggested GH resistance at the receptor level[22] may be as a result of increased circulating levels of glucocorticoids.[24] It is possible that the decrease in plasma IGF-I and local GHR is part of an adaptive mechanism by the body to shunt calories away from nonessential processes, including growth, during periods of malnutrition.[25]

Ghrelin

Nutritional status also affects levels of Ghrelin, a 28-amino acid peptide identified less than a decade ago that serves as the endogenous ligand for the GH secretagogue receptor (GHSR).[26] Ghrelin is mainly expressed in the stomach, but also in other tissues, such as the hypothalamus and placenta. Its major function is the central regulation of food intake: ghrelin levels increase preprandially and under cachectic conditions and significantly decrease within 1 hour after eating. It has therefore been named "the hunger hormone." Ghrelin not only induces an increase in food consumption, it also apparently shifts food preference toward high-fat diets.[27]

In vivo and in vitro studies showed that ghrelin, in its acylated form, releases GH by binding to its hypothalamic receptor, GHSRα 1. Interestingly, this receptor has significant ligand-independent activity.[28–30] Its physiologic importance was suggested by findings that natural mutations segregated with short stature in several families.[31,32] Functional analysis revealed a disruption of the constitutive activity of the receptor, with no effect on binding of the ligand.[29,31,32] The short stature in these cases may have been caused by reduced activity at the hypothalamic-pituitary-GH axis. Recently mutations in GHSR were identified in children with constitutional delay of growth and puberty. These mutations showed a reduction in cell surface expression, with the p.Ser84Ile mutation also associated with a defect in ghrelin potency.[33] However, a large genetic study in a French population failed to find evidence of a major contribution of common variants of the ghrelin and GHSR genes to height variations.[34] Moreover, in several animal models, knock out of either ghrelin or its receptor genes was not associated with any attenuation of growth.[35–38]

GHSR levels are stimulated by fasting,[29,39,40] and high levels of IGF-I inhibit pituitary GHSR mRNA levels.[41] By contrast, neither total nor octanoylated ghrelin increased during fasting in parallel to the massive increase in GH secretion.[42]

Although specific ghrelin activity in the growth plate has not yet been identified, a direct effect was suggested by findings that ghrelin is synthesized by growth plate chondrocytes.[43]

Leptin

We summarized the role of leptin in growth in a recent publication[44]; thus, only a brief review is presented here.

Leptin, a hormone predominantly produced by adipocytes, was first identified as the product of the Ob gene in 1994, in studies of leptin-deficient obese (Ob/Ob) mice.[45] It was originally described as a circulating hormone involved in feeding behavior and energy homeostasis.[46,47] However, the wide distribution of the Ob receptor (ObR; LEPR) in different tissues indicated that besides body weight regulation, leptin had numerous peripheral effects, including bone growth and remodeling.[22,44,48–51]

In children, the involvement of leptin in growth was supported by a series of studies suggesting that periods of fast growth such as fetal life[52] and adolescence[53,54] require a certain level of leptin.

A direct link between leptin and linear growth was suggested by findings that leptin administration to Ob/Ob mice corrected their metabolic abnormalities and also led to a significant increase in femoral length.[55,56] Leptin was also found to directly stimulate GH secretion.[57,58] Others reported lower levels of GH in both leptin-deficient Ob/Ob mice and humans with a mutation of the leptin receptor.[59,60] In addition, in an animal model of catch-up growth consisting of 40% food restriction for 10 days followed by food replenishment, we observed that weight gain associated with an increase in the level of serum leptin preceded tibial catch-up growth.[22]

To address the role of leptin on linear growth, several groups followed its effects in vivo and ex vitro and noted a stimulatory effect on growth-plate cartilage proliferation and differentiation.[50,61–63] In our studies, leptin was shown to exert its effects on chondrocytes in the EGP through its active, long-form, receptor[50,62,64] and possibly through the activation of the PTHrP/Ihh axis.[51]

In mice models, leptin administration led to reduced food consumption and reduced body weight. However, normal mice treated with repeated subcutaneous leptin injections had longer tibia than pair-fed controls. Leptin stimulation of the EGP was balanced, positively affecting both proliferation and differentiation, so that the ratio between proliferating and hypertrophic chondrocytes remained constant.[50,51] These results were supported by the study of Martin and colleagues[65] wherein leptin stimulated femoral length and the midshaft cortical area independently of peripheral IGF-I. Furthermore, leptin administration to rat with intrauterine growth retardation significantly improved structural properties and elongation rate of bones.[66]

Fasting experiments performed in rodents reported a drop in GH and IGF-I serum levels in response to a reduction in food consumption.[25] Leptin administration to the fasted rats restored their blunted GH secretion[67,68] but failed to increase their serum IGF-I levels.[50,69] These results again indicate that leptin can act as a metabolic signal connecting adipocyte tissues with the GH axis and that its stimulatory effect on growth under conditions of food restriction is not dependent on circulating IGF-I.

Although leptin-deficient mice have impaired linear growth, Farooqi and colleagues[70] described a family with a mutation in leptin in which the index patient and her affected cousin were both tall. These observations may suggest that the effect of leptin in humans is different from that observed in rodents. At the same time, the scarce information on human subjects with leptin abnormalities should be taken into account.

Insulin

Insulin, a 51-amino acid beta-cell–specific hormone, is secreted from the pancreas in response to increased glucose levels and binds to its receptors on peripheral cells and tissues to enable the assimilation of glucose into cells. Insulin was the first hormone in the central nervous system that was implicated in the control of body weight.[71] Findings of severe IUGR in babies with pancreatic agenesis[72] or mutations in the insulin receptor gene suggest an essential role for insulin signaling in normal intrauterine growth.[14,73] Extreme insulin resistance as a result of a mutation in the insulin receptor leads to leprechaunism, a congenital disorder characterized by insulin resistance, fasting hypoglycemia, and severe pre- and postnatal growth retardation.[74] The outcome may be caused by an insufficient energy supply to the cells or lack of insulin activity on chondrocytes of the growth plate.

Other evidence for the role of insulin in fetal growth comes from children with mutations in the gene encoding for glucokinase (GCK), which catalyzes the rate-limiting step in glycolysis and serves as a pancreatic β-cell glucose sensor. Mutations in GCK result in altered glucose sensing and decreased insulin secretion. Children with a mutation in GCK are approximately 500 g smaller than unaffected siblings.[75]

In children with type I diabetes, the lack of adequate insulin levels may lead to growth failure if the disease is chronically under poor control. However, the growth failure in general is modest, and it probably represents a combination of calorie wasting, chronic acidosis, and increased glucocorticoid production characteristic of other chronic diseases as well.[76] In most cases, there is no correlation between glycemic control and skeletal growth, and many children with apparently marginal control appear to grow well.

ENERGY/CALORIES/PROTEIN

Protein-energy malnutrition (PEM) is the most important nutritional disease in developing countries because of its high prevalence and its relationship with child mortality rates and impaired physical growth and higher cognitive development. Children with chronic PEM were found to perform poorly on tests of attention, working memory, learning and memory, and visuospatial ability; only scores on tests of motor speed and coordination were not affected.[77]

Children with marasmus (a form of malnutrition caused by long-lasting insufficient caloric intake) and kwashiorkor (a form of malnutrition caused mainly by insufficient protein consumption) had significantly lower body weight and height than healthy subjects, as well as reduced levels of serum leptin, insulin, and IGF-I.[78,79]

Animal studies clearly demonstrated the deleterious effects of PEM on linear growth, but in humans, it was somewhat difficult to dissociate the effect of the nutritional and other environmental factors or to ascertain the irreversibility of the nutritional damage. In the presence of infection, PEM induced greater loss of nutrients or led to metabolic alterations.[80] In children with idiopathic short stature from developed countries, where plenty of variable food is available, calorie intake was positively correlated with growth velocity both before GH treatment and during the first year of GH treatment.[81] Children with eating disorders from developed countries were on average shorter than controls; this effect was independent of age of onset.[82] Several specific amino acids, such as the amino acids arginine and lysine, which are known to stimulate GH\IGF-I secretion, might have an important role in linear growth. Unfortunately, studies exploring the role of specific amino acids in growth are sparse. One recent observational study,[83] which explored the association between arginine and lysine intake and linear growth in children, found that high arginine intake was positively associated with linear growth among girls. No such association was found for lysine.

Anorexia nervosa (AN), characterized by voluntary marked food restriction, could potentially serve as an excellent model to follow the effect of PEM on growth. AN has a female predominance, with an estimated prevalence of 1% in young women. Adolescents may present with short stature and delayed pubertal development or secondary amenorrhea.[84,85] These abnormalities normalize with weight gain, although the effect of AN on final height is not clear. In a study performed in male adolescents, who account for 5% to 10% of all patients with AN, growth failure was a prominent feature, and weight restoration resulted in accelerated growth in all those with growth retardation.[86] Weight gain was necessary for catch-up growth, but the weight had to be gained before the ability to grow was lost with age.[87] By contrast, in two studies performed in girls, height potential was preserved. Some authors suggested that the discrepancy among studies was attributable to AN-associated hypogonadism[88] or to the fact that by the time of disease onset in girls, that is, around age 13 to 14 or 17 to 18, most have already or nearly completed growth.[89]

In several animal models, even short-term (48- to 72-hour) fasting caused a decrease in the rate of longitudinal bone growth.[20,21] The height of the growth plate, the number of proliferative and hypertrophic chondrocyte per column, and the height of terminal hypertrophic chondrocytes were all reduced, with no disorganization

(**Fig. 3**). This immediate growth cessation may have important implications also for children, although in most cases recovery was rapid.

MOLECULAR MECHANISMS REGULATING THE INTERACTION BETWEEN NUTRITION AND GROWTH

Regulatory factors involved in the translation of energy within cells may be important for linear growth. These include hypoxia-inducible factor (HIF) 1, mammalian target of rapamycin (mTOR),[90] epigenetic mechanism, and microRNAs (miRNAs). The involvement of the last two in regulation of growth is only suggested and was not shown in growth plates yet. It will be interesting to follow upcoming developments in these fascinating new fields.

Hypoxia-inducible Factor 1

To study the effect of food restriction on gene expression, analyses were performed on a diversity of animals and tissues. Although no common gene affected by food restriction was identified across the different species, several shared factors were found, including metabolism and cell growth, regulation of transcription, energy metabolism, and stress and immune functions.[91] To the best of our knowledge, the only study that analyzed genes in the EGP itself is our own. We showed that in rats, 40% food restriction for 10 days induced dramatic changes in the expression of several genes. One of them was HIF1α, a key subunit of HIF, which serves as a master transcription factor regulating the expression of several genes that code for proteins involved in angiogenesis, cell metabolism, proliferation, motility, adhesion, and survival.[23]

HIF1α is responsible for the adaptation of chondrocytes to the low oxygen pressure of the avascular and relatively hypoxic tissue in which they are located. Its significance to chondrocyte survival, especially in the hypoxic regions of the embryonic EGF, and its involvement in chondrocyte proliferation, differentiation, and growth arrest, are well recognized.[92,93] These studies demonstrated the importance of tight regulation of HIF1 levels during development of the prenatal growth plate. HIF1 was also found to be a major factor in anaerobic glycolysis, which supplies most of the energy requirements of the chondrocytes. In addition it is required for extracellular matrix production

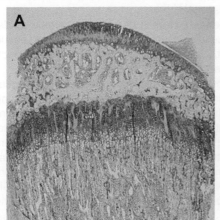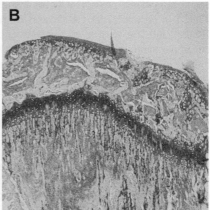

Fig. 3. The effect of nutritional restriction on the height of the growth plate. (*A*) EGP taken from 34-day-old rats fed ad libitum. (*B*) EGP taken from 34-day-old rats subjected for the preceding 10 days to 40% food restriction.

which is essential for proper growth and development, in cultured proliferating chondrocytes, by up-regulating the expression of the cartilage transcription factor Sox9 and by regulating the enzymes responsible for the hydroxylation of collagen prolines (P4HaI and P4HaII), and the enzyme lysyl oxidase, which is responsible for the formation of cross links between collagen molecules.[94]

These findings indicate that nutrition has a profound effect on the level of gene expression within the growth plate during longitudinal growth and that HIF1α plays an important role in growth of the mature plate growth in response to nutritional manipulation.[23]

Mammalian Target of Rapamycin

Cells have a complex sensing system designed to ensure that they do not undergo periods of growth unless adequate levels of nutrients are available to produce the energy necessary to support that growth. mTOR is an evolutionarily conserved serine/threonine protein kinase, which, like HIF1, serves as a key regulator of cell metabolism. It is activated in the presence of adequate levels of nutrients (glucose, amino acids, lipoproteins, minerals), turning on the cell's translational machinery for the synthesis of proteins that are essential for its growth and other functions.[95] Activated mTOR stimulates angiogenesis, which increases the number of blood vessels through which nutrients can reach the cell. In addition, it increases the production of nutrient transporter proteins, which enhance the cell's ability to import essential nutrients, and stimulates HIF1α expression and glycolysis. When nutrient levels are inadequate, mTOR is inactivated, protein synthesis is inhibited, cell growth is arrested, and autophagic protein degradation takes place.

mTOR is found in the form of two multiprotein complexes, mTOR Complex 1 (TORC1)[96,97] and mTOR Complex 2 (TORC2). TORC1 is sensitive to the cellular nutritional state, and it targets the phosphorylation of proteins that regulate protein translation, gene expression, and autophagy.[98] TORC2, by contrast, does not respond to changes in nutritional conditions but has been implicated in cytoskeleton regulation.[99,100]

Among the most studied substrates of TORC1 are the eukaryotic initiation factor 4E (eIF4E), binding protein (4E-BP), and ribosomal protein S6 kinase (S6K).[101] 4E-BP is a translational inhibitor that is deactivated by TORC1 phosphorylation; S6K is a positive translational effector activated on phosphorylation. By activating ribosomal S6K and inhibiting 4E-BP, mTOR initiates translation.[102,103]

TORC1 is regulated by insulin and nutrients, including glucose and amino acids, particularly leucine, as well as a variety of cellular stresses. In some cell types, amino acids can activate mTOR alone; in others, they collaborate with growth factors, such as insulin.[104] In the absence of amino acids, growth factors are helpless.

Modulation of mTOR signaling was shown to stimulate chondrocyte differentiation.[105] TOR, together with HIF1α, is also involved in the autophagy of the maturing chondrocytes of the EGP. Autophagy is induced under energy-restricted environmental conditions and inhibited by nutrient sufficiency. It plays a role in the control of several physiologic processes.[106] Specifically, in response to nutrient deprivation, the cells degrade the cytosolic content by the formation of a double-walled vesicular structure that eventually fuses with lysosomes, so that energy can be generated from the cells' own protein and lipid stores. Nutrient-stimulated activation of the TOR protein kinase leads to the phosphorylation and inactivation of components of the autophagy pathway.[107]

Vps34 (vacuolar protein sorting 34), a member of the PI3K family of lipid kinases, also participates in nutrient signaling to mTOR.[108] It is inhibited by amino acid deprivation and up-regulated with mTOR signaling.

In a recent study, maturing chondrocytes were found to exhibit an autophagic phase.[90,109] Its regulation was dependent on the activities of mTOR and AMP kinase in response to the AMP/ATP ratio in the cells.[110] When AMP kinase activity was blocked, autophagy could not be activated. Thus, nutrient insufficiency may increase the autophagic response in the growth plate chondrocytes, reducing the size of the cells and growth plate and leading to growth attenuation. When the restriction is short, this process may be reversible, but when it is prolonged, cell number may be reduced and growth stunted.

The involvement of the following two systems was not shown in growth plate yet; however, we hypothesize that these systems may serve as potential links translating nutrition to growth.

Sirtuins

Sirtuins, class III histone deacetylases (HDAC), are highly conserved enzymes that use nicotinamide adenine dinucleotide (NAD+) to deacetylate a number of histone and nonhistone substrates. The founding member of this family, silent information regulator 2 (Sir2), promotes longevity in yeast by repressing gene expression and stabilizing chromatin. Mammals have seven Sir2 homologs (SIRT1 to SIRT7), which are involved in regulating cell survival and stress response. Specifically, SIRT1 and SIRT6 are implicated in the response to calorie restriction (CR).[111,112] Studies found that SIRT1 was induced in vitro by nutrient deprivation and in vivo after long-term CR.[111] Cells cultured in the presence of serum from CR rats showed an attenuation of stress-induced apoptosis and an increase in SIRT1 expression. The enzymatic activity of SIRT1 appears to be positively regulated by NAD+, which increases during CR and fasting. Mice overexpressing SIRT1 exhibited similar physiologic properties to mice on a CR regimen. SIRT1 may regulate cell proliferation, senescence, and apoptosis by regulating several transcription factors that govern metabolism and endocrine signaling, including PPAR-γ,[113] PGC-1α,[114] FOXOs,[115,116] and p53.[117] Levels of SIRT6, whose absence in mice causes genome instability and the premature appearance of aging-related pathologies,[118] were also found to increase in rats subjected to prolonged CR, in mice after 24 hours of fasting, and in cell culture after nutrient depletion.[112] The role of sirtuins in the EGP has not been reported.

MicroRNAs

On completion of the Genome Project, researchers recognized that a large part of the genome is not translated into proteins. This noncoding, so-called "junk" DNA, has recently been found to be highly relevant to the regulation of gene expression and the maintenance of genomic stability. Some of it is transcribed into small non–protein-coding RNAs, or microRNAs (miRNAs), measuring approximately 19 to 23 nucleotides in length, which negatively regulate the expression of a large portion of the protein-encoding and non–protein-encoding genes at the posttranscriptional level (**Fig. 4**). Each miRNA can regulate one to several mRNA transcripts, and conversely, a single mRNA may be regulated by one to several miRNA sequences.[119,120] Genomic computational analysis indicates that as many as 50,000 miRNAs may exist in the genome. Cumulative laboratory data have confirmed the presence of hundreds of these miRNAs in the genomes of animals, plants, and viruses.

The miRNAs are transcribed by RNA polymerase II–producing primary (pri)-miR-NAs, which vary greatly in size, from a few hundred bases to tens of thousands.[121] Mature miRNAs are derived from two major processing events driven by sequential cleavages by the RNAse-III enzymes, Drosha and Dicer. The result is a small double-stranded (ds) miRNA duplex that is quickly unwound by a helicase and the

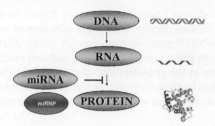

Fig. 4. The role of microRNA in protein synthesis regulation.

single mature strand is asymmetrically incorporated into the RNA-induced silencing complex (RISC) to guide it to its target. This is accomplished by base-pairing of the mRNAs with their complementary miRNA binding sites, most of which are thought to lie in the 3′ untranslated region (UTR) of the target. RISC then acts by translational repression (cleavage-incompetent RISC) or mRNA degradation (cleavage-competent Slicer containing RISC). The degree of inhibition is often correlated with the number of miRNA binding sites. The major advantage of the miRNA regulatory system is its tiny size: it is much more rapidly expressed than a typical protein-coding primary transcript, and it is not further delayed by splicing and translation.[122] In mammals, miRNAs have been shown to regulate numerous systems, among them adipocyte differentiation,[123] insulin secretion and B-cell development,[124] neural stem cell fate, immune function and cellular metabolism[125]; miRNA dysregulation is associated with several diseases, including cancer.[126,127]

Recently it was shown that miRNA-375, a beta-cell–specific microRNA, regulates glucose-induced insulin secretion, suggesting a link between nutrition and micro-RNA.[128] Others identified miR-140 to be chondrocyte-specific in zebrafish.[129] In mice, miRNA-140 was detected specifically in cartilaginous tissues of the developing limbs, ribs, vertebrae, sternum, and skull.[130] Binding sites for miRNA-140 were predicted in numerous genes, including some known to play a role in chondrogenesis, such as vascular endothelial growth factor A, matrix metalloproteinase (MMP) 13, basic fibroblast growth factor 2, platelet-derived growth factor[125,131] and many more.[132] In addition, miRNA-140 is known to target HDAC4, an essential element in chondrocyte hypertrophy in mice limbs.[130] Roles for Dicer,[133,134] and several additional miRNA including miR-1, miRNA-196, miR-199a, and miR-675 in skeletal morphogenesis have also been reported.[135–138]

These results show that miRNA may be responsive to nutritional cues and that micro-RNAs are involved in chondrogenesis; thus, it seems reasonable to suggest that micro-RNA may serve as mediators translating nutritional signals to processes in the EGP.

EFFECT OF SPECIFIC NUTRITIONAL FACTORS

The role played by amino acids and glucose in growth has been extensively studied. What about other components of our daily meals? Do specific food ingredients have specific beneficial effects, or are they all alike?

Vitamins

Vitamin D

Vitamin D is known to be involved in calcium homeostasis. Calcium is required for normal growth and development and maintenance of the skeleton. Vitamin D regulates endochondral ossification in a cell-maturation–dependent manner via nuclear vitamin D receptor (VDR) as well as ERp60, a membrane-associated $1\alpha25$ $(OH)_2D_3$-binding protein.[139] Both resting zone and growth-zone cells possess enzymes involved in the metabolism of $25(OH)D_3$, and they produce and secrete the $24R,25(OH)_2D_3$ metabolite and the $1\alpha25(OH)_2D_3$ metabolite into their extracellular environment.[140] They also harbor nuclear receptors for $1\alpha25(OH)_2D_3$ and respond to it by a decrease in number and proliferation. Cells in the resting zone respond primarily to $24R,25(OH)_2D_3$, and cells in the prehypertrophic and upper hypertrophic zones respond primarily to the $1\alpha25(OH)_2D_3$. The vitamin D hormone $1\alpha25(OH)_2D_3$ binds with high affinity to the VDR, which recruits its retinoid X receptor heterodimeric partner to recognize the vitamin D–responsive elements in target genes.[141] VDR also selectively binds certain omega3/omega6 polyunsaturated fatty acids (PUFA) with low affinity, leading to transcriptionally active VDR-RXR complexes. The cell maturation–specific actions of the metabolites affects ECM synthesis and turnover, including matrix composition with release and activation of latent factors such as TGF-β, all of which fine tune the rate and extent of chondrocyte proliferation and hypertrophy.[5]

Numerous association studies have dealt with single-nucleotide polymorphisms (SNPs) in the coding and intronic regions of the human VDR gene; however, only one study showed a clinical association between two SNPs located upstream of the transcriptional start site of the main human VDR gene promoter and height. These authors found that adolescent girls with a CC/GG genotype had lower circulating levels of 25-(OH)D, with no detectable consequence on calcium metabolism, in addition to lower serum levels of IGF-I and shorter stature from age 11 years to achievement of adult height.[142] Interestingly, however, in the absence of vitamin D or in the presence of a malfunctioning receptor, rickets rather than short stature is described. Furthermore, a recent study shows that pharmaceutical doses (given for example to children with CKD) of calcitriol, the 1,25 vitamin D inhibited intra-cortical bone formation and elongation.[143]

Vitamin A

Vitamin A and its derivative, retinoic acid, were suggested to promote the differentiation of pituitary cells to secret GH.[144] At the same time, retinoic acid was shown to inhibit the growth of metatarsals in vitro, by inhibiting chondrocyte proliferation, hypertrophy, and matrix synthesis.[145] Results of epidemiologic studies are also confusing: some observational studies reported significant correlations between vitamin A status and stunting,[146–148] a recent study shows that six months of vitamin A, iron and zinc supplementation induces growth acceleration in short children born SGA with subnormal nutrients intake similar to growth hormone therapy.[149] In contarst but others concluded that vitamin A supplementation had little or no impact on linear growth.[150,151] A recent study in mice also failed to demonstrate any effect of vitamin A deficiency on longitudinal growth.[152] Further studies are required to fully unravel the role of vitamin A in growth.

Micronutrients

Several micronutrients have been investigated for their potential influence on linear growth, namely, zinc, iron, copper, iodine, calcium, phosphorous, and magnesium. Observational or animal studies suggested that children with stunted growth are deficient in these micronutrients, but there is as yet no confirmatory evidence-based data for any of them, apart from zinc and iron.[150]

Zinc

Studies of zinc have so far provided the most conclusive evidence linking the intake of a specific micronutrient to child growth. However, the mechanism by which zinc deficiency impairs growth has not been elucidated. Some authors reported that zinc supplementation led to a highly significant increase in height and weight, with a greater growth response in children with initially low Z-scores for weight or height,[153] especially those known to be zinc deficient.[154,155] By contrast, when zinc was administered to children with idiopathic short stature and normal serum zinc levels there was no effect on height or weight SDS.[156] In addition, treatment of infants with nonorganic failure to thrive was associated with an increase in serum IGF-I levels, but not with an improvement in growth parameters.[157]

Researchers speculated that the effect of zinc on growth was mediated by its effect on IGF-I levels. Zinc deficiency reduces IGF-I production and may also decrease cellular IGF-I responsiveness,[158] and transient partial GH deficiency due to zinc deficiency was reported in children.[159] Zinc supplementation was found to increase basal levels of IGF-I, IGFBP-3, alkaline phosphatase, and osteocalcin, without changing GH levels or increasing subjects' sensitivity to exogenous GH. Others reported that Zinc supplementation led to a significant increase in growth rate and GH levels.[160] Additionally, through its influence on the GH/IGF-I system, zinc deficiency has been observed to affect bone metabolism.[156,161] In our study, zinc increased levels of IGF-I but not of IGFBP3.[157]

Zinc deficiency was shown to cause morphologic and pathologic changes in the growth plate, leading to disorganization of the chondrocytes of the EGP and shorter tibias and femurs in rats.[162] This effect may be attributable to malfunctioning of zinc-containing nucleoproteins, transcription factors, or MMPs. The latter are a group of zinc-dependent endopeptidases that play an important role in catabolism and turnover of the matrix and are crucial during bone growth and development.[163] Deficiency of either of the most abundant MMPs (MMP-9, 13, 14) in mice led to phenotypes of severe skeletal dysplasia.[164] Both MMP-9 and VEGF are regulated by vitamin D.[165] Thus a balanced regulation of MMPs is essential for proper EGP growth.

In conclusion, zinc appears to be an important linear-growth–limiting micronutrient. Further studies are needed to clarify the underlying mechanism of its action in this setting.

Iron

Several observational studies documented a relationship between iron-deficiency anemia and impaired physical growth.[166,167] The proposed mechanisms include its effect on immunity, appetite, thermogenesis, and thyroid hormone metabolism.[168,169] However, a clear causal inference was precluded in these studies owing to the presence of several confounders, as follows: (1) Coexistent parasitic infections, which cause iron deficiency, may also impair growth. (2) Children who grow rapidly may have more depleted iron stores, whereas those with slow growth may appear iron-replete.[81] (3) Concomitant deficiencies of other macronutrients and micronutrients, such as zinc, may also affect linear growth.[170] Two recent reviews of the literature concluded that iron interventions had no significant effect on child growth, with similar results obtained across categories of age, duration of intervention, mode and dosage of intervention, and baseline anthropometric status.[151,170] Some authors suggested that the effect of iron on growth was supported by the findings that zinc has a positive stimulatory effect on growth only when iron levels are adequate.[171,172] However, others failed to show a beneficial effect of these supplements on growth, possibly because of concurrent deficiencies of other micronutrients.[173] The fact that most of the studies were conducted in developing countries, where food supply is limited, should be considered when interpreting the clinical meaning of the results.[151,170,174]

Combinations of Micronutrients

The treatment of children with a mixture of micronutrients for 1 year had small but significant impact, with a greater benefit in those of low and medium socioeconomic status.[151,175,176] The supplements contained at least vitamin A, iron, zinc, B vitamins, and folic acid, in addition to iodine,[177,178] vitamin C,[178,179] vitamin E,[178,179] calcium,[179-181] potassium,[179,180] copper,[177,180] and other trace vitamin and minerals.[177]

Milk

The unique role of milk in newborns led many researchers to study its effect on linear growth also in older children. Milk is an important source of nutrients supporting growth, such as high-quality proteins containing all essential amino acids, high lactose content which seems to support growth due to a pro-biotic effect and improved absorption of minerals, and minerals, such as potassium, magnesium, phosphorus and zinc. Whole milk is also a good source of energy and has a good balance between energy and protein, which is important for optimal utilization of proteins.[182,183] An extensive review by Hoppe and colleagues[1] suggested that milk has a significant growth-stimulating effect. Their conclusion was based on observational[184,185] and interventional[186,187] studies in developing countries, as well as observational studies of well-nourished populations.[188-190] However, in the well-nourished populations, the association between milk and linear growth was less clear, and some interventional studies had negative findings.[191,192] The effect of milk on growth may not be the same in all age groups. In a study using data from the NHANES 1999-2002, milk consumption was a predictor of height in age groups 12-18 years but not in age group 5-11 years.[190] Cow's milk may have the strongest effects in children with existing undernutrition.[1]

According to one hypothesis, milk promotes linear growth by stimulating circulating IGF-I levels. However, although some studies reported supportive findings,[193-195] others did not.[196]

SUMMARY

Common knowledge is based on the wisdom of hundreds of generations. It is clear that malnutrition impairs linear growth. However, the specific nutrients or combination of nutrients that play a role remain controversial. Malnourished children in developing countries, where most of the studies exploring the relationship between nutrients and linear growth were performed, are likely to have multiple deficiencies, so supplementation with an individual micronutrient can be expected to have only a limited impact. Further, well-designed studies are needed. In spite of the enormous effort of pediatric endocrinologists, dieticians, and scientists working on this question, our understandings of the interaction of energy, protein, macronutrients, and micronutrients intake in linear growth in children is still lacking. In addition, the exact mechanism by which the body signals the growth plate to grow or attenuate growth is still unclear, although several possible mediators are beginning to emerge. It will be fascinating to follow this research in the next years to improve our understanding of events at this level and to translate this new knowledge to the development of therapeutic regimens for children with short stature. When mothers tell their children to eat to grow properly, they are right, but we still don't know exactly why.

ACKNOWLEDGMENTS

We thank Dr Liora Lazar for critical reading of the review and Gloria Ginzach for English editing.

REFERENCES

1. Hoppe C, Molgaard C, Michaelsen KF. Cow's milk and linear growth in industrialized and developing countries. Annu Rev Nutr 2006;26:131–73.
2. Thibault H, Souberbielle JC, Taieb C, et al. Idiopathic prepubertal short stature is associated with low body mass index. Horm Res 1993;40(4):136–40.
3. Wudy SA, Hagemann S, Dempfle A, et al. Children with idiopathic short stature are poor eaters and have decreased body mass index. Pediatrics 2005;116(1):e52–7.
4. van der Eerden BC, Karperien M, Wit JM. Systemic and local regulation of the growth plate. Endocr Rev 2003;24(6):782–801.
5. Boyan BD, Wong KL, Fang M, et al. 1alpha,25(OH)$_2$D$_3$ is an autocrine regulator of extracellular matrix turnover and growth factor release via ERp60 activated matrix vesicle metalloproteinases. J Steroid Biochem Mol Biol 2007;103(3–5):467–72.
6. Baker J, Liu JP, Robertson EJ, et al. Role of insulin-like growth factors in embryonic and postnatal growth. Cell 1993;75(1):73–82.
7. Liu JP, Baker J, Perkins AS, et al. Mice carrying null mutations of the genes encoding insulin-like growth factor I (Igf-1) and type 1 IGF receptor (Igf1r). Cell 1993;75(1):59–72.
8. Woods KA, Camacho-Hubner C, Savage MO, et al. Intrauterine growth retardation and postnatal growth failure associated with deletion of the insulin-like growth factor I gene. N Engl J Med 1996;335(18):1363–7.
9. Walenkamp MJ, de Muinck Keizer-Schrama SM, de Mos M, et al. Successful long-term growth hormone therapy in a girl with haploinsufficiency of the insulin-like growth factor-I receptor due to a terminal 15q26.2 → qter deletion detected by multiplex ligation probe amplification. J Clin Endocrinol Metab 2008; 93(6):2421–5.
10. Abuzzahab MJ, Schneider A, Goddard A, et al. IGF-I receptor mutations resulting in intrauterine and postnatal growth retardation. N Engl J Med 2003;349(23): 2211–22.
11. Raile K, Klammt J, Schneider A, et al. Clinical and functional characteristics of the human Arg59Ter insulin-like growth factor I receptor (IGF1R) mutation: implications for a gene dosage effect of the human IGF1R. J Clin Endocrinol Metab 2006;91(6):2264–71.
12. Inagaki K, Tiulpakov A, Rubtsov P, et al. A familial insulin-like growth factor-I receptor mutant leads to short stature: clinical and biochemical characterization. J Clin Endocrinol Metab 2007;92(4):1542–8.
13. Peoples R, Milatovich A, Francke U. Hemizygosity at the insulin-like growth factor I receptor (IGF1R) locus and growth failure in the ring chromosome 15 syndrome. Cytogenet Cell Genet 1995;70(3–4):228–34.
14. Walenkamp MJ, Wit JM. Single gene mutations causing SGA. Best Pract Res Clin Endocrinol Metab 2008;22(3):433–46.
15. Hunziker EB, Wagner J, Zapf J. Differential effects of insulin-like growth factor I and growth hormone on developmental stages of rat growth plate chondrocytes in vivo. J Clin Invest 1994;93(3):1078–86.
16. Cruickshank J, Grossman DI, Peng RK, et al. Spatial distribution of growth hormone receptor, insulin-like growth factor-I receptor and apoptotic chondrocytes during growth plate development. J Endocrinol 2005;184(3):543–53.

17. Mosier HD Jr, Jansons RA. Growth hormone during catch-up growth and failure of catch-up growth in rats. Endocrinology 1976;98(1):214–9.
18. Hermanussen M, Rol de Lama MA, Romero AP, et al. Differential catch-up in body weight and bone growth after short-term starvation in rats. Growth Regul 1996;6(4):230–7.
19. Fontana L, Weiss EP, Villareal DT, et al. Long-term effects of calorie or protein restriction on serum IGF-1 and IGFBP-3 concentration in humans. Aging Cell 2008;7(5):681–7.
20. Heinrichs C, Colli M, Yanovski JA, et al. Effects of fasting on the growth plate: systemic and local mechanisms. Endocrinology 1997;138(12):5359–65.
21. Farnum CE, Lee AO, O'Hara K, et al. Effect of short-term fasting on bone elongation rates: an analysis of catch-up growth in young male rats. Pediatr Res 2003;53(1):33–41.
22. Gat-Yablonski G, Shtaif B, Abraham E, et al. Nutrition-induced catch-up growth at the growth plate. J Pediatr Endocrinol Metab 2008;21(9):879–93.
23. Even-Zohar N, Jacob J, Amariglio N, et al. Nutrition-induced catch-up growth increases hypoxia inducible factor 1alpha RNA levels in the growth plate. Bone 2008;42(3):505–15.
24. Robson H, Phillip M, Wit JM. The Second European Growth Plate Working Group Symposium 25th September 2002, Madrid, Spain. J Pediatr Endocrinol Metab 2003;16(3):461–6.
25. Lowe WL Jr, Adamo M, Werner H, et al. Regulation by fasting of rat insulin-like growth factor I and its receptor. Effects on gene expression and binding. J Clin Invest 1989;84(2):619–26.
26. Kojima M, Hosoda H, Date Y, et al. Ghrelin is a growth-hormone-releasing acylated peptide from stomach. Nature 1999;402(6762):656–60.
27. Shimbara T, Mondal MS, Kawagoe T, et al. Central administration of ghrelin preferentially enhances fat ingestion. Neurosci Lett 2004;369(1):75–9.
28. Holst B, Cygankiewicz A, Jensen TH, et al. High constitutive signaling of the ghrelin receptor—identification of a potent inverse agonist. Mol Endocrinol 2003;17(11):2201–10.
29. Holst B, Schwartz TW. Constitutive ghrelin receptor activity as a signaling setpoint in appetite regulation. Trends Pharmacol Sci 2004;25(3):113–7.
30. Costa T, Cotecchia S. Historical review: negative efficacy and the constitutive activity of G-protein-coupled receptors. Trends Pharmacol Sci 2005;26(12):618–24.
31. Holst B, Schwartz TW. Ghrelin receptor mutations—too little height and too much hunger. J Clin Invest 2006;116(3):637–41.
32. Pantel J, Legendre M, Cabrol S, et al. Loss of constitutive activity of the growth hormone secretagogue receptor in familial short stature. J Clin Invest 2006;116(3):760–8.
33. Pugliese-Pires PN, Fortin JP, Arthur T, et al. Novel inactivating mutations in the GH secretagogue receptor gene in patients with constitutional delay of growth and puberty. Eur J Endocrinol 2011;165(2):233–41.
34. Gueorguiev M, Lecoeur C, Benzinou M, et al. A genetic study of the ghrelin and growth hormone secretagogue receptor (GHSR) genes and stature. Ann Hum Genet 2008;73(1):1–9.
35. Sun Y, Ahmed S, Smith RG. Deletion of ghrelin impairs neither growth nor appetite. Mol Cell Biol 2003;23(22):7973–81.
36. Wortley KE, Anderson KD, Garcia K, et al. Genetic deletion of ghrelin does not decrease food intake but influences metabolic fuel preference. Proc Natl Acad Sci U S A 2004;101(21):8227–32.

37. Wortley KE, del Rincon JP, Murray JD, et al. Absence of ghrelin protects against early-onset obesity. J Clin Invest 2005;115(12):3573–8.
38. Zigman JM, Nakano Y, Coppari R, et al. Mice lacking ghrelin receptors resist the development of diet-induced obesity. J Clin Invest 2005;115(12):3564–72.
39. Petersenn S, Rasch AC, Penshorn M, et al. Genomic structure and transcriptional regulation of the human growth hormone secretagogue receptor. Endocrinology 2001;142(6):2649–59.
40. Park S, Sohn S, Kineman RD. Fasting-induced changes in the hypothalamic-pituitary-GH axis in the absence of GH expression: lessons from the spontaneous dwarf rat. J Endocrinol 2004;180(3):369–78.
41. Kamegai J, Tamura H, Shimizu T, et al. Insulin-like growth factor-I down-regulates ghrelin receptor (growth hormone secretagogue receptor) expression in the rat pituitary. Regul Pept 2005;127(1–3):203–6.
42. Avram AM, Jaffe CA, Symons KV, et al. Endogenous circulating ghrelin does not mediate growth hormone rhythmicity or response to fasting. J Clin Endocrinol Metab 2005;90(5):2982–7.
43. Caminos JE, Gualillo O, Lago F, et al. The endogenous growth hormone secretagogue (ghrelin) is synthesized and secreted by chondrocytes. Endocrinology 2005;146(3):1285–92.
44. Gat-Yablonski G, Phillip M. Leptin and regulation of linear growth. Curr Opin Clin Nutr Metab Care 2008;11(3):303–8.
45. Zhang Y, Proenca R, Maffei M, et al. Positional cloning of the mouse obese gene and its human homologue. Nature 1994;372(6505):425–32.
46. Pelleymounter MA, Cullen MJ, Baker MB, et al. Effects of the obese gene product on body weight regulation in ob/ob mice. Science 1995;269(5223):540–3.
47. Campfield LA. Metabolic and hormonal controls of food intake: highlights of the last 25 years—1972–1997. Appetite 1997;29(2):135–52.
48. Hoggard N, Mercer JG, Rayner DV, et al. Localization of leptin receptor mRNA splice variants in murine peripheral tissues by RT-PCR and in situ hybridization. Biochem Biophys Res Commun 1997;232(2):383–7.
49. Cohen MM Jr. Role of leptin in regulating appetite, neuroendocrine function, and bone remodeling. Am J Med Genet A 2006;140(5):515–24.
50. Gat-Yablonski G, Ben-Ari T, Shtaif B, et al. Leptin reverses the inhibitory effect of caloric restriction on longitudinal growth. Endocrinology 2004;145(1):343–50.
51. Gat-Yablonski G, Shtaif B, Phillip M. Leptin stimulates parathyroid hormone related peptide expression in the endochondral growth plate. J Pediatr Endocrinol Metab 2007;20(11):1215–22.
52. Grisaru-Granovsky S, Samueloff A, Elstein D. The role of leptin in fetal growth: a short review from conception to delivery. Eur J Obstet Gynecol Reprod Biol 2008;136(2):146–50.
53. Apter D. The role of leptin in female adolescence. Ann N Y Acad Sci 2003;997:64–76.
54. Maqsood AR, Trueman JA, Whatmore AJ, et al. The relationship between nocturnal urinary leptin and gonadotrophins as children progress towards puberty. Horm Res 2007;68(5):225–30.
55. Steppan CM, Crawford DT, Chidsey-Frink KL, et al. Leptin is a potent stimulator of bone growth in ob/ob mice. Regul Pept 2000;92(1–3):73–8.
56. Iwaniec UT, Boghossian S, Lapke PD, et al. Central leptin gene therapy corrects skeletal abnormalities in leptin-deficient ob/ob mice. Peptides 2007;28(5):1012–9.

57. Jin L, Burguera BG, Couce ME, et al. Leptin and leptin receptor expression in normal and neoplastic human pituitary: evidence of a regulatory role for leptin on pituitary cell proliferation. J Clin Endocrinol Metab 1999;84(8):2903–11.
58. Accorsi PA, Munno A, Gamberoni M, et al. Role of leptin on growth hormone and prolactin secretion by bovine pituitary explants. J Dairy Sci 2007;90(4):1683–91.
59. Clement K, Vaisse C, Lahlou N, et al. A mutation in the human leptin receptor gene causes obesity and pituitary dysfunction. Nature 1998;392(6674): 398–401.
60. Luque RM, Huang ZH, Shah B, et al. Effects of leptin replacement on hypothalamic-pituitary growth hormone axis function and circulating ghrelin levels in ob/ob mice. Am J Physiol Endocrinol Metab 2007;292(3):E891–9.
61. Kume K, Satomura K, Nishisho S, et al. Potential role of leptin in endochondral ossification. J Histochem Cytochem 2002;50(2):159–69.
62. Maor G, Rochwerger M, Segev Y, et al. Leptin acts as a growth factor on the chondrocytes of skeletal growth centers. J Bone Miner Res 2002;17(6):1034–43.
63. Nakajima R, Inada H, Koike T, et al. Effects of leptin to cultured growth plate chondrocytes. Horm Res 2003;60(2):91–8.
64. Ben-Eliezer M, Phillip M, Gat-Yablonski G. Leptin regulates chondrogenic differentiation in ATDC5 cell-line through JAK/STAT and MAPK pathways. Endocrine 2007;32(2):235–44.
65. Martin A, David V, Malaval L, et al. Opposite effects of leptin on bone metabolism: a dose-dependent balance related to energy intake and insulin-like growth factor-I pathway. Endocrinology 2007;148(7):3419–25.
66. Bar-El Dadon S, Shahar R, Katalan V, et al. Leptin administration affects growth and skeletal development in a rat intrauterine growth restriction model: Preliminary study. Nutrition 2011;27(9):973–7.
67. Carro E, Senaris R, Considine RV, et al. Regulation of in vivo growth hormone secretion by leptin. Endocrinology 1997;138(5):2203–6.
68. LaPaglia N, Steiner J, Kirsteins L, et al. Leptin alters the response of the growth hormone releasing factor-growth hormone–insulin-like growth factor-I axis to fasting. J Endocrinol 1998;159(1):79–83.
69. Underwood LE, Clemmons DR, Maes M, et al. Regulation of somatomedin-C/insulin-like growth factor I by nutrients. Horm Res 1986;24(2–3):166–76.
70. Farooqi IS, Keogh JM, Kamath S, et al. Partial leptin deficiency and human adiposity. Nature 2001;414(6859):34–5.
71. Schwartz MW, Woods SC, Porte D Jr, et al. Central nervous system control of food intake. Nature 2000;404(6778):661–71.
72. Baumeister FA, Engelsberger I, Schulze A. Pancreatic agenesis as cause for neonatal diabetes mellitus. Klin Padiatr 2005;217(2):76–81.
73. Taylor SI. Lilly Lecture: molecular mechanisms of insulin resistance. Lessons from patients with mutations in the insulin-receptor gene. Diabetes 1992; 41(11):1473–90.
74. Krook A, O'Rahilly S. Mutant insulin receptors in syndromes of insulin resistance. Baillieres Clin Endocrinol Metab 1996;10(1):97–122.
75. Hattersley AT, Beards F, Ballantyne E, et al. Mutations in the glucokinase gene of the fetus result in reduced birth weight. Nat Genet 1998;19(3):268–70.
76. Rosenfeld R, Cohen P. Disorders of growth hormone/insulin like growth factor secretion and action in pediatric endocrinology. In: Sperling M, editor. Pediatric endocrinology. Philadelphia: Saunders; 2002. p. 211–88.
77. Kar BR, Rao SL, Chandramouli BA. Cognitive development in children with chronic protein energy malnutrition. Behav Brain Funct 2008;4:31–42.

78. Soliman AT, ElZalabany MM, Salama M, et al. Serum leptin concentrations during severe protein-energy malnutrition: correlation with growth parameters and endocrine function. Metabolism 2000;49(7):819–25.

79. Kilic M, Taskin E, Ustundag B, et al. The evaluation of serum leptin level and other hormonal parameters in children with severe malnutrition. Clin Biochem 2004;37(5):382–7.

80. Torun B, Chew F. Protein energy malnutrition. In: Shils ME, Olson J, Shike M, Ross C, editors. Modern nutrition in health and disease. 8th edition. Philadelphia: Lippincott Williams & Wilkins; 1994. p. 950–66.

81. Zadik Z, Sinai T, Zung A, et al. Effect of nutrition on growth in short stature before and during growth-hormone therapy. Pediatrics 2005;116(1):68–72.

82. Favaro A, Tenconi E, Degortes D, et al. Association between low height and eating disorders: cause or effect? Int J Eat Disord 2007;40(6):549–53.

83. van Vught AJ, Heitmann BL, Nieuwenhuizen AG, et al. Association between intake of dietary protein and 3-year-change in body growth among normal and overweight 6-year-old boys and girls (CoSCIS). Public Health Nutr 2010; 13(5):647–53.

84. Pugliese MT, Lifshitz F, Grad G, et al. Fear of obesity. A cause of short stature and delayed puberty. N Engl J Med 1983;309(9):513–8.

85. Danziger Y, Mukamel M, Zeharia A, et al. Stunting of growth in anorexia nervosa during the prepubertal and pubertal period. Isr J Med Sci 1994;30(8):581–4.

86. Modan-Moses D, Yaroslavsky A, Novikov I, et al. Stunting of growth as a major feature of anorexia nervosa in male adolescents. Pediatrics 2003;111(2):270–6.

87. Swenne I. Weight requirements for catch-up growth in girls with eating disorders and onset of weight loss before menarche. Int J Eat Disord 2005;38(4):340–5.

88. Prabhakaran R, Misra M, Miller KK, et al. Determinants of height in adolescent girls with anorexia nervosa. Pediatrics 2008;121(6):e1517–23.

89. Misra M, Prabhakaran R, Miller KK, et al. Weight gain and restoration of menses as predictors of bone mineral density change in adolescent girls with anorexia nervosa-1. J Clin Endocrinol Metab 2008;93(4):1231–7.

90. Srinivas V, Bohensky J, Shapiro IM. Autophagy: a new phase in the maturation of growth plate chondrocytes is regulated by HIF, mTOR and AMP kinase. Cells Tissues Organs 2009;189(1–4):88–92.

91. Han ES, Hickey M. Microarray evaluation of dietary restriction. J Nutr 2005; 135(6):1343–6.

92. Schipani E, Ryan HE, Didrickson S, et al. Hypoxia in cartilage: HIF-1alpha is essential for chondrocyte growth arrest and survival. Genes Dev 2001;15(21): 2865–76.

93. Schipani E. Hypoxia and HIF-1 alpha in chondrogenesis. Semin Cell Dev Biol 2005;16(4–5):539–46.

94. Schipani E. Posttranslational modifications of collagens as targets of hypoxia and Hif-1alpha in endochondral bone development. Annals of the New York Academy of Sciences 2010;1192:317–21.

95. Tokunaga C, Yoshino K, Yonezawa K. mTOR integrates amino acid- and energy-sensing pathways. Biochem Biophys Res Commun 2004;313(2):443–6.

96. Kim DH, Sarbassov DD, Ali SM, et al. mTOR interacts with raptor to form a nutrient-sensitive complex that signals to the cell growth machinery. Cell 2002;110(2):163–75.

97. Kim DH, Sarbassov DD, Ali SM, et al. GbetaL, a positive regulator of the rapamycin-sensitive pathway required for the nutrient-sensitive interaction between raptor and mTOR. Mol Cell 2003;11(4):895–904.

98. Wullschleger S, Loewith R, Hall MN. TOR signaling in growth and metabolism. Cell 2006;124(3):471–84.

99. Sarbassov DD, Ali SM, Kim DH, et al. Rictor, a novel binding partner of mTOR, defines a rapamycin-insensitive and raptor-independent pathway that regulates the cytoskeleton. Curr Biol 2004;14(14):1296–302.

100. Frias MA, Thoreen CC, Jaffe JD, et al. mSin1 is necessary for Akt/PKB phosphorylation, and its isoforms define three distinct mTORC2s. Curr Biol 2006; 16(18):1865–70.

101. Hay N, Sonenberg N. Upstream and downstream of mTOR. Genes Dev 2004; 18(16):1926–45.

102. Pullen N, Thomas G. The modular phosphorylation and activation of p70s6k. FEBS Lett 1997;410(1):78–82.

103. Saitoh M, Pullen N, Brennan P, et al. Regulation of an activated S6 kinase 1 variant reveals a novel mammalian target of rapamycin phosphorylation site. J Biol Chem 2002;277(22):20104–12.

104. Backer JM. The regulation and function of Class III PI3Ks: novel roles for Vps34. Biochem J 2008;410(1):1–17.

105. Phornphutkul C, Wu KY, Auyeung V, et al. mTOR signaling contributes to chondrocyte differentiation. Dev Dyn 2008;237(3):702–12.

106. Klionsky DJ. The correct way to monitor autophagy in higher eukaryotes [comment]. Autophagy 2005;1(2):65.

107. Levine B, Klionsky DJ. Development by self-digestion: molecular mechanisms and biological functions of autophagy. Dev Cell 2004;6(4):463–77.

108. Byfield MP, Murray JT, Backer JM. hVps34 is a nutrient-regulated lipid kinase required for activation of p70 S6 kinase. J Biol Chem 2005;280(38):33076–82.

109. Srinivas V, Shapiro IM. Chondrocytes embedded in the epiphyseal growth plates of long bones undergo autophagy prior to the induction of osteogenesis. Autophagy 2006;2(3):215–6.

110. Savabi F. Interaction of creatine kinase and adenylate kinase systems in muscle cells. Mol Cell Biochem 1994;133–134:145–52.

111. Kanfi Y, Peshti V, Gozlan YM, et al. Regulation of SIRT1 protein levels by nutrient availability. FEBS Lett 2008;582(16):2417–23.

112. Kanfi Y, Shalman R, Peshti V, et al. Regulation of SIRT6 protein levels by nutrient availability. FEBS Lett 2008;582(5):543–8.

113. Picard F, Kurtev M, Chung N, et al. Sirt1 promotes fat mobilization in white adipocytes by repressing PPAR-gamma. Nature 2004;429(6993):771–6.

114. Rodgers JT, Lerin C, Haas W, et al. Nutrient control of glucose homeostasis through a complex of PGC-1alpha and SIRT1. Nature 2005;434(7029):113–8.

115. Nemoto S, Fergusson MM, Finkel T. Nutrient availability regulates SIRT1 through a forkhead-dependent pathway. Science 2004;306(5704):2105–8.

116. Jing E, Gesta S, Kahn CR. SIRT2 regulates adipocyte differentiation through FoxO1 acetylation/deacetylation. Cell Metab 2007;6(2):105–14.

117. Cheng HL, Mostoslavsky R, Saito S, et al. Developmental defects and p53 hyperacetylation in Sir2 homolog (SIRT1)-deficient mice. Proc Natl Acad Sci U S A 2003;100(19):10794–9.

118. Mostoslavsky R, Chua KF, Lombard DB, et al. Genomic instability and aging-like phenotype in the absence of mammalian SIRT6. Cell 2006;124(2):315–29.

119. Chen K, Rajewsky N. The evolution of gene regulation by transcription factors and microRNAs. Nat Rev Genet 2007;8(2):93–103.

120. He L, Hannon GJ. MicroRNAs: small RNAs with a big role in gene regulation. Nat Rev Genet 2004;5(7):522–31.

121. Saini HK, Griffiths-Jones S, Enright AJ. Genomic analysis of human microRNA transcripts. Proc Natl Acad Sci U S A 2007;104(45):17719–24.

122. Ruvkun G, Wightman B, Ha I. The 20 years it took to recognize the importance of tiny RNAs. Cell 2004;116(Suppl 2):S93–6, 92 p following S96.

123. Esau C, Kang X, Peralta E, et al. MicroRNA-143 regulates adipocyte differentiation. J Biol Chem 2004;279(50):52361–5.

124. Lovis P, Gattesco S, Regazzi R. Regulation of the expression of components of the exocytotic machinery of insulin-secreting cells by microRNAs. Biol Chem 2008;389(3):305–12.

125. Krutzfeldt J, Stoffel M. MicroRNAs: a new class of regulatory genes affecting metabolism. Cell Metab 2006;4(1):9–12.

126. McManus MT. MicroRNAs and cancer. Semin Cancer Biol 2003;13(4):253–8.

127. Wilson AJ, Byun DS, Nasser S, et al. HDAC4 promotes growth of colon cancer cells via repression of p21. Mol Biol Cell 2008;19(10):4062–75.

128. Poy MN, Eliasson L, Krutzfeldt J, et al. A pancreatic islet-specific microRNA regulates insulin secretion. Nature 2004;432(7014):226–30.

129. Wienholds E, Kloosterman WP, Miska E, et al. MicroRNA expression in zebrafish embryonic development. Science 2005;309(5732):310–1.

130. Tuddenham L, Wheeler G, Ntounia-Fousara S, et al. The cartilage specific microRNA-140 targets histone deacetylase 4 in mouse cells. FEBS Lett 2006; 580(17):4214–7.

131. Eberhart JK, He X, Swartz ME, et al. MicroRNA Mirn140 modulates Pdgf signaling during palatogenesis. Nat Genet 2008;40(3):290–8.

132. Nicolas FE, Pais H, Schwach F, et al. mRNA expression profiling reveals conserved and non-conserved miR-140 targets. RNA Biol 2011;8(4).

133. Harfe BD, McManus MT, Mansfield JH, et al. The RNaseIII enzyme Dicer is required for morphogenesis but not patterning of the vertebrate limb. Proc Natl Acad Sci U S A 2005;102(31):10898–903.

134. Kobayashi T, Lu J, Cobb BS, et al. Dicer-dependent pathways regulate chondrocyte proliferation and differentiation. Proc Natl Acad Sci U S A 2008;105(6): 1949–54.

135. Sumiyoshi K, Kubota S, Ohgawara T, et al. Identification of miR-1 as a micro RNA that supports late-stage differentiation of growth cartilage cells. Biochemical and biophysical research communications 2010; 402(2):286–90.

136. Hornstein E, Mansfield JH, Yekta S, et al. The microRNA miR-196 acts upstream of Hoxb8 and Shh in limb development. Nature 2005;438(7068): 671–4.

137. Lin EA, Kong L, Bai XH, et al. miR-199a, a bone morphogenic protein 2-responsive MicroRNA, regulates chondrogenesis via direct targeting to Smad1. The Journal of biological chemistry 2009;284(17):11326–35.

138. Dudek KA, Lafont JE, Martinez-Sanchez A, et al. Type II collagen expression is regulated by tissue-specific miR-675 in human articular chondrocytes. The Journal of biological chemistry 2010;285(32):24381–7.

139. Boyan BD, Schwartz Z. Rapid vitamin D-dependent PKC signaling shares features with estrogen-dependent PKC signaling in cartilage and bone. Steroids 2004;69(8–9):591–7.

140. Schwartz Z, Sylvia VL, Luna MH, et al. The effect of 24R,25-(OH) (2)D(3) on protein kinase C activity in chondrocytes is mediated by phospholipase D whereas the effect of 1alpha,25 (OH) (2)D(3) is mediated by phospholipase C. Steroids 2001;66(9):683–94.

141. Jurutka PW, Bartik L, Whitfield GK, et al. Vitamin D receptor: key roles in bone mineral pathophysiology, molecular mechanism of action, and novel nutritional ligands. J Bone Miner Res 2007;22(Suppl 2):V2–10.

142. d'Alesio A, Garabedian M, Sabatier JP, et al. Two single-nucleotide polymorphisms in the human vitamin D receptor promoter change protein-DNA complex formation and are associated with height and vitamin D status in adolescent girls. Hum Mol Genet 2005;14(22):3539–48.

143. Idelevich A, Kerschnitzki M, Shahar R, et al. 1,25(OH)(2)D(3) Alters growth plate maturation and bone architecture in young rats with normal renal function. PLoS ONE 2011;6(6):e20772.

144. Djakoure C, Guibourdenche J, Porquet D, et al. Vitamin A and retinoic acid stimulate within minutes cAMP release and growth hormone secretion in human pituitary cells. J Clin Endocrinol Metab 1996;81(8):3123–6.

145. De Luca F, Uyeda JA, Mericq V, et al. Retinoic acid is a potent regulator of growth plate chondrogenesis. Endocrinology 2000;141(1):346–53.

146. Kurugol Z, Egemen A, Keskinoglu P, et al. Vitamin A deficiency in healthy children aged 6–59 months in Izmir Province of Turkey. Paediatr Perinat Epidemiol 2000;14(1):64–9.

147. Fuchs GJ, Ausayakhun S, Ruckphaopunt S, et al. Relationship between vitamin A deficiency, malnutrition, and conjunctival impression cytology. Am J Clin Nutr 1994;60(2):293–8.

148. Fawzi WW, Herrera MG, Willett WC, et al. Dietary vitamin A intake in relation to child growth. Epidemiology 1997;8(4):402–7.

149. Zadik Z, Sinai T, Zung A, et al. "Functional food" for acceleration of growth in short children born small for gestational age. J Pediatr Endocrinol Metab 2010;23(5):435–41.

150. Bhandari N, Bahl R, Taneja S. Effect of micronutrient supplementation on linear growth of children. Br J Nutr 2001;85(Suppl 2):S131–7.

151. Ramakrishnan U, Aburto N, McCabe G, et al. Multimicronutrient interventions but not vitamin A or iron interventions alone improve child growth: results of 3 meta-analyses. J Nutr 2004;134(10):2592–602.

152. Sagazio A, Piantedosi R, Alba M, et al. Vitamin A deficiency does not influence longitudinal growth in mice. Nutrition 2007;23(6):483–8.

153. Brown KH, Peerson JM, Rivera J, et al. Effect of supplemental zinc on the growth and serum zinc concentrations of prepubertal children: a meta-analysis of randomized controlled trials. Am J Clin Nutr 2002;75(6):1062–71.

154. Hakimi SM, Hashemi F, Valaeei N, et al. The effect of supplemental zinc on the height and weight percentiles of children. Arch Iran Med 2006;9(2):148–52.

155. Gibson RS, Manger MS, Krittaphol W, et al. Does zinc deficiency play a role in stunting among primary school children in NE Thailand? Br J Nutr 2007;97(1):167–75.

156. Imamoglu S, Bereket A, Turan S, et al. Effect of zinc supplementation on growth hormone secretion, IGF-I, IGFBP-3, somatomedin generation, alkaline phosphatase, osteocalcin and growth in prepubertal children with idiopathic short stature. J Pediatr Endocrinol Metab 2005;18(1):69–74.

157. Hershkovitz E, Printzman L, Segev Y, et al. Zinc supplementation increases the level of serum insulin-like growth factor-I but does not promote growth in infants with nonorganic failure to thrive. Horm Res 1999;52(4):200–4.

158. Cole CR, Lifshitz F. Zinc nutrition and growth retardation. Pediatr Endocrinol Rev 2008;5(4):889–96.

159. Nishi Y, Hatano S, Aihara K, et al. Transient partial growth hormone deficiency due to zinc deficiency. J Am Coll Nutr 1989;8(2):93–7.

160. Collipp PJ, Castro-Magana M, Petrovic M, et al. Zinc deficiency: improvement in growth and growth hormone levels with oral zinc therapy. Ann Nutr Metab 1982; 26(5):287–90.

161. Nishi Y. Zinc and growth. J Am Coll Nutr 1996;15(4):340–4.

162. Yu XD, Yan CH, Yu XG, et al. [Effect of zinc deficiency on femoral pathological and morphological changes in growth-term rats]. Wei Sheng Yan Jiu 2005;34(2): 178–80 [in Chinese].

163. Haeusler G, Walter I, Helmreich M, et al. Localization of matrix metalloproteinases, (MMPs) their tissue inhibitors, and vascular endothelial growth factor (VEGF) in growth plates of children and adolescents indicates a role for MMPs in human postnatal growth and skeletal maturation. Calcif Tissue Int 2005;76(5):326–35.

164. Holmbeck K, Bianco P, Caterina J, et al. MT1-MMP-deficient mice develop dwarfism, osteopenia, arthritis, and connective tissue disease due to inadequate collagen turnover. Cell 1999;99(1):81–92.

165. Lin R, Amizuk N, Sasaki T, et al. 1Alpha,25-dihydroxyvitamin D3 promotes vascularization of the chondro-osseous junction by stimulating expression of vascular endothelial growth factor and matrix metalloproteinase 9. J Bone Miner Res 2002;17(9):1604–12.

166. Owen GM, Lubin AH, Garry PJ. Preschool children in the United States: who has iron deficiency? J Pediatr 1971;79(4):563–8.

167. Rao KV, Radhaiah G, Raju SV. Association of growth status and the prevalence of anaemia in preschool children. Indian J Med Res 1980;71:237–46.

168. Beard J, Haas J, Gomez LH. The relationship of nutritional status to oxygen transport and growth in highland Bolivian children. Hum Biol 1983;55(1): 151–64.

169. Lawless JW, Latham MC, Stephenson LS, et al. Iron supplementation improves appetite and growth in anemic Kenyan primary school children. J Nutr 1994; 124(5):645–54.

170. Sachdev H, Gera T, Nestel P. Effect of iron supplementation on physical growth in children: systematic review of randomised controlled trials. Public Health Nutr 2006;9(7):904–20.

171. Perrone L, Salerno M, Gialanella G, et al. Long-term zinc and iron supplementation in children of short stature: effect of growth and on trace element content in tissues. J Trace Elem Med Biol 1999;13(1–2):51–6.

172. Fahmida U, Rumawas JS, Utomo B, et al. Zinc-iron, but not zinc- alone supplementation, increased linear growth of stunted infants with low haemoglobin. Asia Pac J Clin Nutr 2007;16(2):301–9.

173. Rosado JL, Lopez P, Munoz E, et al. Zinc supplementation reduced morbidity, but neither zinc nor iron supplementation affected growth or body composition of Mexican preschoolers. Am J Clin Nutr 1997;65(1):13–9.

174. Beckett C, Durnin JV, Aitchison TC, et al. Effects of an energy and micronutrient supplement on anthropometry in undernourished children in Indonesia. Eur J Clin Nutr 2000;54(Suppl 2):S52–9.

175. Sandstead HH, Penland JG, Alcock NW, et al. Effects of repletion with zinc and other micronutrients on neuropsychologic performance and growth of Chinese children. Am J Clin Nutr 1998;68(Suppl 2):470S–5S.

176. Rosado JL. Separate and joint effects of micronutrient deficiencies on linear growth. J Nutr 1999;129(Suppl 2S):531S–3S.

177. Rivera JA, Gonzalez-Cossio T, Flores M, et al. Multiple micronutrient supplementation increases the growth of Mexican infants. Am J Clin Nutr 2001;74(5): 657–63.
178. Ash DM, Tatala SR, Frongillo EA Jr, et al. Randomized efficacy trial of a micronutrient-fortified beverage in primary school children in Tanzania. Am J Clin Nutr 2003;77(4):891–8.
179. Abrams SA, Mushi A, Hilmers DC, et al. A multinutrient-fortified beverage enhances the nutritional status of children in Botswana. J Nutr 2003;133(6): 1834–40.
180. Lartey A, Manu A, Brown KH, et al. A randomized, community-based trial of the effects of improved, centrally processed complementary foods on growth and micronutrient status of Ghanaian infants from 6 to 12 mo of age. Am J Clin Nutr 1999;70(3):391–404.
181. Liu DS, Bates CJ, Yin TA, et al. Nutritional efficacy of a fortified weaning rusk in a rural area near Beijing. Am J Clin Nutr 1993;57(4):506–11.
182. Michaelsen KF, Nielsen AL, Roos N, et al. Cow's milk in treatment of moderate and severe undernutrition in low-income countries. Nestle Nutr Workshop Ser Pediatr Program 2011;67:99–111 .
183. Molgaard C, Larnkjaer A, Arnberg K, et al. Milk and growth in children: effects of whey and casein. Nestle Nutr Workshop Ser Pediatr Program 2011;67:67–78.
184. Allen LH, Backstrand JR, Stanek EJ 3rd, et al. The interactive effects of dietary quality on the growth and attained size of young Mexican children. Am J Clin Nutr 1992;56(2):353–64.
185. Takahashi E. Secular trend in milk consumption and growth in Japan. Hum Biol 1984;56(3):427–37.
186. Baker IA, Elwood PC, Hughes J, et al. A randomised controlled trial of the effect of the provision of free school milk on the growth of children. J Epidemiol Community Health 1980;34(1):31–4.
187. Du X, Zhu K, Trube A, et al. School-milk intervention trial enhances growth and bone mineral accretion in Chinese girls aged 10–12 years in Beijing. Br J Nutr 2004;92(1):159–68.
188. Berkey CS, Rockett HR, Willett WC, et al. Milk, dairy fat, dietary calcium, and weight gain: a longitudinal study of adolescents. Arch Pediatr Adolesc Med 2005;159(6):543–50.
189. Black RE, Williams SM, Jones IE, et al. Children who avoid drinking cow milk have low dietary calcium intakes and poor bone health. Am J Clin Nutr 2002; 76(3):675–80.
190. Wiley AS. Does milk make children grow? Relationships between milk consumption and height in NHANES 1999–2002. Am J Human Biol 2005;17(4):425–41.
191. Cook J, Irwig LM, Chinn S, et al. The influence of availability of free school milk on the height of children in England and Scotland. J Epidemiol Community Health 1979;33(3):171–6.
192. Rona RJ, Chinn S. School meals, school milk and height of primary school children in England and Scotland in the eighties. J Epidemiol Community Health 1989;43(1):66–71.
193. Cadogan J, Eastell R, Jones N, et al. Milk intake and bone mineral acquisition in adolescent girls: randomised, controlled intervention trial. BMJ 1997;315(7118): 1255–60.
194. Hoppe C, Molgaard C, Juul A, et al. High intakes of skimmed milk, but not meat, increase serum IGF-I and IGFBP-3 in eight-year-old boys. Eur J Clin Nutr 2004; 58(9):1211–6.

195. Hoppe C, Udam TR, Lauritzen L, et al. Animal protein intake, serum insulin-like growth factor I, and growth in healthy 2.5-y-old Danish children. Am J Clin Nutr 2004;80(2):447–52.

196. Hoppe C, Molgaard C, Thomsen BL, et al. Protein intake at 9 mo of age is associated with body size but not with body fat in 10-y-old Danish children. Am J Clin Nutr 2004;79(3):494–501.

Growth Hormone: The Expansion of Available Products and Indications

Sherry L. Franklin, MD[a],*, Mitchell E. Geffner, MD[b]

KEYWORDS

- Growth hormone • Indications • ISS • SHOX
- Turner syndrome • Prader-Willi syndrome
- Small for gestational age

Growth hormone (GH) first was isolated from the human pituitary gland in 1956, but its biochemical structure was not elucidated until 1972. The most famous person to exemplify the appearance of untreated congenital GH deficiency (GHD) was Charles Sherwood Stratton (1838–1883), who was exhibited by P.T. Barnum as General Tom Thumb and who married Lavinia Warren.[1] Pictures of the couple show the typical adult features of untreated severe GHD along with proportional limbs and trunks. By the middle of the 20th century, endocrinologists understood the clinical features of GHD. The first report of successful treatment of human GHD was in 1958, so that GH therapy now is celebrating its 51st anniversary. Raben, an endocrinologist at Tufts University School of Medicine in Boston, was able to purify enough GH from the pituitary glands of autopsied bodies to treat a 17-year-old boy who had presumed GHD.[2] A few endocrinologists then began to help parents of children who had severe GHD to make arrangements with local pathologists to collect human pituitary glands after removal at autopsy. Parents then would contract with a biochemist to purify enough GH to treat their child. Supplies of this cadaveric GH were limited, and only the most severely deficient children were treated. From 1963 to 1985, about 7700 children in the United States and 27,000 children worldwide were given GH extracted from human pituitary glands to treat severe GHD. Physicians trained in the relatively new specialty of pediatric endocrinology provided most of this care, but, in the late 1960s, there were only

Portions of this article were previously published in the *Endocrinology and Metabolism Clinics of North America*, 38:3.

[a] University of California San Diego School of Medicine, Rady Childrens Hospital of San Diego, 7910 Frost Street, Suite 435, San Diego, CA 92123, USA

[b] Keck School of Medicine of the University of Southern California, Saban Research Institute of Childrens Hospital of Los Angeles, 4650 Sunset Boulevard, Mailstop 61, Los Angeles, CA 90027, USA

* Corresponding author.

E-mail address: sfranklin@rchsd.org

Pediatr Clin N Am 58 (2011) 1141–1165

doi:10.1016/j.pcl.2011.07.006

pediatric.theclinics.com

100 such physicians in a few dozen of the largest university medical centers around the world. To maximize procurement, purification, distribution, and clinical investigation, the National Institutes of Health and the College of American Pathologists formed the National Pituitary Agency (NPA) in 1960.[3] Treatment was reserved for only the most severe cases of GHD and, because of scarce supplies, was discontinued when girls reached 5 ft and boys reached 5.5 ft. Identification of the biochemical structure of GH in 1972 became the catalyst for the development of recombinant DNA-derived human GH, the gene for which first was cloned in 1979. The discovery was fortuitous considering the identification in 1985 of four young adults in the United States with the fatal, slow viral (prion-mediated) Creuzfeldt-Jacob Disease (CJD), who had been treated with GH from the NPA in the 1960s.[4] The connection was recognized within a few months, and use of human pituitary GH rapidly ceased. Between 1985 and 2003, 26 (out of 7700 patients treated) cases of CJD occurred in adults in the United States who had received NPA GH before 1977; 135 other cases were identified around the world. As of 2003, there had been no cases identified in people who received only GH purified by the improved 1977 methods.

A new American biotechnology company, Genentech (San Francisco, California), developed in 1981 the first recombinant human GH (rhGH) by a biosynthetic process called inclusion body technology.[5] Later, an improved process to develop rhGH was developed called protein secretion technology.[6] This is currently the most common method used to synthesize rhGH, known generically as somatotropin. Discontinuation of human cadaveric GH led to rapid US Food and Drug Administration (FDA) approval of Genentech's synthetic methionyl GH, which was introduced in the United States in 1985 for the therapy of severe childhood GHD. Although this previously scarce commodity was suddenly available in bucketfuls, the price of treatment ($10,000 to 30,000 per year) was extraordinary for a pharmaceutical at that time.

With the development of rhGH, an unlimited commercial source became available, allowing for an ever-growing list of FDA-approved indications for GH use in non-GH deficient children and for additional indications in adults:

- Children with chronic renal insufficiency (CRI) in 1993
- Turner syndrome (TS) in 1996 to 1997
- Prader-Willi syndrome (PWS) in 2000
- A history of small for gestational age (SGA) in 2001
- Idiopathic short stature (ISS) in 2003
- Short stature homeobox (SHOX) gene deficiency in 2006, Noonan syndrome (NS) in 2007
- Adults with severe GHD and for HIV wasting in 1996
- Short bowel syndrome in 2003.

APPROVED BRANDS AND INDICATIONS
Introduction

The first available rhGH, Protropin, was a polypeptide hormone produced by inclusion body recombinant DNA technology. Protropin had 192 amino acid residues and a molecular weight of about 22,000 d. The product contained the identical sequence of 191 amino acids constituting pituitary-derived human GH and an additional amino acid, methionine (MET), on the N-terminus of the molecule. Protropin was synthesized in a special laboratory strain of *Escherichia coli*, which had been modified by the addition of the gene for human growth hormone (hGH). This Met-GH was not a pure GH and, therefore, caused some patients to produce antibodies against the product.[7]

All GH preparations used today in clinical practice and in clinical trials contain the identical 191 amino acid sequence found in pituitary-derived hGH. Brands of rhGH available in the United States include: Accretropin (Cangene), Genotropin (Pharmacia), Humatrope (Eli Lilly, Indianapolis, IN, USA), Norditropin (NovoNordisk, Princeton, NJ, USA), Nutropin (Genentech, San Francisco, CA, USA), Omnitrope (Sandoz Holzkirchen, Germany), Saizen (EMD Serono, Boston, MA, USA), Serostim (EMD Serono), Tevtropin (Gate Pharmaceuticals, a division of Teva Pharmaceuticals USA, Rehovot, Isreal), and Zorbtive (EMD Serono, Boston, MA, USA). There are also brands not approved for use in the United States that are used more commonly in Asia, including: Ansomone (Anke Bio), Fitropin (Kexing), Hypertropin (Neogenica BioScienche Limited), Jintropin (Gene Science Pharmaceuticals), and Zomacton (Ferring Pharmaceuticals). Valtropin (Bio-Partners) has been approved for use in Europe. Although all current rhGH products are the same molecule, manufacturers have pursued varying FDA-approved indications for their products in the United States (**Table 1**). This may be a consideration when looking at the prospect of off-label prescribing. Reconstitution, delivery devices, storage, preservatives, and time to expiration also differ across product lines. The dose range of GH depends on age, gender, and the disease being treated. In adults, rhGH usually is administered at much lower doses with titration of doses to serum insulin-like growth factor (IGF)-1 concentrations.

Indications for Growth Hormone Therapy in Children

Growth hormone deficiency (1985)

GHD may result from a disruption of the GH axis in the hypothalamus or pituitary gland. This etiology of the dysfunction may be congenital or acquired in etiology. Congenital GHD results from genetic abnormalities (molecular defects of the GH-releasing hormone [GHRH] receptor, GH gene,[8] and abnormalities in pituitary transcription factors[9]) or anatomic malformations (midline cranial defects such as anencephaly or prosencephaly, optic nerve hypoplasia/septo-optic dysplasia, and vascular malformations[10]). Acquired GHD results from:

- Neoplasms[11] (craniopharyngioma, glioma, and pituitary adenomas)
- Cysts (Rathke cleft cyst or arachnoid cleft cyst)
- Inflammatory processes (autoimmune hypophysitis,[12] infectious diseases[13] inducing meningitis or encephalitis)
- Infiltrative processes such as sarcoidosis,[14] histiocytosis X,[15] and hemochromotasis[16]
- Head trauma[17]
- Surgery
- Radiation[18]
- Chemotherapy[19]
- Psychosocial deprivation.[20]

In spite of this expansive list of etiologies, the cause of GHD in most children is idiopathic. The classical presentation of severe GHD is characterized by short stature, slow growth, and delayed skeletal maturation, with reduced secretion of GH in response to provocative stimulation.

GH has a pulsatile and mainly sleep-entrained (nyctohemeral) pattern of secretion, occurring mainly during deep sleep (stage 3 to 4 electroencephalogram sleep). Random measurements are typically low and, therefore, of limited clinical application in the diagnosis of GHD.[21] Surrogate markers of GH action (ie, IGF-1 and insulin-like growth factor binding protein-3 [IGFBP-3]) have been used as screening tests for

Table 1
Growth hormone products and indications in the United States (2008)

Growth Hormone product	Indication
Accretropin (Cangene)	2008: Childhood growth hormone deficiency (GHD)—0.18–0.3 mg/kg/wk 2008: Turner syndrome (TS)—0.36 mg/kg/wk
Genotropin (Pfizer, Strangnas, Sweden) Cartridge—5.8 mg, 13.8 mg MiniQuick—0.2–2 mg	1995: Childhood GHD—0.16–0.24 mg/kg/wk 1997: Adult GHD 2000: Prader-Willi syndrome (PWS)—0.24 mg/kg/wk 2001: Small for gestational age (SGA)—0.48 mg/kg/wk 2008: Idiopathic short stature (ISS)—0.47 mg/kg/wk
Humatrope (Eli Lilly, Indianapolis, Indiana) Vials—5 mg/5 mL Cartridge kits—6 mg/3 mL, 12 mg/3 mL, and 24 mg/3 mL	1987: Childhood GHD—0.18–0.3 mg/kg/wk 1996: Adult GHD—0.006–0.0125 mg/kg/d 1997: TS—up to 0.375 mg/kg/wk 2003: ISS—up to 0.37 mg/kg/wk 2006: Short stature homeobox (SHOX) deficiency—0.35 mg/kg/wk 2009: SGA—up to 0.47 mg/kg/wk
Norditropin (NovoNordisk, Princeton, New Jersey) NordiPen cartridges—5 or 15 mg/1.5 mL NordiFlex pens—5, 10, or 15 mg/1.5 mL Vials—4 mg or 8 mg/5 mL	1997: Childhood GHD—0.034 mg/kg/d 2004: Adult GHD—0.004–0.125 mg/kg/d 0.15–0.3 mg/d 2007: Noonan syndrome (NS)—up to 0.066 mg/kg/d 2007: TS—up to 0.067 mg/kg/d 2008: SGA—up to 0.067 mg/kg/d
Nutropin and Nutropin AQ (Genentech, San Francisco, California) Nutropin vials—5 or 10 mg/2 mL Nutropin AQ vials—10 mg/2 mL Nutropin AQ pen cartridge—10 or 20 mg/2 mL	1993: Chronic renal insufficiency (CRI)—0.35 mg/kg/wk 1994: Childhood GHD—0.3 mg/kg/wk 1996: TS—0.375 mg/kg/wk 1997: Adult GHD—0.006–0.025 mg/kg/d 2005: ISS—0.3 mg/kg/wk 2006: Pubertal GHD dosing—up to 0.7 mg/kg/wk
Omnitrope (Sandoz, Holzkirchen, Germany) Vials—5.8 mg Cartridge—5 mg/1.5 mL, 10 mg/1.5 mL	2006: Childhood GHD—0.15–0.24 mg/kg/wk 2006: Adult GHD—0.04–0.08 mg/kg/wk
Saizen (EMD Serono, Boston, Massachusettes) Vials—5 mg, 8.8 mg Cartridges for Easypod, Cool.click, and One.click = – 8.8 mg	1996: Childhood GHD—0.06 mg/kg 2004: Adult GHD—0.005–0.01 mg/kg/d
Serostim (EMD Serono, Boston, Massachusettes)	1996 accelerated approval, 2003 full approval: HIV-associated wasting (adults)—0.1 mg/kg 3 times per week (up to 6 mg/d) for 12 weeks
Tev-Tropin (Gate/Teva Pharmaceuticals, Rehovot, Isreal) Vials—5 mg	2005: Childhood GHD—0.1 mg/kg 3 × per week
Zorbtive (EMD Serono, Boston, Massachusettes) Vials—4 mg, 5 mg, 6 mg, 8.8 mg	2003: Short bowel syndrome—0.1 mg/kg/d to a maximum of 8 mg/d for 4 weeks

First column with brand of somatotropin, company producing, and delivery formulation information. Second column with US Food and Drug Administration approval year, indication, and dosing.

childhood GHD. Because random GH levels are low during the day, provocative tests of GH release were introduced to determine GH status. The first established pharmacologic stimulus introduced for assessment of GH status was insulin hypoglycemia (ie, the insulin tolerance test [ITT]). The main advantages of this test include the concurrent ability to assess the corticotropin (ACTH)–adrenal axis while at the same time providing a powerful stimulus for the release of GH.[22] The main disadvantages of this test include the lack of normative data in children, a characteristic it shares with all other pharmacologic tests, and the risk of severe hypoglycemia.[23] Since the development of the ITT, a growing awareness that any normal child might fail any single GH provocative test led to the strategy of submitting a child to two GH provocative tests. Thus, a series of other pharmacologic stimuli were introduced into the GH diagnostic investigational arena including l-dopa (combined with propranolol), arginine, glucagon, clonidine, and GHRH.[24] Various combinations of these tests have been used and, in some centers, they are administered sequentially on the same day while, in other centers, they are administered on different days. A normal GH response to provocative testing is defined arbitrarily as greater than 10 ng/mL. This definition has been criticized as provocative tests have been shown to have poor reproducibility, and there are numerous false-positive results. Furthermore, as many as 70% of children diagnosed with idiopathic, isolated GHD, upon retesting as young adults after completion of treatment and conclusion of growth, have normal stimulated GH secretory responses, suggesting that current GH testing paradigms may be flawed.[25]

Sex steroid priming with estrogen or androgen administered before the GH provocative test is an additional maneuver designed to distinguish between genuine GHD and constitutional delay in growth and puberty (CDGP) and to improve the value of GH testing.[26] At puberty, in normal children, there is a marked amplitude-modulated increase in GH secretion directly caused by the marked rise in estrogen concentrations. Teen-aged children who have CDGP often exhibit very low GH secretion while still prepubertal or in early puberty, but show a normal increase in GH secretion with progress through puberty. Their GH responses to unprimed provocative stimuli mirror the physiologic changes in spontaneous GH secretion. Thus, in a child of peripubertal age who has slow growth disorder, CDGP is a much more common cause than is GHD. In such a child, priming with sex steroids before performing GH provocative tests will help to differentiate severe GHD (minimal GH response) from CDGP (normal GH response).

GH treatment of GHD in children is, to a certain extent, standardized worldwide.[27] Recombinant 22-kDa GH is injected once daily by the subcutaneous route, usually in the evening to simulate normal physiology. The amount of GH injected (calculated per kilogram body weight) in prepubertal children mimics the known production rate of 0.02 mg/kg/d.[27] There is a wide variation, however, in dosage used (0.17 to 0.3 mg/kg/wk), the reasons for which are partly unknown and partly because of national traditions and regimens imposed by authorities regulating reimbursement. Final height evaluations range in the -0.5 to -1.5 SDs from the mean.[28] The situation during puberty is more variable, even though a higher dose range (up to 0.7 mg/kg/wk) is approved in the United States to mimic normal physiology. The results of these approaches, in terms of adult height outcome, are not always satisfactory. To achieve optimal height development during childhood, strategies must be developed to individualize GH dosing according to set therapeutic goals taking into account efficacy, safety, and cost. A few such strategies have included higher pubertal dosing and IGF-1 based dosing.[29] The goal of therapy is to allow children who have GHD to achieve adult heights within the normal range for the population and, if possible, for the family. Although most pediatric endocrinologists currently provide therapy until adult height is achieved, there are new data to suggest that patients may be able to discontinue therapy during puberty if retesting at that time indicates normalization of the GH response to provocative testing.[30]

Serious adverse effects with GH therapy are rare but include benign intracranial hypertension (pseudotumor cerebri), slipped capital femoral epiphysis (SCFE), and type 2 diabetes. More common adverse effects include injection site reactions, transient peripheral edema, arthralgias, myalgias, and mild gynecomastia in boys. There have been many concerns about the potential role of GH in the development of cancer.[31] Long-term surveillance, however, has not supported this relationship.[32]

Chronic renal insufficiency (1993)

Children suffering from chronic kidney disease (CKD) are prone to develop severe growth failure. In a recent analysis of the North American Pediatric Renal Trials and Collaborative Studies (NAPRTCS), 37%, 47%, and 43% of children on conservative treatment, dialysis, and transplantation, respectively, presented with severe short stature (standardized height less than -2 SDs).[33] The etiology of uremic growth failure is multifactorial, including energy malnutrition, water and electrolyte disturbances, metabolic acidosis, anemia, and hormonal disturbances affecting the somatotropic and gonadotropic hormone axes.[34] In addition, children who have CKD suffer from various underlying renal diseases and may undergo different modes of renal replacement therapy at certain time points during their growth period. GH treatment in CRI has improved final height by 0.5 to 1.7 SD scores (SDS) in various studies.[35]

Abnormalities in GH and the IGF-1 axis appear to play a major role in growth failure in CKD (**Fig. 1**). Random fasting serum levels of GH are normal or increased in children and adults who have CKD, depending on the extent of renal failure. The half-life of GH is prolonged because of decreased metabolic clearance secondary to decreased functional renal mass in proportion to the degree of renal dysfunction. A high normal calculated GH secretion rate and amplified numbers of GH secretory bursts have been reported in prepubertal children with end-stage renal disease, likely because of attenuated IGF-1 feedback.[36] This has led to the concept of GH insensitivity or resistance in uremia. One mechanism for GH resistance is a reduced density of GH receptors (GHRs) in target organs.[37] Determination of the concentration of serum GH binding protein (GHBP), which is the cleaved extracellular binding domain of the GHR, may be used to assess GHR density in tissues, particularly liver, because GHBP is derived mainly, but not exclusively, from the liver. GHBP is low in children who have CKD and proportionate to the degree of renal dysfunction. Serum GHBP correlates with spontaneous growth rate and response to GH therapy, and it is an indirect indicator of sensitivity to exogenous and endogenous GH. There is controversy, however, as to the reliability of serum GHBP levels as a marker of GHR levels in specific tissues. Another mechanism for GH resistance in uremia is a defect in postreceptor GH-activated Janus kinase/signal transducer and activator of transcription (JAK/STAT) signaling.[38] GH action is mediated by the binding of GH to the GHR, resulting in its dimerization and the auto-phosphorylation of the tyrosine kinase, Janus kinase 2 (JAK2), which, in turn, stimulates phosphorylation of the signaling proteins, STAT1, STAT3, and STAT5. Upon activation, these STAT proteins translocate to the nucleus and activate GH-regulated genes. An intact JAK2-STAT5b signaling pathway is essential for GH stimulation of IGF-1 gene expression. In uremia, a defect in postreceptor GH-activated JAK2 signal transducer and STAT transduction is described as one of the mechanisms causing GH resistance. The JAK2/STAT pathway is regulated by, among other factors, suppressor of cytokine signaling (SOCS) proteins, which are induced by GH. These proteins bind to JAK2 and inhibit STAT phosphorylation.

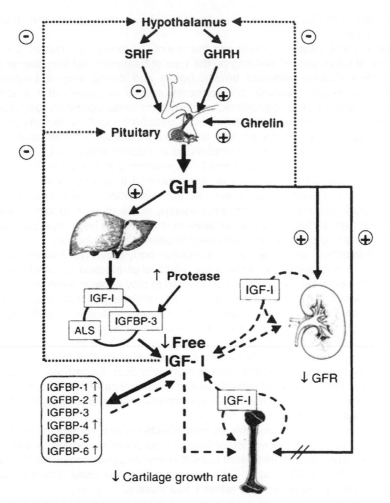

Fig. 1. Growth hormone (GH)/insulin-like growth factor (IGF)-1 axis in chronic kidney disease (CKD). The GH/IGF-I axis in corticotropin-releasing factor (CRF) is changed markedly, compared with the normal axis shown here. In CKD, the total concentrations of the hormones in the GH/IGF-I axis are not reduced, but there is reduced effectiveness of endogenous GH and IGF-I, which probably plays a major role in reducing linear bone growth. The reduced effectiveness of endogenous IGF-I likely is caused by decreased levels of free, bioactive IGF-I, as levels of circulating inhibitory IGF binding proteins (IGFBPs) are increased. In addition, less IGF-I is circulating in the complex with acid-labile subunit (ALS) and insulin-like growth factor binding protein-3 (IGFBP-3) as a result of increased proteolysis of IGFBP-3. Together, these lead to decreased IGF-I receptor activation and a decreased feedback to the hypothalamus and pituitary. Low free IGF-I and high IGFBP-1 and IGFBP-2 levels probably contribute to reduced renal function and lead to reduced stature. The direct effects of GH on bone, which are understood poorly, also are blunted. (*From* Roelfsema V, Clark RG. The growth hormone and insulin-like growth factor axis: its manipulation for the benefit of growth disorders in renal failure. J Am Soc Nephrol 2005;12:1297–306; with permission.)

Upregulation of SOCS has been described in inflammatory states and may play a similar role in CKD.

The factors that influence growth and the use of GH therapy in children who have chronic renal failure vary, depending on the type of treatment that they are receiving for their renal disease. Whereas growth before and during dialysis treatment is affected by nutritional, metabolic, and endocrine alterations, growth after renal transplantation is affected by glucocorticoid and other immunosuppressive therapies and graft failure.[39] Among children treated with GH, treatment usually is discontinued after transplantation (in line with the product label), but it sometimes is reinstituted if the growth rate remains low. Doses recommended in children who have CKD (0.35 mg/kg/wk) are higher (because of presumed GH resistance in this population) than in patients who have GHD.[40] Therapy is recommended if growth failure persists for longer than 6 months and is continued until transplantation is performed. The most important predictive factor for successful therapy is the growth velocity in the first year of treatment. Better outcomes are seen in children who begin treatment earlier, who are younger, and who have milder deterioration in renal function.

Although treatment with rhGH clearly stimulates body growth in children who have renal failure, it is possible that rhGH may affect renal function adversely in some situations. For example, GH has been suggested to play a role in the development of glomerulosclerosis in mice,[41] but there is no proof in children that rhGH has deleterious effects on renal function or, when given before renal transplantation, on graft function.[42]

rhGH therapy also has been proposed for treating growth failure after renal transplantation, as catch-up growth does not occur in up to 75% of these patients. Guest and colleagues[43] showed in a prospective randomized study that rhGH therapy after renal transplantation tended to increase the number of acute biopsy-proven rejections (9 rejections in 44 rhGH-treated patients vs 4 of 46 control patients), although this was related to a previous history of rejection. rhGH treatment after renal transplantation still must be considered experimental.

Special considerations for possible adverse effects of GH treatment in children who have CKD include an increased risk of benign intracranial hypertension and type 2 diabetes, indicating that rhGH-treated patients deserve close monitoring.[44] It seems prudent in pediatric CKD to start GH treatment with a half dose, which should be ramped up to the therapeutic dose within 1 to 2 months.

Turner syndrome (1996 to 1997)

TS is a sporadic disorder in females defined by the complete or partial absence of the second X chromosome. X monosomy is the most commonly occurring sex chromosome anomaly (1% to 2% of all female conceptions), although 90% or more of Turner conceptions spontaneously are aborted. TS has an incidence of about 1 in 2000 to 2500 live female births.

An almost universal feature of TS is severe short stature. The consequence of childhood growth failure is marked short stature in adulthood; the average height of untreated women with TS is 143 cm (4 ft 8 in) or approximately 20 cm (8 in) below that of adult women in the general United States population.[45] The short stature characteristic of individuals who have TS is believed to result, at least in part, from haploinsufficiency of the short stature homeobox-containing gene (located in the pseudoautosomal region) on the X chromosome.[46] Other features of TS are listed in **Box 1**.

Some of the features may be secondary to lymphedema during gestation. Girls who have TS may present in childhood with short stature, declining growth velocity, mildly elevated levels of follicle-stimulating hormone (FSH), or any grouping of TS stigmata described previously (**Fig. 2**). On average, the height of girls who have TS is less

Box 1
Features of Turner syndrome

- Ptosis
- Down-slanting palpebral fissures
- Epicanthal folds
- Low-set or malformed ears
- Hearing deficits
- Retrognathia
- High-arched palate
- Short and webbed neck
- Low posterior hairline
- Broad shield-like chest
- Hypoplastic nipples
- Left-sided cardiac anomalies (marked tortuosity or ectasia of the aortic arch, nonstenotic isolated bicuspid aortic valve, coarctation of the aorta, and hypoplastic left heart syndrome)
- Cubitus valgus
- Brachymetacarpia/brachymetatarsia
- Nail hypoplasia and hypercovexity

than the fifth percentile for 5 years before the diagnosis made and, more specifically, 50% of girls are less than the fifth percentiles by 1.5 years, and 75% are less than the fifth percentile by 4 years. Early growth failure occurs with all karyotypes, but the timing of growth failure is more variable with an iso-X chromosome or with a mosaic karyotype.

In girls who have TS, rhGH has been the mode of therapy used to achieve the goal of attaining as normal a height for age by as young an age as is possible; however, the magnitude of the benefit has varied greatly depending upon study design and treatment parameters. Factors predictive of taller adult stature include a relatively tall height at initiation of therapy, tall parental heights, young age at initiation of therapy, a long duration of therapy, and a higher GH dose than traditionally is used in GHD. Based on the data from the Toddler Turner Study, in which 88 girls with a mean age of 2 years were randomized to receive GH or no GH therapy (regardless of height), GH therapy was shown to be effective beginning as early as 9 months of age.[47] From these results, it can be inferred that treatment with GH should be considered even before growth failure is demonstrated.

GH therapy in the United States generally is initiated at the FDA-approved dose of 0.375 mg/kg/wk. For girls less than approximately 9 years of age, therapy usually is started with GH alone. In older girls, or those who have extreme short stature, consideration can be given to adding a nonaromatizable anabolic steroid, such as oxandrolone (0.05 mg/kg/d) with careful attention paid to hepatic transaminases.[48] Higher doses of oxandrolone are likely to result in virilization and rapid skeletal maturation. Therapy with rhGH may be continued until a satisfactory height has been attained or until little growth potential remains (bone age greater than or equal to 14 years and growth velocity less than 2 cm/y), and it should be monitored closely at quarterly to semiannual intervals.

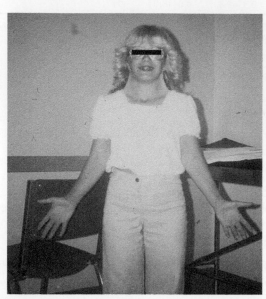

Fig. 2. A 16-year-old patient with Turner syndrome (TS). She demonstrates some of the characteristic stigmata of TS (eg, short stature, webbed neck, low-set ears, and cubitus valgus). (*From* Geffner ME. Disorders of puberty. In: Kliegman RM, Greenbaum LA, Lye PS, editors. Practical Strategies in Pediatric Diagnosis and Therapy. Harcout Health Sciences, 2005; with permission.)

Girls who have TS have a higher frequency of adverse effects that may be associated with GH therapy.[49] The National Cooperative Growth Study (NCGS) has collected safety and efficacy data for close to 6000 children with TS treated with rhGH for over 20 years. Based on a report in 2008 regarding the long-term safety data for GH in this population, there was an increased incidence of intracranial hypertension, slipped capital femoral epiphysis (SCFE), scoliosis, and diabetes. At the time, there were 12 cases of intracranial hypertension that were reported in patients who had TS, representing an incidence of 0.23% in the TS population, compared with 0.11% in non-TS patients. The incidence of SCFE in the TS population was 0.24%, compared with 0.15% for the non-TS patient population. The incidence of scoliosis in TS patients was 0.69%, compared with 0.39% among non-TS patients. Of the 36 reports of scoliosis in TS patients, 16 were considered to be a progression of pre-existing scoliosis. In the remaining 20 cases, scoliosis was described as new in onset, or a prior history was not specified. The incidence of diabetes mellitus in patients who had TS was 0.19%, compared with 0.10% for the non-TS population. Of the 10 TS patients affected, eight represented type 1 diabetes mellitus, and two represented type 2 diabetes mellitus. Additional reports of glucose intolerance or hyperglycemia were received. A comparison of the incidence of type 1 diabetes mellitus in patients who had TS with that of the age-matched general population indicates a higher risk in patients who have TS.

Prader-Willi syndrome (2000)

PWS, with a prevalence rate of 1 in 16,000 people, is the first human disorder attributed to genomic imprinting in which genes are expressed differentially based on the parent of origin. PWS results from the loss of imprinted genomic material within the paternal 15q11.2-13 locus. The loss of maternal genomic material at the 15q11.2-13 locus results in Angelman syndrome. The molecular events underlying the disorder include interstitial deletions (70%), uniparental disomy (25%), imprinting center defects (less than 5%), and rarely chromosomal translocations (less than 1%).[50] Characteristic facial features include narrow bifrontal diameter, almond-shaped palpebral fissures, narrow nasal bridge, and a down-turned mouth. Infants typically have poor muscle tone, delayed development, and failure-to-thrive. By age 2 years, these children develop profound polyphagia and often progress to morbid obesity.

Mild prenatal growth retardation is common, with a median birth weight SDS of -1.37 (range -2.81 to +0.15), with 20% having SDS less than -2.0, and median birth length SDS of -0.46 (range -2.14 to +1.40).[51] During the first year, children who have PWS grow nearly normally in length; thereafter, short stature is present in approximately 50% of patients. Between 3 and 13 years of age, the 50th percentile for height in PWS is roughly identical with the third percentile in healthy controls. Body weight is normal during the first 2 years, although excess fat is already present based on quantitative body composition analyses. Thereafter, rapid weight gain ensues; after age 10 years, the weight-for-height index in nearly all patients exceeds the normal range. The extent of pubertal growth also is reduced in patients who have PSW. Mean adult height in one cohort indicated 161.6 plus or minus 8.1 cm for men and 150.2 plus or minus 5.5 cm for women.[52]

Spontaneous GH secretion is reduced during pharmacologic stimulation in 70% of children who have PWS.[53] Even though it is difficult to ultimately prove GHD in PWS because of the nonspecific effects of obesity to suppress GH secretion in response to all secretagogues, the diagnosis is suggested by low levels of IGF-1. This situation differs from that in simple obesity, in which IGF-1 levels are usually normal to elevated, and children may grow in excess of their genetic potential.[54] Decreasing growth velocity, progressive obesity, decreased muscle-to-fat mass ratio, small hands and feet, and reduced GH/IGF-1 levels, and the positive (and sometimes dramatic) effect of GH treatment on these parameters, support the presence of hypothalamic GHD in patients who have PWS. The goals of GH treatment in children who have PWS in the United States are to improve growth during childhood and improve adult height (FDA-approved dose is 0.24 mg/kg/wk). There is controversy in the United States, although not in Europe, regarding the additional goal to improve metabolic parameters. There are clear data through randomized controlled studies showing a significant increase in height and growth velocity, with a corresponding decrease in percent body fat during the first year of GH treatment followed by stabilization during the second year.[55] Lean body mass increased significantly during the first 2 years of GH treatment compared with that seen in untreated children who had PWS. After the initial 2 years of treatment, GH therapy for an additional 2 years had continued beneficial effects on body composition. Only a few studies have reported data on adult height. In the Kabi International Growth Study database, 21 boys and 12 girls reached adult height, two thirds of whom were greater than −2 SDS; the median adult height was 11 SDS for height after a mean treatment duration of 8.4 years.[51] In a recent report, including 13 boys and 8 girls, the mean adult height was -0.3 SDS after a mean duration of 7.9 years of GH treatment.[56] Improvements in strength and agility during GH treatment were documented in prior studies and are speculated to positively contribute to a higher quality of life and reduced levels of depression in patients who have PWS.[57]

The benefits of starting GH treatment as early as 2 years are well-established in young children who have PWS, but there is suggested evidence of additional benefit in starting therapy between 6 and 12 months of age, particularly in terms of motor development, muscle, head circumference, and possibly cognition.[58] Starting GH treatment early could be difficult in the United States, where GH treatment is labeled solely for short stature (in patients who have chromosomally-proven PWS). In Europe, growth retardation is not required in children who have PWS for initiation of GH treatment.

Hypothyroidism has been reported in children who have PWS[59] and may be of central or peripheral origin, requiring screening with TSH and free T_4 measurements before and on GH treatment.

Since October 2002, several reports of unexpected death in infants and children with PWS have been published. Most of them, whether in patients with or without GH treatment, were related to a complicated course of a relatively mild respiratory tract infection, sleep apnea, adenoidal or tonsillar hypertrophy, hypoventilation, and aspiration; many were related to obesity. A recent review including 64 children (42 boys and 22 girls, 28 on GH treatment) suggested a high-risk period of death during the first 9 months of GH treatment.[60] For this reason, it has been advised that GH treatment should be started at a low dose for the first few weeks to months and titrated to the standard dose of 0.24 mg/kg/wk, while closely monitoring for any adverse respiratory effects (new or worsening of snoring, headache, excessive daytime sleeping, or lethargy). There are some clinicians who recommend a sleep study just before and 1 month after initiating GH therapy in patients who have PWS.

Other special considerations regarding risks of GH therapy in children who have PWS include glucose intolerance and dyslipidemia related to insulin resistance, and the development or progression of scoliosis. Studies, however, do not support metabolic deterioration in treated patients. Rather, there seems to be an improvement in overall body composition, resulting in an improved metabolic profile.[61] It is for this reason that GH is approved for adults who have PWS in Europe.

Small for gestational age (2001)

Nearly 3% of infants are born SGA, defined as birth weight or length at least 2 SDS below the mean for gestational age.[62] Independently of whether these children are born prematurely or at term, most SGA infants experience postnatal growth sufficient to normalize their height by 2 years of age. This is referred to as catch-up growth. It is estimated, however, that approximately 8% of SGA children remain short (height below -2 SDS) throughout childhood. Although most of these children do not exhibit GH deficiency, the International Small for Gestational Age Advisory Board has suggested that GH deficiency should be ruled out in these patients.[63] Several international studies have shown that most of these children benefit from GH therapy by normalizing height during childhood, maintaining a normal growth velocity during the prepubertal years and through puberty, and attaining a normal adult height. Because of presumed GH resistance contributing to the lack of catch-up growth in the former SGA population and results of heightened efficacy at high doses, GH therapy in the United States is FDA-approved at a dose of 0.48 mg/kg/wk.

Children who are born SGA have a higher incidence of insulin resistance, hypertension, dyslipidemia, type 2 diabetes mellitus, and cardiovascular disease later in life. These metabolic abnormalities occur, even at the same body mass index (BMI) as other adults. Individuals born SGA have been found to have a higher fat-to-muscle mass ratio and a higher visceral adiposity than do age- and weight-matched controls. Theoretically, the use of GH in a patient who already has insulin resistance is of concern. Studies have demonstrated worsening of elevated insulin levels (presumably reflecting insulin resistance) during therapy. The studies, however, have not demonstrated any actual changes in fasting glucose, postglucose load, or lipids during GH administration and resolution of hyperinsulinemia after conclusion of GH treatment.[64]

Idiopathic short stature (2003)

ISS is defined by the FDA as a condition in which the height of an individual is greater than or equal to 2.25 SDS below the corresponding mean height for a given age, sex, and population group (equivalent to the 1.2nd percentile). The predicted adult height (based on bone age) is less than 5 ft 3 in and less than 4 ft 11 in for men and women, respectively, and there is no evidence of systemic, endocrine, nutritional, or chromosomal abnormalities.[65] Specifically, children who have ISS have normal birth weight and length, are GH-sufficient, and do not have any other clearly identifiable diagnosis that predisposes them to poor growth or short stature (eg, celiac disease, inflammatory bowel disease, juvenile rheumatoid arthritis, systemic lupus erythematosus, or chronic steroid use). Based on a consensus statement published in 2008, ISS should be distinguished from constitutional delay of growth and development and from familial short stature.[66] Most patients who have ISS do not have a delayed bone age and are inappropriately short compared with their parents. The expected mean gain in height in children who have ISS is 3 in based on subjects from the seminal Lilly study who were, on average, 9 years old at the start of treatment and who received GH (0.37 mg/kg/wk) for an average treatment period of 5 years.[67]

In the United States, the current FDA-approved dose for GH in children who have ISS is 0.37 mg/kg/wk. In the future, growth prediction models may improve GH dosing strategies. IGF-1 levels may be helpful in assessing compliance and GH sensitivity. Levels that are elevated consistently (greater than +2.5 SDS) should prompt consideration of reduction in GH dose. Recent studies on IGF-1 based dose adjustments in ISS demonstrated increased short-term growth when higher IGF-I targets were selected, but this strategy has not been validated in long-term studies with respect to safety, cost-effectiveness, or adult height.[68] There have been no unusual GH safety issues in patients who have ISS.

Short stature homeobox-containing gene deficiency (2006)

SHOX, discovered during the search for genes responsible for the growth deficit of TS, is located in the pseudoautosomal region 1 on the distal end of both the X and Y chromosomes at Xp22.3 and Yp11.3, respectively.[46] Because genes in this region do not undergo X inactivation, healthy individuals express two copies of the SHOX gene, one from each of the sex chromosomes in both males and females. The SHOX gene encodes a homeodomain transcription factor expressed during early fetal life in developing skeletal tissue of the radius and ulna, the tibia and distal femur, and the first and second pharyngeal arches. The protein is expressed specifically in the growth plate in hypertrophic chondrocytes undergoing apoptosis and appears to play an important role in regulating chondrocyte differentiation and proliferation.

Because they lack all or part of their second X chromosome, individuals who have TS have only a single copy of the SHOX gene. This state of SHOX haploinsufficiency appears to be substantially responsible for the average 20 cm height deficit in women with TS (who receive no growth-promoting therapy) relative to their midparental height and relative to the average height of adult women of the same ethnic background. In addition to its role underlying the growth deficit of TS, SHOX haploinsufficiency is also the primary cause of short stature in most patients who have Léri-Weill dyschondrosteosis, also known as Léri-Weill syndrome (LWS), a pseudoautosomal-dominant condition with greater penetrance in females than in males.[69] In both TS and LWS, there is one missing SHOX allele. In contrast, two defective or absent SHOX alleles result in Langer syndrome, which is characterized by extreme dwarfism and limb deformity. Interesting, in all three conditions there is preferential limb shortening in the middle segments; hence these are all forms of mesomelic dwarfism.

Features suggesting isolated SHOX deficiency include increased BMI (approximately +1 SDS greater than comparably short children without a mutation). This is characterized by a unique stocky body habitus with muscular hypertrophy, along with disproportionate growth, with shortening of limbs compared with the trunk, and bowing of forearms and lower legs. Furthermore, SHOX mutations and deletions also are found in patients who have an unremarkable short stature phenotype.[70] The estimated prevalence of SHOX mutations ranges from 1% to 4% of cases of apparent ISS.

Experience with GH treatment in patients who have SHOX deficiency was limited until a large, randomized clinical controlled study was completed and published in 2007 demonstrating safety and efficacy in this population.[71] FDA-approved GH dosing for SHOX deficiency is 0.35 mg/kg/wk. There have been no unusual safety issues associated with treating SHOX-deficient patients.

Noonan syndrome (2007)

NS is a clinically heterogeneous disorder characterized by proportionate postnatal short stature, dysmorphic facial features (**Fig. 3**), chest deformities, and congenital heart disease (most commonly pulmonary valve stenosis and hypertrophic cardiomyopathy). Mild mental retardation, cryptorchidism, and clotting disorders also may observed in affected individuals. This autosomal-dominant condition is relatively common, with an estimated incidence, based on clinical diagnostic criteria, of 1 of 1000 to 1 of 2500 live births, with an equal male-to-female ratio.

Approximately 50% of cases of NS are caused by gain-of-function mutations in the tyrosine phosphatase, nonreceptor type 11 (PTPN11) gene, which encodes for Src homology protein tyrosine phosphatase-2 (SHP-2).[72] SHP-2 is a ubiquitously expressed cytoplasmic protein, a member of a subfamily of protein tyrosine phosphatases that contains two Src homology 2 (SH2) domains. In addition to tyrosine phosphatase actions, SHP-2 may act as an adapter molecule through phosphorylation of a tyrosine residue at its amino terminal, thus working as a docking site for other SH2-containing molecules. Both functions, adapter molecule and tyrosine phosphatase, are relevant to signal transduction of growth factors and cytokines. The mutations identified in PTPN11 in patients who have NS are predicted to be gain-of- function changes causing a conformational shift in the equilibrium of the molecule favoring an active conformation, thus augmenting the capacity of dephosphorylation. The exact

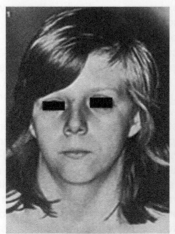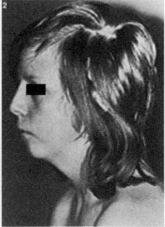

Fig. 3. The cardinal dysmorphic features of a patient with Noonan syndrome are demonstrated in this figure: triangular-shaped face, hypertelorism, down-slanting eyes, ptosis, low-set ears with thickened helices, high nasal bridge, and short webbed neck.

mechanism by which PTPN11 mutations compromise linear growth remains unknown. The GH–IGF-1 axis is essential for normal postnatal growth, and both GH and IGF-1 exert their actions after binding to specific receptors that phosphorylate several tyrosine residues located in the intracellular domain. Activation of these tyrosines is critical for downstream signaling of GH- and IGF-1 stimulated biologic responses, and tyrosine dephosphorylation leads to the physiologic interruption of these pathways. Therefore, in patients who have NS, an increased action of the protein, SHP-2, would be predicted to decrease the actions of endogenous GH[73] and IGF-1.[74] If this theory is correct, limitation in responsiveness to treatment with exogenous GH (or IGF-1) also might be expected. Confirmation of this hypothesis resulted from studies demonstrating better growth responses to GH in patients with NS who were PTPN11-negative (vs those who had a documented mutation), suggesting the presence of GH resistance or a postreceptor signaling defect in the mutation-positive group (but not an insurmountable one).[75] Support for this hypothesis also is demonstrated by the normal GH response to provocative stimulation and low IGF-1 levels seen in patients who have NS.[76]

Of note, the PTPN11 mutation is present in approximately 50% of patients who have NS; additional mutations described involve the SOS1 (20%), RAF1 (10% to 15%), and KRAS (5%) genes. Commercial testing is available and useful, especially if the diagnosis is uncertain on purely clinical grounds.

A beneficial effect of rhGH on height in patients with NS has been demonstrated in several studies. In the seminal studies to adult height leading to regulatory approval in the United States, boys gained an average of 9.9 cm and girls 9.1 cm above their originally predicted respective heights. The FDA-approved dose for patients who have NS is 0.462 mg/kg/wk. A major concern regarding the use of rhGH has been a possible increased risk of alteration in cardiac function, particularly the development or deterioration of left ventricular hypertrophic cardiomyopathy. Suspicions were not confirmed in a multicenter prospective study examining the efficacy and safety of rhGH given in a relatively high dose.[77]

Indications for Growth Hormone Therapy in Adults

Adult growth hormone deficiency (1996)

Adult GHD (AGHD) may result either de novo in adults who sustain hypothalamic or pituitary damage or as the continuation of prior childhood GHD. Pituitary tumors are more common in adults, while lesions involving the hypothalamus and infundibulum are more common in children. A distinct syndrome of AGHD has been described (**Box 2**).[78] This syndrome also appears to be associated with increased cardiovascular mortality, causes for which include increased visceral fat, abnormal lipids, decreased

---

Box 2
Characteristics of adult growth hormone deficiency

- Abnormal body composition (↑ fat mass and ↓ lean body or muscle mass)
- ↓ bone mineral density (with ↑ fracture risk)
- ↓ exercise capacity (perhaps as a result of unfavorable body composition)
- Abnormal serum lipid profile (↑ total cholesterol, ↑ low density lipoprotein [LDL] cholesterol, ↑ lipoprotein a, ↑ apolipoprotein B, and ↑ triglycerides, along with ↓ high density lipoprotein [HDL] cholesterol)
- Impaired quality-of-life (including social isolation, depression, and ↓ sense of well-being)

fibrinolytic activity, excessive number of arterial plaques, increased intima media thickness, endothelial dysfunction, and an altered inflammatory state.[79] This may be exacerbated by the low levels of motivation and exercise associated with the reduced quality-of-life seen in adults who have GHD. Other contributory factors to this increased mortality risk may include radiation (if given), surgery (if performed), and improper replacement of other hormonal deficiencies (if present).

Despite the previously mentioned manifestations of adult GHD and potential serious cardiovascular risk, significant barriers to treatment of adults who have GHD exist for the internist–endocrinologist. These include a lack of awareness or acceptance of data supporting efficacy, concerns regarding cost and need for daily injections potentially for life, nonstandardized strategies for dosing and treatment monitoring, concern regarding the relationship of GH to cancer, and, finally, perceived difficulties in making a secure diagnosis. Because IGF-1 levels are normal in a significant number of adults who have GHD (unlike most of their pediatric counterparts), GH stimulation testing remains paramount in securing the diagnosis of AGHD (**Table 2**).[80] Several additional caveats must be considered when attempting to diagnose GHD in adults. First, stimuli other than insulin or combined arginine-GHRH generally are not recommended in adults. Second, insulin-induced hypoglycemia may pose significant risks in the setting of any known seizure disorder or cardiovascular disease. Third, adults who have GHD may have normal responses to arginine-GHRH, if recently irradiated or in the setting of hypothalamic etiologies. Fourth, the presence of obesity (especially abdominal), which increases with advancing age throughout adulthood, creates significant difficulties in diagnosing AGHD as the obese state is associated with poor GH responsiveness to secretagogues.

The recommended GH dose range to treat AGHD ranges from 0.00625 mg/kg/d (6.35 µg/kg/d) to 0.0125 mg/kg/d (12.5 µg/kg/d), with final dosing guided by attainment of age-adjusted serum IGF-1 levels. Dosing requirements of GH in adults is affected by gender (higher in women), age of treatment (lower with advancing age), age at diagnosis of GHD (higher if childhood-onset), and route of concomitant estrogen administration (if applicable higher on oral than on transdermal replacement). Risk of adverse effects can be minimized by beginning with a low dose of GH (eg, 1 to 2 mg/kg/d in men or in women not receiving any estrogen or receiving it by the transdermal route and 2 to 4 µg/kg/d in younger subjects, those with childhood-onset GHD, or women on oral estrogen). Daily doses should be increased by 100 to 200 µg every 1 to 2 months until target serum IGF-1 levels are reached. Use of GH to treat AGHD is associated with improvements in body composition, muscle strength and endurance, bone density, cardiovascular markers, and quality of life. Adverse effect issues in adults center around those related to fluid retention, including edema, carpal tunnel syndrome, and arthralgias/myalgias, and type 2 diabetes mellitus. To date, there remains no concrete evidence linking GH treatment to new, recurrent, or metastatic cancer.

Table 2 Diagnosis of adult growth hormone deficiency		
Secretagogue	**Dose/Route**	**Cut Point for Normal**
Insulin	0.10–0.15 units/kg intravenously to reduce plasma glucose to <40 mg/dL	>5.1 ng/mL
Glucagon	1.0–1.5 mg IM	>3.0 ng/mL

HIV-associated wasting (1996)

Consideration of GH treatment for HIV-associated wasting stems from the known general anabolic properties of GH and reported derangements in the GH–IGF-1 axis in patients who have HIV wasting. This entity first was recognized as an AIDS-defining illness in 1987 and is defined as the unintentional loss of body weight and lean body mass in patients infected with HIV. The US Centers for Disease Control and Prevention (CDC) specify that there must be a greater than 10% involuntary weight loss along with chronic diarrhea (two loose stools daily for more than 30 days) or chronic weakness and constant or intermittent documented fever for at least 30 days without a cause other than HIV infection. Overt AIDS need not be present. Since the introduction of highly active antiretroviral treatment (HAART) in the early 1990s, the incidence of HIV-associated wasting has fallen dramatically. In the setting of HIV-associated wasting, mortality risk is doubled with or without HAART. Most existing treatments for HIV-associated wasting (other than testosterone and anabolic steroids), if effective, promote weight gain with increased fat mass, but not increased lean body mass, and it is the latter which correlates with survival.[81]

The cause of HIV wasting is likely multifactorial (**Box 3**).[82] Various abnormalities of the GH–IGF-1 axis have been reported, including findings associated with GHD in some studies and of partial GH resistance (characterized by elevated serum levels of GH and reduced levels of IGF-1).[83] The favorable action of GH on body composition promoting accretion of lean body mass and burning of fat make it an attractive candidate for treatment of HIV-associated wasting, assuming that rhGH treatment could overcome any GH resistance that might be present. The GH resistance of HIV-associated wasting seems to resemble that seen in other forms of undernutrition and chronic disease.[84]

The design and outcomes of the seminal study (performed in the pre-HAART era) that led to FDA approval of rhGH for treating HIV-associated wasting are depicted in **Table 3**.[85] Six studies of a total of approximately 500 subjects with HIV-associated wasting treated with GH have been published. All (two before HAART and four after HAART) involved a 12-week high-dose rhGH treatment course (the dosing regimen approved by the FDA) and a placebo arm (and, in one, an anabolic steroid—nandrolone—comparison arm). All reported an increase in lean body mass and some sort of improved functional correlate (exercise tolerance, muscle strength,

Box 3
Causes of HIV-associated wasting
Inadequate nutrient intake
Oral and upper gastrointestinal (GI)
Anorexia
Psychosocial-economic
Malabsorption
Altered metabolism
Uncontrolled HIV infection
Metabolic demands of HAART
Opportunistic infections or malignancies (AIDS-defining conditions)
Hormonal deficiencies/resistance
Cytokine dysregulation

Table 3
Design and outcome of pivotal study leading to US Food and Drug Administration approval of recombinant human growth hormone for treatment of HIV-associated wasting

Design	
178 patients (172 men and 6 women), randomized, double-blind, placebo-controlled study recombinant human growth hormone at a dose of 0.1 mg/kg/d (maximum dose 6 mg/d) for 12 weeks	
Outcomes (vs placebo):	
Weight ↑ by:	1.6 ± 3.7 kg (P = .011)
Lean Body Mass ↑ by:	3.0 ± 3.0 kg (P<.001)
Fat Mass ↓ by:	1.7 ± 1.7 kg (P<.001)
Exercise tolerance (treadmill) ↑ by:	13.2% (P = .039)
Quality-of-life scores:	No significant change

or oxygen extraction) in response to rhGH compared with placebo. Adverse effects relate to fluid retention and type 2 diabetes, with no heightened cancer risk seen (although patients who have histories of malignancies generally have been excluded from these studies). Information on the long-term outcome of adults using rhGH alone for treatment of HIV-associated wasting is sparse.

Three recent randomized, double-blind studies have begun to examine the effect of combined low-dose GH and IGF-1 treatment. Less impressive results have been reported than with GH monotherapy, which may reflect high attrition rates as a result of the requirement for three to four injections per day with dual treatment.[86] Finally, rhGH monotherapy is being studied (not FDA-approved) as a treatment for the HIV-associated lipodystrophy syndrome, with improvements in leady body mass found in most studies.[87]

Short bowel syndrome (2003)

Use of rhGH to treat short bowel syndrome (SBS) in people was based on animal data in which GH promoted intestinal growth in rats and enhanced intestinal growth in GH-transgenic mice. More specifically, GH increased mucosal mass and villi proliferation (absorptive surface) in animals; it also promoted transport of water, electrolytes, and nutrients across the gut and stimulated IGF-1 generation in intestinal mucosa.[88] Based on these data, rhGH was studied in people who had SBS as a means to promote intestinal adaptation and to decrease parenteral nutrition (PN) requirements. SBS is defined as the loss of approximately two thirds of the small intestine, which is normally about 600 to 650 cm in length. The most common causes of SBS are impaired blood flow to the GI tract resulting from thrombosis, trauma, malrotation, or volvulus; inflammatory bowel disease (primarily Crohn's disease); and others, including radiation enteritis, trauma, and cancer.[89] On the basis of data from Europe, PN-dependent SBS occurs in 2 to 3 million people per year, with an estimated prevalence of approximately 4 cases year per million people. Life expectancy is about 75% at 5 years in the total population of SBS patients, with reduced lifespan and quality of life in part caused by PN dependence and its complications and cost. Intestinal transplantation remains an option for some, as does the use of other gut trophic factors such as glucagon-like peptide-2 (GLP-2).[90]

To assess the benefits of GH treatment in patients who had SBS, a 4-week double-blind, controlled, randomized clinical trial of rhGH (0.1 mg/kg/d) in 41 adults was initiated to compare the relative efficacy and safety of rhGH and a specialized diet, with or without glutamine, as a means to improve residual gut absorptive function. The primary endpoint of this trial was reduction in total PN volume. Subjects treated with rhGH achieved a significantly greater reduction in PN than did those receiving a glutamine-supplemented diet alone (**Fig. 4**). Additionally, this response was maintained 12 weeks after the end of rhGH therapy. This reduction in volume and frequency of infusions is considered a major clinical benefit to this PN-dependent patient population. rhGH-related adverse events were expected, well-characterized, and transient (mostly involving fluid retention as occurs in other rhGH-treated adults), and no serious adverse events were considered related to the treatment.

In addition to the previously mentioned study, a recent review of all studies of GH usage in patients who had SBS reported five additional open-label studies in which rhGH significantly increased absorption of energy, protein, and carbohydrates.[91] Four studies of GH treatment also reported significant gains in weight, lean body mass, total body potassium, or total body water. Two other randomized controlled studies, however, showed no effect on energy or fluid absorption. In one other randomized controlled trial and six other open-label trials, rhGH-treated patients, including some with no colon and others who had had major resections, were able to eliminate or markedly reduce PN reliance. Overall, although GH treatment of adult patients who have SBS from an array of causes remains controversial, most published results show that short-term GH treatment, combined with optimized nutrition and glutamine supplementation, allows enhanced bowel absorption and function,

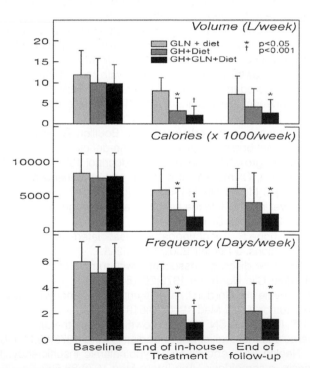

Fig. 4. The volume, caloric content, and frequency of parenteral nutrition (PN) before treatment, after 4 weeks of treatment, and after 3 months of home infusion. (*From* Byrne TA, Wilmore DW, Iyer K, et al. Growth hormone, glutamine, and an optimal diet reduces parenteral nutrition in patients with short bowel syndrome: a prospective, randomized, placebo-controlled, double-blind clinical trial. Ann Surg 2005;242:655–61; with permission.)

permitting reduced PN dependence. Studies of long-term results of short-term GH or longer-term use of GH remain to be done. Additionally, only one of the previously mentioned studies included a subset of children (9 to 13 years of age) with SBS who appeared to benefit comparably with their adult coparticipants.[92]

SUMMARY

In conclusion, GH is a widely used hormone. Although most of the indications cited in this article are of GH-sufficient patients, years of administration have proven safety and efficacy in these populations. There are now reports of the use of GH in cystic fibrosis, inflammatory bowel disease, juvenile rheumatoid arthritis, osteoporosis, and in patients who require chronic glucocorticoid administration. GH is an important growth-promoting factor that also has been shown to also have metabolic, inflammatory, and immunologic importance. As more is learned about GH, it is inevitable that its uses will continue to expand.

REFERENCES

1. McKusick VA, Rimoin DL. General Thom Thumb and other midgits. Sci Am 1967; 217:102–6.
2. Raben MS. Treatment of a pituitary dwarf with human growth hormone. J Clin Endocrinol Metab 1958;18:901–3.
3. Frasier SD. The not-so-good old days: working with pituitary growth hormone in North America, 1956 to 1985. J Pediatr 1997;131:S1–4.
4. Report of the Committee on Growth Hormone Use of the Lawson Wilkins Pediatric Endocrine Society. Degenerative neurologic disease in patients formerly treated with human growth hormone. J Pediatr 1985;107:10–2.
5. Flodh H. Human growth hormone produced with recombinant DNA technology: development and production. Acta Paediatr Scand Suppl 1986;325:1–9.
6. Cronin MJ. Pioneering recombinant growth hormone manufacturing: pounds produced per mile of height. J Pediatr 1997;131:S5–7.
7. Massa G, Vanderschueren-Lodeweyckx M, Bouillon R. Five-year follow-up of growth hormone antibodies in growth hormone-deficient children treated with recombinant human growth hormone. Clin Endocrinol 1993;38:137–42.
8. Takahashi Y, Kaji H, Okimura Y, et al. Short stature caused by a mutant growth hormone. N Engl J Med 1996;334:432–6.
9. Dattani MT. Novel insights into the aetiology and pathogenesis of hypopituitarism. Horm Res 2004;62(Suppl 3):1–13.
10. Traggiai C, Stanhope R. Endocrinopathies associated with midline cerebral and cranial malformations. J Pediatr 2002;140:252–5.
11. Costin G. Endocrine disorders associated with tumors of the pituitary and hypothalamus. Pediatr Clin North Am 1979;26:15–31.
12. Mayfield RK, Levine JH, Gordon L, et al. Lymphoid adenohypophysitis presenting as a pituitary tumor. Am J Med 1980;69:619–23.
13. Bartsocas CS, Pantelakis SN. Human growth hormone therapy in hypopituitarism due to tuberculous meningitis. Acta Paediatr Scand 1973;62:304–6.
14. Stuart CA, Neelon FA, Lebovitz HE. Hypothalamic insufficiency: the cause of hypopituitarism in sarcoidosis. Ann Intern Med 1978;88:589–94.
15. Donadieu J, Rolon MA, Pion I, et al, French LCH Study Group. Incidence of growth hormone deficiency in pediatric-onset Langerhans cell histiocytosis: efficacy and safety of growth hormone treatment. J Clin Endocrinol Metab 2004;89: 604–9.

16. Lewis AS, Courtney CH, Atkinson AB. All patients with idiopathic hypopituitarism should be screened for hemochromatosis. Pituitary 2008;12:273–5.

17. Aimaretti G, Ambrosio MR, Benvenga S, et al. Hypopituitarism and growth hormone deficiency (GHD) after traumatic brain injury (TBI). Growth Horm IGF Res 2004;14(Suppl A):S114–7.

18. Darzy KH, Shalet SM. Pathophysiology of radiation-induced growth hormone deficiency: efficacy and safety of GH replacement. Growth Horm IGF Res 2006;16(Suppl A):S30–40.

19. Roman J, Villaizan CJ, Garcia-Foncillas J, et al. Growth and growth hormone secretion in children with cancer treated with chemotherapy. J Pediatr 1997;131:105–12.

20. Blizzard RM, Bulatovic A. Psychosocial short stature: a syndrome with many variables. Baillieres Clin Endocrinol Metab 1992;6:687–712.

21. Pandian R, Nakamoto JM. Rational use of the laboratory for childhood and adult growth hormone deficiency. Clin Lab Med 2004;24:141–74.

22. Gale EA, Bennett T, MacDonald IA, et al. The physiological effects of insulin-induced hypoglycaemia in man: responses at differing levels of blood glucose. Clin Sci 1983;65:263–71.

23. Shah A, Stanhope R, Matthew D. Hazards of pharmacological tests of growth hormone secretion in childhood. Br Med J 1992;304:173–4.

24. Frasier SD. A review of growth hormone stimulation tests in children. Pediatrics 1974;53:929–37.

25. Bonfig W, Bechtold S, Bachmann S, et al. Reassessment of the optimal growth hormone cut-off level in insulin tolerance testing for growth hormone secretion in patients with childhood-onset growth hormone deficiency during transition to adulthood. J Pediatr Endocrinol Metab 2008;21:1049–56.

26. Rosenfeld RG. Evaluation of growth and maturation in adolescence. Pediatr Rev 1982;4:175–83.

27. Ranke MB, Schweizer R, Wollmann HA, et al. Dosing of growth hormone in growth hormone deficiency. Horm Res 1999;51(Suppl 3):70–4.

28. Cutfield W, Lindberg A, Albertsson Wikland K, et al. Final height in idiopathic growth hormone deficiency: the KIGS experience. KIGS International Board. Acta Paediatr Suppl 1999;88:72–5.

29. Wetterau L, Cohen P. Role of insulin-like growth factor monitoring in optimizing growth hormone therapy. J Pediatr Endocrinol Metab 2000;13(Suppl 6):1371–6.

30. Zucchini S, Pirazzoli P, Baronio F, et al. Effects on adult height of pubertal growth hormone retesting and withdrawal of therapy in patients with previously diagnosed growth hormone deficiency. J Clin Endocrinol Metab 2006;91:4271–6.

31. Giovannuci E, Pollak M. Risk of the cancer after growth hormone treatment. Lancet 2002;360:258–9.

32. Sklar CA. Growth hormone treatment: cancer risk. Horm Res 2004;62:30–4.

33. Seikaly MG, Salhab N, Gipson D, et al. Stature in children with chronic kidney disease: analysis of NAPRTCS database. Pediatr Nephrol 2006;21:793–9.

34. Johannsson G, Ahlmen J. End-stage renal disease: endocrine aspects of treatment. Growth Horm IGF Res 2001;11:59–71.

35. Mehls O, Wuhl E, Tonsshoff B, et al. Growth hormone treatment in short children with chronic kidney disease. Acta Paediatr 2008;97:1159–64.

36. Roelfsema V, Clark RG. The growth hormone and insulin-like growth factor axis: its manipulation for the benefit of growth disorders in renal failure. J Am Soc Nephrol 2001;12:1297–306.

37. Tonshoff B, Cronin MJ, Reichert M, et al. Reduced concentration of serum growth hormone (GH)-binding protein in children with chronic renal failure: correlation

with GH insensitivity. The European Study Group for Nutritional Treatment of Chronic Renal Failure in Childhood. The German Study Group for Growth Hormone Treatment in Chronic Renal Failure. J Clin Endocrinol Metab 1997;82: 1007–13.

38. Rabkin R, Sun DF, Chen Y, et al. Growth hormone resistance in uremia, a role for impaired JAK/STAT signaling. Pediatr Nephrol 2005;20:313–8.

39. Nissel R, Lindberg A, Mehls O, et al. Pfizer International Growth Database (KIGS) International Board. Factors predicting the near final height in growth hormone-treated children and adolescents with chronic kidney disease. J Clin Endocrinol Metab 2008;93:1359–65.

40. Wuhl E, Schaefer F. Effects of growth hormone in patients with chronic renal failure: experience in children and adults. Horm Res 2002;58(Suppl 3):35–8.

41. Doi T, Striker LJ, Quaife C, et al. Progressive glomerulosclerosis develops in transgenic mice chronically expressing growth hormone and growth hormone-releasing factor but not in those expressing insulin-like growth factor-1. Am J Pathol 1988;131:398–403.

42. Fine RN, Sullivan EK, Kuntze J, et al. The impact of recombinant human growth hormone treatment during chronic renal insufficiency on renal transplant recipients. J Pediatr 2000;136:376–82.

43. Guest G, Berard E, Crosnier H, et al. Effects of growth hormone in short children after renal transplantation. French Society of Pediatric Nephrology. Pediatr Nephrol 1998;12:437–46.

44. Cutfield WS, Wilton P, Bennmarker H, et al. Incidence of diabetes mellitus and impaired glucose tolerance in children and adolescents receiving growth hormone treatment. Lancet 2000;355:610–3.

45. Ranke MB, Pfluger H, Rosendahl W, et al. Turner syndrome: spontaneous growth in 150 cases and review of the literature. Eur J Pediatr 1983;141:81–8.

46. Rao E, Weiss B, Fukami M, et al. Pseudoautosomal deletions encompassing a novel homeobox gene cause growth failure in idiopathic short stature and Turner syndrome. Nat Genet 1997;16:54–63.

47. Davenport ML, Quigley CA, Bryant CG, et al. Effect of early growth hormone (GH) treatment in very young girls with Turner syndrome (TS). Presented at the Seventh Joint European Society for Paediatric Endocrinology/Lawson Wilkins Pediatric Endocrine Society Meeting. Lyon, France, September 23, 2005.

48. Rosenfeld RG, Attie KM, Frane J, et al. Growth hormone therapy of Turner's syndrome: beneficial effect on adult height. J Pediatr 1998;132:319–24.

49. Bolar K, Hoffman AR, Maneatis T, et al. Long-term safety of recombinant human growth hormone in turner syndrome. J Clin Endocrinol Metab 2008;93:344–51.

50. Munce T, Simpson R, Bowling F. Molecular characterization of Prader-Willi syndrome by real-time PCR. Genet Test 2008;12:319–24.

51. Tauber M. Effects of growth hormone treatment in children presenting with Prader-Willi syndrome: the KIGS experience. In: Ranke MB, Price DA, Reiter EO, editors. Growth hormone therapy in Pediatrics—20 years of KIGS. Basel: Karger; 2007. p. 377–87.

52. Wollmann HA, Schultz U, Grauer ML, et al. Reference values for height and weight in Prader-Willi syndrome based on 315 patients. Eur J Pediatr 1998;157: 634–42.

53. Corrias A, Bellone J, Beccaria L, et al. IGF-I axis in Prader-Willi syndrome: evaluation of IGF-I levels and of the somatotroph responsiveness to various provocative stimuli. Genetic Obesity Study Group of Italian Society of Pediatric Endocrinology and Diabetology. J Endocrinol Invest 2000;23:84–9.

54. Eiholzer U, Bachmann S, l'Allemand D. Is there growth hormone deficiency in Prader-Willi syndrome? Six arguments to support the presence of hypothalamic growth hormone deficiency in Prader-Willi syndrome. Horm Res 2000;53(Suppl 3): 44–52.

55. Carrel AL, Myers SE, Whitman BY, et al. Benefits of long-term GH therapy in Prader-Willi syndrome: a 4-year study. J Clin Endocrinol Metab 2002;87:1581–5.

56. Angulo MA, Castro-Magana M, Lamerson M, et al. Final adult height in children with Prader-Willi syndrome with and without human growth hormone treatment. Am J Med Genet A 2007;143:1456–61.

57. Whitman BY, Myers S, Carrel A, et al. The behavioral impact of growth hormone treatment for children and adolescents with Prader-Willi syndrome: a 2-year, controlled study. Pediatrics 2002;109:E35.

58. Festen DAM, Wevers M, Lindgren AC, et al. Mental and motor development before and during growth hormone treatment in infants and toddlers with Prader-Willi syndrome. Clin Endocrinol (Oxf) 2008;68:919–25.

59. Festen DA, Visser TJ, Otten BJ, et al. Thyroid hormone levels in children with Prader-Willi syndrome before and during growth hormone treatment. Clin Endocrinol (Oxf) 2007;67:449–56.

60. Tauber M, Diene G, Molinas C, et al. A review of 64 cases of death in children with Prader-Willi syndrome (PWS). Am J Med Genet A 2008;46:881–7.

61. Mogul HR, Lee PD, Whitman BY, et al. Growth hormone treatment of adults with Prader-Willi syndrome and growth hormone deficiency improves lean body mass, fractional body fat, and serum triiodothyronine without glucose impairment: results from the United States multicenter trial. J Clin Endocrinol Metab 2008; 93:1238–45.

62. Hokken-Koelega AC, De Ridder MA, Lemmen RJ, et al. Children born small for gestational age: do they catch up? Pediatr Res 1995;38:267–71.

63. Lee PA, Chernausek SD, Hokken-Koelega AC. International Small for Gestational Age Advisory Board consensus development conference statement: management of short children born small for gestational age, April 24–October 1, 2001. Pediatrics 2003;111:1253–61.

64. Sas T, Mulder P, Aanstoot HJ, et al. Carbohydrate metabolism during long-term growth hormone treatment in children with short stature born small for gestational age. Clin Endocrinol (Oxf) 2001;54:243–51.

65. Ranke MB. Towards a consensus on the definition of idiopathic short stature. Horm Res 1996;45(Suppl 2):64–6.

66. Cohen P, Rogol AD, Deal CL, et al, 2007 Consensus Workshop participants. Consensus statement on the diagnosis and treatment of children with idiopathic short stature: a summary of the Growth Hormone Research Society, the Lawson Wilkins Pediatric Endocrine Society, and the European Society for Paediatric Endocrinology Workshop. J Clin Endocrinol Metab 2008;93:4210–7.

67. Rochiccioli P, Battin J, Bertrand AM, et al. Final height in Turner syndrome patients treated with growth hormone. Horm Res 1995;44:172–6.

68. Cohen P, Rogol AD, Howard CP, et al. Insulin growth factor-based dosing of growth hormone therapy in children: a randomized, controlled study. J Clin Endocrinol Metab 2007;92:2480–6.

69. Belin V, Cusin V, Viot G, et al. SHOX mutations in dyschondrosteosis (Léri-Weill syndrome). Nat Genet 1998;19:67–9.

70. Huber C, Rosilio M, Munnich A, et al, French SHOX GeNeSIS Module. High incidence of SHOX anomalies in patients with short stature. J Med Genet 2006;43: 735–9.

71. Blum WF, Crowe BJ, Quigley CA, et al. Growth hormone is effective in treatment of short stature associated with short stature homeobox-containing gene deficiency: two-year results of a randomized, controlled multicenter trial. J Clin Endocrinol Metab 2007;92:219–28.

72. Tartaglia M, Mehler EL, Goldberg R, et al. Mutations in PTPN11, encoding the protein tyrosine phosphatase SHP-2, cause Noonan syndrome. Nat Genet 2001;29:465–8.

73. Stofega MR, Herrington J, Billestrup N, et al. Mutation of the SHP-2 binding site in growth hormone (GH) receptor prolongs GH-promoted tyrosyl phosphorylation of GH receptor, JAK2, and STAT5B. Mol Endocrinol 2000;14: 1338–50.

74. Maile LA, Clemmons DR. The $_v\beta_3$ integrin regulates insulin-like growth factor I (IGF-I) receptor phosphorylation by altering the rate of recruitment of the Src-homology 2-containing phosphotyrosine phosphatase-2 to the activated IGF-I receptor. Endocrinology 2002;143:4259–64.

75. Ferreira LV, Souza SA, Arnhold IJ, et al. PTPN11 mutations and response to growth hormone therapy in children with Noonan syndrome. J Clin Endocrinol Metab 2005;90:5156–60.

76. Limal JM, Parfait B, Cabrol S, et al. Noonan syndrome: relationships between genotype, growth, and growth factors. J Clin Endocrinol Metab 2006;91: 300–6.

77. Cotterill AM, McKenna WJ, Brady AF, et al. The short-term effects of growth hormone therapy on height velocity and cardiac ventricular wall thickness in children with Noonan's syndrome. J Clin Endocrinol Metab 1996;81:2291–7.

78. Molitch ME, Clemmons DR, Malozowski S, et al. Endocrine Society's Clinical Guidelines Subcommittee. Evaluation and treatment of adult growth hormone deficiency: an Endocrine Society clinical practice guideline. J Clin Endocrinol Metab 2006;91:1621–34.

79. Laursen T, Jørgensen JO, Christiansen JS. The management of adult growth hormone deficiency syndrome. Expert Opin Pharmacother 2008;9:2435–50.

80. Biller BM, Samuels MH, Zagar A, et al. Sensitivity and specificity of six tests for the diagnosis of adult GH deficiency. J Clin Endocrinol Metab 2002;87:2067–79.

81. Mulligan K, Schambelan M. Anabolic treatment with GH, IGF-I, or anabolic steroids in patients with HIV-associated wasting. Int J Cardiol 2002;85:151–9.

82. Morley JE, Thomas DR, Wilson MM. Cachexia: pathophysiology and clinical relevance. Am J Clin Nutr 2006;83:735–43.

83. Heijligenberg R, Sauerwein HP, Brabant G, et al. Circadian growth hormone secretion in asymptomatic human immune deficiency virus infection and acquired immunodeficiency syndrome. J Clin Endocrinol Metab 1996;81:4028–32.

84. Geffner ME, Yeh DY, Landaw EM, et al. In vitro insulin-like growth factor-I, growth hormone, and insulin resistance occurs in symptomatic human immunodeficiency virus-1-infected children. Pediatr Res 1993;34:66–72.

85. Schambelan M, Mulligan K, Grunfeld C, et al. Recombinant human growth hormone in patients with HIV-associated wasting. A randomized, placebo-controlled trial. Serostim Study Group. Ann Intern Med 1996;125:873–82.

86. Gelato M, McNurlan M, Freedland E. Role of recombinant human growth hormone in HIV-associated wasting and cachexia: pathophysiology and rationale for treatment. Clin Ther 2007;29:2269–88.

87. Macallan DC, Baldwin C, Mandalia S, et al. Treatment of altered body composition in HIV-associated lipodystrophy: comparison of rosiglitazone, pravastatin, and recombinant human growth hormone. HIV Clin Trials 2008;9:254–68.

88. Lund PK, Ulshen MH, Rountree DB, et al. Molecular biology of gastrointestinal peptides and growth factors: relevance to intestinal adaptation. Digestion 1990;46(Suppl 2):66–73.
89. Guarino A, De Marco G, Italian National Network for Pediatric Intestinal Failure. Natural history of intestinal failure, investigated through a national network-based approach. J Pediatr Gastroenterol Nutr 2003;37:136–41.
90. Pereira PM, Bines JE. New growth factor therapies aimed at improving intestinal adaptation in short bowel syndrome. J Gastroenterol Hepatol 2006;21:932–40.
91. Messing B, Blethen S, Dibaise JK, et al. Treatment of adult short bowel syndrome with recombinant human growth hormone: a review of clinical studies. J Clin Gastroenterol 2006;40(Suppl 2):S75–84.
92. Weiming Z, Ning L, Jieshou L. Effect of recombinant human growth hormone and enteral nutrition on short bowel syndrome. JPEN J Parenter Enteral Nutr 2004;28: 377–81.

Strategies for Maximizing Growth in Puberty in Children with Short Stature

Nelly Mauras, MD[a,b],*

KEYWORDS

- Short stature • Aromatase • Aromatase inhibitors
- Anastrozole • Letrozole • GnRH analogues

The management of the growth-retarded child who is in the midst of puberty is an area of common difficulty in pediatric endocrinology practice. Regardless of the etiology of the growth retardation, attempts to increase height potential during puberty often are complicated by the inexorable tempo of epiphyseal fusion caused by the pubertal sex steroids, greatly limiting the time available for linear growth. Several strategies have evolved that attempt to increase height potential in growth hormone (GH)- deficient children who are in puberty, or in those who have idiopathic short stature, some of which are summarized in this article.

HIGH-DOSE GROWTH HORMONE

During human puberty, there is an approximate doubling of GH production rates,[1] with peak production coinciding with peak height velocity.[2] This increase in GH secretory rates is mediated, at least in part, through sex steroid hormones, and in both testosterone-treated and estradiol-treated prepubertal children, there is an augmentation of the GH production rates, mostly as an amplitude-modulated phenomenon, relatively independent of changes in pulse frequency.[1–5] The author and colleagues performed a randomized study designed to compare the efficacy and safety of standard recombinant human GH therapy (0.3 mg/kg/wk) versus high-dose therapy (0.7 mg/kg/wk) in GH-deficient adolescents previously treated with GH for at least 6 months.[6] Ninety-seven GH-deficient children participated (83 boys, 14 girls), of

Portions of this article were previously published in the *Endocrinology and Metabolism Clinics of North America*, 38:3.
a Division of Endocrinology and Metabolism, Nemours Children's Clinic, Jacksonville, FL 32207, USA
b Mayo College of Medicine, Jacksonville, FL, USA
* Division of Endocrinology and Metabolism, Nemours Children's Clinic, Jacksonville, FL 32207.
E-mail address: nmauras@nemours.org

Pediatr Clin N Am 58 (2011) 1167–1179
doi:10.1016/j.pcl.2011.07.007
0031-3955/11/$ – see front matter © 2011 Elsevier Inc. All rights reserved.

whom 48 completed the study. The author and colleagues observed that a mean of 3 years of high-dose GH therapy to GH-deficient adolescents was associated with a statistically significant increase in near-adult height of 4.6 cm over that observed in children treated with standard doses of GH. In those treated for 4 years, the increase was 5.7 cm. This was not associated with an undue advancement of skeletal maturation, alteration of the tempo of puberty, or greater frequency of adverse events. The mean height SD score at near-adult height was −0.7 plus or minus 0.9 in the standard dose group and 0.0 plus or minus 1.2 in the high-dose group (**Fig. 1**). Median plasma insulin-like growth factor (IGF)-I concentrations at baseline were 427 µg/L (range, 204 to 649) in the standard-dose group and 435 µg/L (range, 104 to 837) in the high-dose group. At 36 months, they were 651 µg/L (range, 139 to 1079) versus 910 µg/L (range, 251 to 1843) in the standard- and high-dose groups, respectively (P = not significant [NS]). There were no differences in any measures of carbohydrate metabolism. No difference in change in bone age was detected between groups at any interval.

The author and colleagues concluded from these data that high-dose GH therapy, administered during a finite window of time, may be beneficial and safe for increasing the final adult height of youngsters with GH-deficiency who are in the midst of puberty. Although these data led to the US Food and Drug Administration (FDA) approval of high-dose GH in puberty, the results were not meant to imply the need for an automatic increase in the dose of GH when the child reaches puberty (ie, if a child is growing well, there should be no need to increase the dose of GH). High-dose GH may be particularly useful, however, in selected cases of those most growth-retarded at the start of puberty. This strategy warrants careful monitoring of IGF-I and glucose concentrations and continued surveillance for adverse events.

GNRH ANALOG

Because the principal culprit for epiphyseal fusion is the presence of pubertal sex steroids, the use of GnRH analogs has been tried in an effort to slow down fusion of the growth plate. Abundant data show that suppressing the production of sex steroidal hormones delays epiphyseal fusion and ultimately can render youngsters with precocious puberty taller than they would be otherwise.[7,8] The use of GnRH

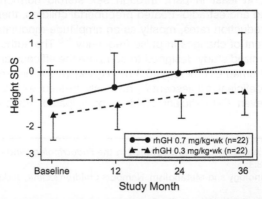

Fig. 1. Mean (plus or minus SD) height SD score (SDS) in pubertal growth hormone deficiency patients treated with standard versus high dose growth hormone (GH). (*From* Mauras N, Attie KM, Reiter EO, et al. High-dose recombinant human growth hormone (GH) treatment of GH-deficient patients in puberty increases near-final height: a randomized, multicenter trial. J Clin Endocrinol Metab 2000;85:3659; with permission. Copyright © 2000, The Endocrine Society.)

analogs in precocious puberty subjects accomplishes a biochemical castration and ultimately renders patients taller by delaying the timing of bone fusion. This strategy has been tried not only in children with sexual precocity but in those with GH-deficiency who are in physiologic puberty and even in those with short stature not caused by GH-deficiency who are also in puberty, with mixed results.[9–14] In the patients treated with both GH and GnRH analog, improvements in height predictions (as determined by bone ages) have ranged from 7.9 cm to 14 cm when the children were treated for 2 to 4 years.[9,11,14] This therapy has been less successful in augmenting final height when used alone in children with normal variant short stature and normally timed puberty,[10,13] and a recent consensus conference on the use of GnRH analogs could not recommend the routine use of GnRH analogs in such setting.[15]

The consequences of this approach, as it pertains to bone accretion/bone density, and the psychological impact of suppressing the timely course of puberty in an already short child, have not been studied appropriately, however. Even 10 W of GnRH analog therapy in healthy young adult males is associated with substantial changes in body composition and intermediate metabolism, with increased adiposity, decreased rates of protein synthesis, decreased lipid oxidation, decreased energy expenditure, and decreased muscle strength.[16] Using stable tracers of calcium, the author's group's studies in GnRH analog-treated males show a marked increase in urinary calcium losses and bone calcium resorption rates, indicating the crucial role of sex steroidal hormones in bone mineralization, even in the male.[17] Hence in physiologically timed, normal puberty, GnRH analogs should not be used as monotherapy.[18]

AROMATASE INHIBITORS

A large body of experimental and human data has shown that estrogen, in both females and males, is a principal regulator of epiphyseal fusion. This is evidenced by detailed studies of male patients with point mutations either in the estrogen receptor gene[19] or in the aromatase enzyme gene,[20,21] who grew to significantly tall heights because of the lack of estrogen effect. When an estrogen receptor blocker was given to estrogen-treated mice, the acceleration in bone maturation caused by estrogen was blocked, supporting further the effect of estrogen on bone maturation.[22] Animal data suggest that the estrogen receptor β (ERβ) is the principal physiologic inhibitor of axial and appendicular growth.[23] The availability of aromatase inhibitors now allows the possibility of studying their use in growth disorders in greater detail.

Pharmacology

Aromatase inhibitors are a class of compounds that block aromatase, a microsomal P450 enzyme product of the CYP19 gene, which catalyzes the rate-limiting step in the production of estrogens (ie, the conversion of testosterone to estradiol and androstenedione to estrone). Enzyme activity is present in many tissues, including the ovary, breast, brain, muscle, liver, and adipose tissues among others. Over the last decades, several aromatase inhibitors have been developed with relatively weak suppression of the enzyme and hence variable clinical response. These compounds (eg, testolactone, fedrozole) also had some significant adverse effects. A third generation of aromatase inhibitors has been developed with much more potent blockade of the aromatase enzyme and greater safety profiles. There are three of these drugs on the market in the United States for treating breast cancer in postmenopausal women, including anastrozole, letrozole, and exemestane (**Fig. 2**). The author and colleagues have conducted studies on the pharmacokinetic properties of exemestane,[24] and more recently anastrozole in young males,[25] and they have found

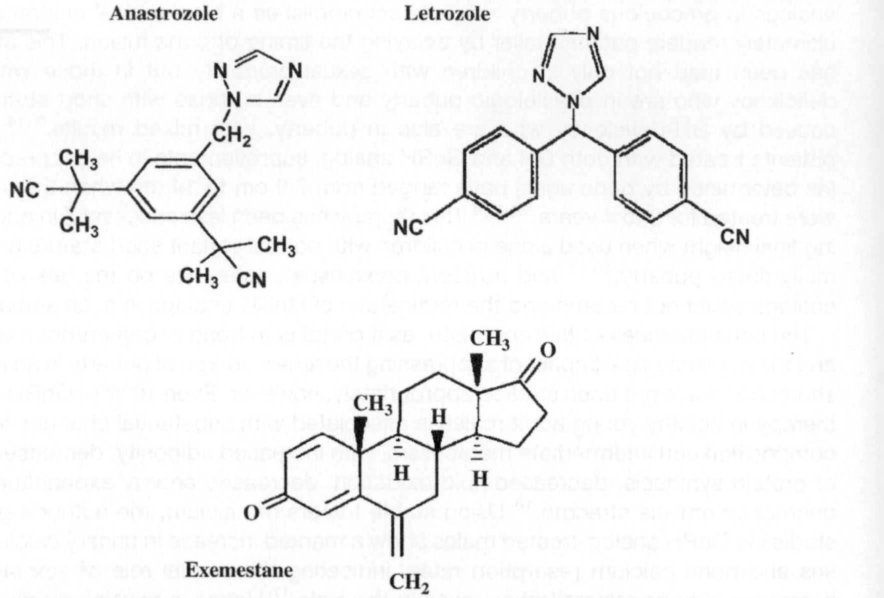

Anastrozole   Letrozole

Exemestane

Fig. 2. Chemical structures of commercially available aromatase inhibitors.

similar properties as those in post menopausal women. These aromatase inhibitors are absorbed after oral administration and are given once daily, with a terminal half-life of approximately 45hrs (30–60) and either hepatic or renal clearance. Anastrozole (compounded as 1 mg tablets) and letrozole (2.5 mg tablets) are reversible inhibitors of the enzyme and are nonsteroidal, whereas aromasin (25 mg tablets) is a steroid analog of androstenedione and an irreversible inhibitor of aromatase. Neither anastrozole nor letrozole absorption are affected significantly by food, so they can be taken at any time. Exemestane's absorption, however, is enhanced by food intake, particularly fatty foods, so it is best to have patients take the drug with a meal.

Physiologic Studies

To better characterize the metabolic effects of estrogen suppression in males, the author and colleagues administered 10 weeks of 1 mg of anastrozole to young healthy men ages 18 to 25 years.[26] The author observed no negative effects of estrogen suppression on a host of metabolic measures, including lipid concentrations, liver profiles, complete blood cell counts (CBCs), bone formation markers, and body composition measures, as well as measures of whole-body protein synthesis and calcium turnover. This was despite a 50% reduction in circulating estradiol concentrations measured by a recombinant cell bioassay. This is in sharp contrast to the deleterious effects of GnRH analog therapy described by the author's group in males,[16,17] suggesting that at least during a finite window of intervention, aromatase inhibitors did not have catabolic effects like GnRH analogs (**Fig. 3**).

Studies in Boys with Disorders of Growth

A group of boys in Finland who had history of constitutional growth delay were treated for 5 months with intramuscular testosterone and either letrozole (2.5 mg) or placebo tablets daily for 12 months.[27] Six months after discontinuation of the tablets, bone ages were examined to predict adult height, and there was a statistically significant

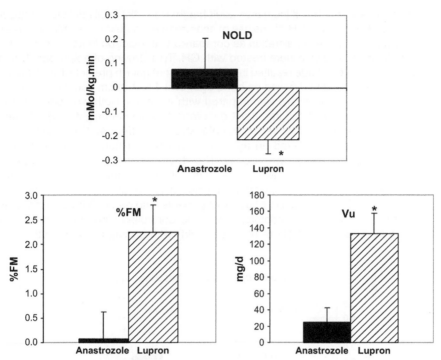

Fig. 3. Comparison of the changes observed after 10 weeks of anastrozole treatment (n = 8) versus GnRH analog therapy with Lupron (n = 6) in healthy boys and young men for whole-body protein synthesis rates (NOLD), percentage of fat mass measured by DEXA, and urinary calcium excretion (Vu) measured by calcium tracers. Data are expressed as the absolute change from baseline. Comparisons were made using analysis of variance (ANOVA) between the groups. (*From* Mauras N, O'Brien KO, Oerter Klein K, et al. Estrogen suppression in males: metabolic effects. J Clin Endocrinol & Metab 2000;85:2374; with permission. Copyright © 2000, The Endocrine Society.)

increase in predicted adult height above that of those treated with placebo of +5.9 cm (*P* = .04). These boys have been followed to final adult height, and the projected height increase was found to hold after treatment discontinuation.[28] There were significant increases in circulating testosterone concentrations due to the rise in gonadotropins caused by the aromatase blockade, some of which were supraphysiological.

The same group of investigators extended their use of letrozole given as monotherapy for 2 years to a group of boys who had idiopathic short stature.[29] They recruited 31 boys, 27 of whom were prepubertal at study entry, and treated with either letrozole (2.5 mg) or placebo. The investigators observed a significant slowing of bone age acceleration, an increase in height predictions, and taller height standard deviation score (SDS) for bone age in the letrozole group compared with the placebo group.[29] Testosterone concentrations increased significantly more in the letrozole group; however, the investigators reported no advancement in the timing of puberty onset. The drug was tolerated well, but IGF-I concentrations were lower in the letrozole group. The latter is an important marker to follow, especially in those subjects using this class of drugs as monotherapy. Bone mineral density accrual was reported to be comparable in both groups.

Recently, we reported the results of a double-blind, randomized, placebo-controlled clinical trial in the United States to investigate whether treatment with a selective and potent aromatase inhibitor (anastrozole) could delay the rate of bone age maturation and whether it increases adult height potential in GH deficient adolescent boys also treated with GH.[30] The use of anastrozole resulted in a significant delay in the tempo of bone age acceleration as compared with placebo in adolescent boys with GH deficiency who also were treated with GH. This slowing of epiphyseal fusion caused by estrogen blockade resulted in a significant net gain in predicted adult height from baseline, as calculated based on bone age, of +4.5 (1.2) cm and +6.7 (1.4) cm after 2 and 3 years respectively, as compared with +1 cm at both time points in the placebo group. This translated into a net gain from baseline in height SDS adjusted for bone age in the anastrozole versus the placebo group (**Fig. 4**).[30] The author and colleagues intentionally targeted an age range in which a natural deceleration of growth occurs after peak growth velocity. The decrease in growth velocity during the course of these studies was also greater in the placebo group than in the anastrozole group at 36 months. Bone mineral density accrual by dual energy x-ray absorptiometry (DEXA) was comparable in a subset of patients who had DEXAs performed. In a prospective, double-blind, randomized, placebo-controlled clinical trial, investigators in Iran studied 91 boys (12.6–14.6 years old) with constitutional growth delay

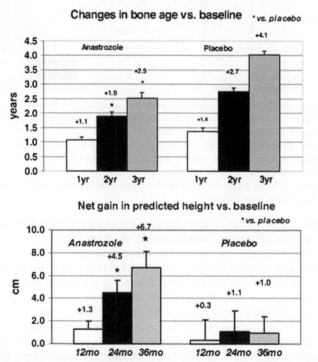

Fig. 4. Top panel shows changes in bone age compared with baseline at 12, 24, and 36 months in the anastrozole and placebo groups. *Insets* indicate mean change from baseline. *, *P* value is significant versus placebo group at 24 and 36 months (*P*<.001 both times). Bottom panel shows changes in predicted adult height based on Bayley Pinneau tables compared with baseline in the anastrozole and placebo groups. *, *P* value is significant versus placebo group at 24 (*P* = .04) and 36 months (*P* = .004). (*From* Mauras N, Gonzalez de Pijem L, Hsiang HY, et al. Anastrozole increases predicted adult height of growth hormone deficient adolescent males treated with growth hormone: a randomized, double-blind, placebo-controlled multicenter trial for up to three years. J Clin Endocrinol Metab 2008;93:827–8; with permission. Copyright © 2008, The Endocrine Society.)

and predicted adult short stature treated with either letrozole (2.5 mg/day), oxandro-lone (2.5 mg/day), or placebo for 2 years.[31] They reported that letrozole differed from oxandrolone and placebo in significantly increasing predicted adult height, and slightly but significantly decreasing HDL-cholesterol. However, both oxandrolone, and to a lesser degree letrozole, significantly increased the height standard deviation score and bone age compared to placebo. Letrozole had a good safety profile over 2 years. In aggregate, data thus far suggest that aromatase inhibitors are effective in slowing down bone age progression and increasing adult height potential. These cohorts need to be followed to adult height. Ongoing trials will hopefully provide more informa-tion regarding efficacy in adult height promotion in this patient population.

Gonadotropin-independent Precocity

Estrogen blockers have been used in precocious puberty in two forms of gonadotropin-independent precocious puberty (GIP), in girls with McCune Albright syndrome (MAS) and in boys with testotoxicosis. Both are complex and very difficult conditions to treat and are not responsive to GnRH analogs, as puberty is independent of gonadotropin activation. MAS is caused by a gene mutation that causes constitu-tive activation of the guanine nucleotide regulatory subunit of adenyl cyclase, hence turning on ovarian estrogen production independent of gonadotropins. In MAS, the use of an estrogen receptor blocker (Tamoxifen) was associated with a modest reduc-tion in vaginal bleeding in these youngsters, although the trial was not long enough to assess impact in long-term growth and bone age changes.[32] A pilot study in 9 girls with MAS treated with letrozole at variable doses and for 12–36 months showed decreased rates of growth and bone age advance but no substantial improvement in ovarian cyst formation.[33] An uncontrolled open-label trial using anastrozole in 28 girls with MAS showed no beneficial effect in decreasing vaginal bleeding or promoting growth.[34]

On the other hand, promising results have been observed in boys who have GIP caused by testotoxicosis or familial male-limited precocious puberty. These young-sters have mutations in the luteinizing hormone (LH) receptor gene causing constitu-tive activation of the LH receptor and massive testosterone production at a very young age independent of LH production. In these patients, the reduction in estrogen caused by the use of aromatase inhibitors results in a significant increase in testos-terone, which is already high because of the primary disease process. The latter necessitates the coadministration of androgen receptor blockers to minimize a wors-ening of the androgen effects. The author and colleagues performed a multicenter, open-label, single-arm, 12-month phase 2 trial involving 14 boys aged 2 years and older with testotoxicosis.[35] Patients received daily doses of a nonsteroidal androgen receptor blocker, bicalutamide (12.5, 25, 50, and 100 mg), and anastrozole (0.5 and 1 mg). The daily dose of bicalutamide and anastrozole were titrated independently in each patient until steady state; then patients were monitored monthly for 12 months. Although we cannot comment about long-term efficacy, the combination treatment was tolerated well, and no safety concerns have been noted in this group of very young patients.[35] The author has used anastrozole in combination with a relatively weak androgen receptor blocker (Aldactone) and observed excellent responses in suppression of bone age and increased height potential in three boys who had GIP followed for more than 10 years (Nelly Mauras, MD, unpublished data, 2009).

Potency

Regarding the issue of potency of the available aromatase inhibitors, anastrozole, letrozole, and exemestane all significantly block tissue aromatase and are used for treating postmenopausal women who have breast cancer. Studies done in these women have shown that total-body aromatization was suppressed slightly better with letrozole than anastrozole (estrone suppression: 81% vs 84% [P = .019], estradiol suppression: 84.9% vs 87.8% [P = NS]).[36] Mean residual estradiol concentrations were 10.1% for anastrozole and 5.9% for letrozole in a recent study also in breast cancer,[37] and findings also have been confirmed in other conditions.[38] Neither compound affects growth velocity, and the increases in predicted adult height have been comparable using either compound. In boys, the increase in gonadotropins and testosterone concentrations in the letrozole-treated groups[27,29] has been much greater than that observed with anastrozole.[30] No studies directly comparing clinical efficacy in treating the primary conditions in the same patient population have been conducted, and it is unclear whether greater estrogen suppression would be necessarily beneficial in treating growth disorders in puberty. Further studies are needed.

Estradiol Assay

A common difficulty in interpreting the degree of estrogen suppression in treating these subjects has been the great variability of the estradiol assays used. Immunoassays for plasma or serum estradiol (E_2) are sufficiently sensitive for clinical assessment of E_2 levels (40 to 600 pg/mL) in premenopausal women but lack the sensitivity and specificity necessary for accurate detection in postmenopausal women and in pre- and early pubertal children (less than 10 pg/mL). More importantly, these assays lack the ability to measure very low E_2 accurately in patients receiving aromatase inhibitors. The author and colleagues previously had used highly sensitive, yeast- or HeLa cell based- recombinant DNA bioassays for quantitation of aromatase inhibitors suppression, but these methods have inherent variability and are not widely available. The gas chromatography-mass spectrometry (GC-MS)/MS and LC-MS/MS assays yielded levels of E_2 that were two- to threefold lower than with measurements by RIA in all groups.[39] Because of this, sensitive LC-MS/MS or GC-MS/MS assays should be used to monitor patients using this class of compounds. These are widely available commercially.

Doses and Safety

The dose of anastrozole used in the previously mentioned studies was 1 mg/d; that of letrozole was 2.5 mg/d. The author and colleagues have used exemestane in males to study its pharmacokinetics in doses of 25 mg/d. Long-term experience (up to 3 years of continuous use) using anastrozole has been excellent, with a good safety profile when used in combination with GH in short boys and as monotherapy in cases of GIP, with normal liver, CBC, and bone markers. Their use has been associated with decreased HDL-C[30,40] however the levels remain within the normal range. Cognitive function is not impaired with their use.[41] The use of anastrozole or letrozole in the pediatric studies thus far has shown the same bone mineral accrual as the control groups. It is important to emphasize that it takes at least 2 to 3 years of daily treatment to observe positive effects in height prognosis. Assessment of bone mineral density should be performed at baseline and at least 2 years after initiating treatment. Liver profiles, testosterone, estradiol and IGF-I concentrations, in my view, should be followed periodically.

Estrogen treatment in an aromatase deficient man increased bone mass[42] yet in boys with idiopathic short stature treated with letrozole alone who were in puberty, letrozole treatment seemed to stimulate cortical bone growth by presumably increasing the testosterone-to-estradiol ratio.[43] The same investigators in Finland reported in males with idiopathic short stature, mild vertebral body deformities in 5 of 11 letrozole-treated subjects, on lateral spine MRIs obtained after completion of treatment, whereas in the placebo group no deformities were detected.[44] In the cohort of males with constitutional delay of puberty, a high prevalence of endplate and intervertebral disk abnormalities was observed in both the letrozole- and the placebo-treated groups; subjects were asymptomatic.[44] These subjects were either pre-pubertal or early pubertal at study entry and the investigators concluded that aromatase inhibitor therapy during prepuberty or early puberty may predispose to vertebral deformities, which they postulate probably reflect impaired vertebral body growth rather than impaired bone quality and compression fractures.[44] We recalled a number of available subjects in our own randomized controlled trial of GH and anastrozole or placebo several years after discontinuation of treatment and obtained lateral spine films. We observed a variety of asymptomatic vertebral findings (mild disc space narrowing and end plate irregularity) both in those treated with aromatase inhibitors and also those who took placebo (Mauras N, unpublished observations). Nonetheless, we have now incorporated lateral spine films (either X rays or through the lateral DEXA images) in subjects treated with aromatase inhibitors at both baseline and after 2 years. We have also restricted the use of this class of drugs to pubertal children.

The role of estrogen in spermatogenesis and sperm function has been studied in experimental animals and in people. There is a significant difference between timed aromatase blockade and congenital deficiencies in the aromatase enzyme or the estrogen receptor. In people, the man reported to have a mutation in the estrogen receptor β (ERKO) had 25 mL testes and sperm counts of 25 million/mL, but only 18% were viable.[19] The man reported by Morishima and colleagues[21] with a mutation in the aromatase gene (ARKO) was fully virile, had 34 mL testes, but no sperm counts were reported. Another adult male reported by Carani and colleagues[20] with ARKO had very small 8 mL testes, less than 1 million sperm/mL, and 100% were immotile. Identical findings, however, were observed in the subject's brother, who had a normal aromatase gene; hence the infertility was thought to be unrelated to the estrogen deficiency.[20] Chronic administration of anastrozole to adult male rats for 1 year showed essentially normal spermatogenesis after treatment,[45] and administering exemestane for up to 250 mg/kg/d (100 times the human dose) did not affect the mating behavior or fertility of adult male rats.[46]

In human studies, timed aromatase blockade has been used in males with oligospermia and has been shown to increase sperm concentrations and motility index in the ejaculates.[47] Whether this could serve as an adjunct to improve fertility in males awaits further study[48] and clinical trials in this patient population are ongoing. The author and colleagues also studied a group of late adolescents who had GH deficiency treated with GH and anastrozole or GH alone in an open-label pilot trial for 1 year[49] and examined their sperm several years after discontinuation of anastrozole. They compared their data with age-matched normal controls.[50] The author's group observed similar sperm concentrations and motility in all three groups regardless of previous treatment with anastrozole.

Aromatase inhibitors are banned in high level athletic competition by the World Anti Doping Agency (WADA) as they increase endogenous testosterone and are hence considered ergogenic. GH use is also banned. It is hence important for adolescents using any of these agents to be advised regarding these restrictions if they are interested in high level athletics. Full disclosure with coaches regarding their medicinal use is warranted. [For a full list of banned substances go to: http://www.wada-ama.org/en/World-Anti-Doping-Program/.]

The use of aromatase inhibitors in young females has not been studied except in girls with MAS. This is because of the theoretical concern of increased ovarian cyst formation; this also requires more study. Overall, further longitudinal follow-up is needed to better characterize the long-term safety of the use of aromatase inhibitors in children with growth retardation who are also in puberty. So far, most of the data available restrict its use to males who have disordered growth.

SUMMARY

The approach to the child with growth retardation who is in puberty remains an important clinical challenge. The use of high-dose GH, suppression of puberty with GnRH analogs in combination with GH, and the use of selective inhibitors of the aromatase enzyme with aromatase inhibitors (also in combination with GH) are therapeutic choices that have been studied. Aromatase blockade effectively blocks estrogen production in males with a reciprocal increase in testosterone, and a new generation of aromatase inhibitors, including anastrozole, letrozole, and exemestane is being investigated in adolescent subjects who have severe growth retardation. This class of drugs, if judiciously used for a window of time, offers promise as an adjunct treatment of growth delay in pubertal patients with GH deficiency, idiopathic short stature, testotoxicosis, and other disorders of growth.

Because the effect slowing down epiphyseal fusion is mediated by means of estrogen blockade, it is reasonable to continue these studies predominantly in those children who stand to derive the most potential benefit (ie, those who are growth retarded and in the midst puberty and not prepubertal children). The use of aromatase inhibitors to promote growth in girls should be pursued only in the context of a clinical trial. It is important to emphasize that these evolving uses of aromatase inhibitors represent off-label use of the product and that definitive data on their efficacy are not available for each of the previously described conditions. Safety issues regarding bone health also require further study.

REFERENCES

1. Mauras N, Blizzard RM, Link K, et al. Augmentation of growth hormone secretion during puberty: evidence for a pulse amplitude-modulated phenomenon. J Clin Endocrinol Metab 1987;64:596–601.
2. Martha PMJ, Rogol AD, Veldhuis JD. Alterations in the pulsatile properties of circulating growth hormone concentrations during puberty in boys. J Clin Endocrinol Metab 1989;69:563–70.
3. Rose SR, Municchi G, Barnes KM, et al. Spontaneous growth hormone secretion increases during puberty in normal girls and boys. J Clin Endocrinol Metab 1991; 73:428–35.
4. Mauras N, Rogol AD, Veldhuis JD. Specific time-dependent actions of low-dose ethinyl estradiol administration on the episodic release of GH, FSH and LH in prepubertal girls with Turner's syndrome. J Clin Endocrinol Metab 1989;69:1053–8.
5. Mauras N, Rogol AD, Veldhuis JD. Increased hGH production rate after low-dose estrogen therapy in prepubertal girls with Turner's syndrome. Pediatr Res 1990; 28:626–30.
6. Mauras N, Attie KM, Reiter EO, et al. High-dose recombinant human growth hormone (GH) treatment of GH-deficient patients in puberty increases near-final height: a randomized, multicenter trial. J Clin Endocrinol Metab 2000;85:3653–60.
7. Paul D, Conte FA, Grumbach MM, et al. Long-term effect of gonadotropin-releasing hormone agonist therapy on final and near-final height in 26 children

with true precocious puberty treated at a median age of less than 5 years. J Clin Endocrinol Metab 1995;80:546–51.

8. Kletter GB, Kelch RP. Clinical review 60: effects of gonadotropin-releasing hormone analog therapy on adult stature in precocious puberty. J Clin Endocrinol Metab 1994;79:331–4.

9. Pasquino AM, Municchi G, Pucarelli I, et al. Combined treatment with gonadotropin-releasing hormone analog and growth hormone in central precocious puberty. J Clin Endocrinol Metab 1996;81:948–51.

10. Balducci R, Toscano V, Mangiantini A, et al. Adult height in short normal adolescent girls treated with GnRHa and GH. J Clin Endocrinol Metab 1995;80:3596–600.

11. Cassorla F, Mericq V, Eggers M, et al. Effects of luteinizing hormone-releasing hormone analog-induced pubertal delay in growth hormone (GH)-deficient children treated with GH: preliminary results. J Clin Endocrinol Metab 1997;82:3989–92.

12. Adan L, Souberbielle JC, Zucker JM, et al. Adult height in 24 patients treated for GH deficiency and early puberty. J Clin Endocrinol Metab 1997;82:229–33.

13. Lanes R, Gunczler P. Final height after combined growth hormone and gonadotropin-releasing hormone analogue therapy in short healthy children entering into normally timed puberty. Clin Endocrinol (Oxf) 1998;49:197–202.

14. Cara JF, Kreiter ML, Rosenfield RL. Height prognosis of children with true precocious puberty and growth hormone deficiency: effect of combination therapy with gonadotropin-releasing hormone agonist and growth hormone. J Pediatr 1992;120:709–15.

15. Carel JC, Eugster EA, Rogol A, et al. Consensus statement on the use of gonadotropin-releasing hormone analogs in children. Pediatrics 2009;123:e752–62.

16. Mauras N, Hayes V, Welch S, et al. Testosterone deficiency in young men: marked alterations in whole body protein kinetics, strength, and adiposity. J Clin Endocrinol Metab 1998;83:1886–92.

17. Mauras N, Hayes V, Yergey AL. Profound hypogonadism has significant negative effects on calcium balance in males: a calcium kinetic study. J Bone Miner Res 1999;14:577–82.

18. Yanovski JA, Rose SR, Municchi G, et al. Treatment with a luteinizing hormone-releasing hormone agonist in adolescents with short stature. N Engl J Med 2003;348:908–17.

19. Smith EP, Boyd J, Frank GR. Estrogen resistance caused by a mutation in the estrogen receptor gene in a man. N Engl J Med 1994;331:1056–61.

20. Carani C, Qin K, Simoni M. Effect of testosterone and estradiol in man with aromatase deficiency. N Engl J Med 1997;1337:91–5.

21. Morishima A, Grumbach MM, Simpson ER, et al. Aromatase deficiency in male and female siblings caused by a novel mutation and the physiological role of estrogens. J Clin Endocrinol Metab 1995;80:3689–98.

22. Gunther DF, Calikoglu AS, Underwood LE. The effects of the estrogen receptor blocker, Faslodex (ICI 182,780), on estrogen-accelerated bone maturation in mice. Pediatr Res 2000;46:269–73.

23. Chagin AS, Lindberg MK, Andersson N, et al. Estrogen receptor-beta inhibits skeletal growth and has the capacity to mediate growth plate fusion in female mice. J Bone Miner Res 2004;19:72–7.

24. Mauras N, Lima J, Patel D, et al. Pharmacokinetics and dose finding of a potent aromatase inhibitor, aromasin (exemestane), in young males. J Clin Endocrinol Metab 2003;88:5951–6.

25. Mauras N, Bishop K, Merinbaum D, et al. Pharmacokinetics and pharmacody-namics of anastrozole in pubertal boys with recent onset gynecomastia. J Clin Endocrinol Metab, in press.
26. Mauras N, O'Brien KO, Oerter Klein K, et al. Estrogen suppression in males: metabolic effects. J Clin Endocrinol Metab 2000;85:2370–7.
27. Wickman S, Sipila I, Ankarberg-Lindgren C, et al. A specific aromatase inhibitor and potential increase in adult height in boys with delayed puberty: a randomized controlled trial. Lancet 2001;357:1743–8.
28. Hero M, Wickman S, Dunkel L. Treatment with the aromatase inhibitor letrozole during adolescence increases near-final height in boys with constitutional delay of puberty. Clin Endocrinol 2006;64:510–3.
29. Hero M, Norjavaara E, Dunkel L. Inhibition of estrogen biosynthesis with a potent aromatase inhibitor increases predicted adult height in boys with idiopathic short stature: a randomized controlled trial. J Clin Endocrinol Metab 2005;90: 6396–402.
30. Mauras N, Gonzalez de Pijem L, Hsiang HY, et al. Anastrozole increases pre-dicted adult height of growth hormone deficient adolescent males treated with growth hormone: a randomized, double-blind, placebo-controlled multicenter trial for up to three years. J Clin Endocrinol Metab 2008;93:823–31.
31. Salehpour S, Alipour P, Razzaghy-Azar M, et al. A double-blind, placebo-controlled comparison of letrozole to oxandrolone effects upon growth and puberty of children with constitutional delay of puberty and idiopathic short stature. Horm Res Paediatr 2010;74:428–35.
32. Eugster EA, Rubin SD, Reiter EO, et al. Tamoxifen treatment for precocious puberty in McCune-Albright syndrome: a multicenter trial. J Pediatr 2003;143: 60–6.
33. Feuillan P, Calsi K, Hill S, et al. Letrozole treatment of precocious puberty in girls with the McCune-albright syndrome: a pilot study. J Clinical Endocrinol Metab 2007;92:2100–6.
34. Mieszczak J, Lowe ES, Plourde P, et al. The aromatase inhibitor anastrozole is ineffective in the treatment of precocious puberty in girls with McCune-Albright syndrome. J Clin Endocrinol Metab 2008;93:2751–4.
35. Reiter E, Mauras N, McCormick K, et al. Bicalutamide (B) plus anastrozole (A) for the treatment of gonadotropin-independent precocious puberty in boys with tes-totoxicosis: a phase II, open-label pilot study (BATT). J Pediatr Endocrinol Metab 2010;23:999–1009.
36. Geisler J, Haynes B, Anker G, et al. Influence of letrozole and anastrozole on total body aromatization and plasma estrogen levels in postmenopausal breast cancer patients evaluated in a randomized, cross-over study. J Clin Oncol 2002;20:3039–40.
37. Dixon JM, Renshaw L, Young O, et al. Letrozole suppresses plasma estradiol and estronesulphate more completely than anastrozole in postmenopausal women with breast cancer. J Clin Onc 2008;26:1671–6.
38. Al-Omari WR, Sulaiman WR, Al-Hadithi N. Comparison of two aromatase inhibi-tors in women with clomiphene-resistant polycystic ovary syndrome. Int J Gynae-col Obstet 2004;85:289–91.
39. Santen RJ, Lee JS, Wang S, et al. Potential role of ultrasensitive estradiol assays in estimating the risk of breast cancer and fractures. Steroids 2008;73:1318–21.
40. Hero M, Ankarberg-Lindgren C, Taskinen MR, et al. Blockade of oestrogen biosynthesis in peripubertal boys: effects on lipid metabolism, insulin sensitivity, and body composition. Eur J Endocrinol 2006;155:453–60.

41. Hero M, Maury S, Luotoniemi E, et al. Cognitive effects of aromatase inhibitor therapy in peripubertal boys. Eur J Endocrinol 2010;163:149–55.
42. Bilezikian JP, Morishima A, Bell J, et al. Increased bone mass as a result of estrogen therapy in a man with aromatase deficiency. N Engl J Med 1998;339: 599–603.
43. Hero M, Makitie O, Kroger H, et al. Impact of aromatase inhibitor therapy on bone turnover, cortical bone growth. and vertebral morphology in pre- and peripubertal boys with idiopathic short stature. Horm Res 2009;71:290–7.
44. Hero M, Toiviainen-Salo S, Wickman S, et al. Vertebral morphology in aromatase inhibitor-treated males with idiopathic short stature or constitutional delay of puberty. J Bone Miner Res 2010;25:1536–43.
45. Turner KJ, Morley M, Atanassova N, et al. Effect of chronic administration of an aromatase inhibitor to adult male rats on pituitary and testicular function and fertility. J Endocrinol 2000;164:225–38.
46. Beltrame D, di Salle E, Giavini E, et al. Reproductive toxicity of exemestane, an antitumoral aromatase inactivator, in rats and rabbits. Reprod Toxicol 2001;15: 195–213.
47. Raman JD, Schlegel PN. Aromatase inhibitors for male infertility. J Urol 2002;167: 624–9.
48. Kim HH, Schlegel PN. Endocrine manipulation in male infertility [review]. Urol Clin North Am 2008;35:303–18.
49. Mauras N, Welch S, Rini A, et al. An open-label 12-month pilot trial on the effects of the aromatase inhibitor anastrozole in growth hormone (GH)-treated GH-deficient adolescent boys. J Pediatr Endocrinol Metab 2004;17:1597–606.
50. Mauras N, Bell J, Snow BG, et al. Sperm analysis in growth hormone-deficient adolescents previously treated with an aromatase inhibitor: comparison with normal controls. Fertil Steril 2005;84:239–42.

Etiology and Treatment of Hypogonadism in Adolescents

Vidhya Viswanathan, MD*, Erica A. Eugster, MD

KEYWORDS

- Hypergonadotropic hypogonadism
- Hypogonadotropic hypogonadism • Adolescents
- Delayed puberty • Treatment

Factors that mitigate the onset of puberty have yet to be fully elucidated. Gonadarche refers to the onset of gonadal sex steroid production during puberty. Gonadarche results from pulsatile gonadotropin releasing hormone (GnRH) secretion from the hypothalamus. GnRH secretion occurs every 60 to 90 minutes,[1] and there is subsequent release of the pituitary gonadotropins luteinizing hormone (LH) and follicle stimulating hormone (FSH) initially during sleep,[2] which leads to gonadal stimulation. LH stimulates Leydig cell hyperplasia in males and subsequent testosterone release. FSH has little effect in males until the onset of spermarche (sperm maturation). In females, FSH stimulates the production of estradiol via ovarian follicular development. Testosterone and estradiol secretion lead to the development of secondary sexual characteristics. Adequate functioning at all levels of the hypothalamic-pituitary-gonadal axis is necessary for normal gonadal development and subsequent sex steroid production. Deficiencies at any level of the axis can lead to a hypogonadal state.

In boys, hypogonadism can manifest as a complete lack of secondary sexual development or failure of normal pubertal progression. In girls, it can present with failure of pubertal initiation, failure of pubertal progression, or menstrual irregularities. Abnormalities within the hypothalamus or pituitary lead to *hypogonadotropic hypogonadism* whereas primary gonadal failure is characterized as *hypergonadotropic hypogonadism*.

HYPOGONADOTROPIC HYPOGONADISM

Hypogonadotropic hypogonadism can be attributed to a variety of congenital origins including single gene mutations, idiopathic forms, and genetic syndromes. Acquired

Portions of this article were previously published in the *Endocrinology and Metabolism Clinics of North America*, 38:4.

Section of Pediatric Endocrinology, Department of Pediatrics, Riley Hospital for Children, Indiana University School of Medicine, Room 5960, 702 Barnhill Drive, Indianapolis, IN 46202, USA
* Corresponding author.
E-mail address: vviswana@iupui.edu

doi:10.1016/j.pcl.2011.07.009
0031-3955/11/$ – see front matter © 2011 Elsevier Inc. All rights reserved.
pediatric.theclinics.com

causes of hypogonadotropic hypogonadism include central nervous system (CNS) insults such as trauma, irradiation, and intracranial tumors. By far the most common cause of hypogonadotropic hypogonadism is transient, and is termed constitutional delay of growth and puberty (CDGP). Each of these causes is briefly discussed here, and the molecular genetic causes of hypogonadotropic hypogonadism are shown in **Table 1**.

Constitutional Delay of Growth and Puberty

CDGP is a variation of normal development that can be difficult to differentiate from pathologic hypogonadotropic hypogonadism. In this condition, puberty and the pubertal growth spurt occur at or later than the extreme upper end of the normal age. The diagnosis is made more often in boys than girls, likely due to referral bias, and has a strongly familial pattern.[3] Skeletal maturation is delayed in comparison with chronologic age. CDGP results in delayed but *normal* puberty; thus puberty progresses through the normal stages but starts at a later time. Children with CDGP achieve their genetic potential for height,[4] and laboratory evaluation is normal. Some patients benefit from short-term treatment to augment secondary sexual development and boost linear growth.[5]

Congenital Origins

Gene defects
Nuclear receptor mutations Nuclear receptors influence gene transcription at multiple levels, and exert their effects in a time- and dosage-specific fashion. An important nuclear receptor involved in gonadotropin secretion is steroidogenic factor-1 (SF-1), a key regulator of genes involved in sexual differentiation, steroidogenesis, and reproduction. SF-1 knockout mice show marked abnormalities in the development of the hypothalamus and impaired development of pituitary gonadotropes, with decreased levels of serum gonadotropins as well as gonadal dysgenesis.[6] Target genes of SF-1 within the hypothalamus and pituitary include the gonadotropin releasing hormone receptor (GnRHR) and the β subunit of LH. Both heterozygous and homozygous mutations in the DNA binding domain of SF-1 result in complete XY sex reversal, testicular dysgenesis, and adrenal failure in genotypic males. A milder phenotype has also been described in which there is impaired gonadal but intact adrenal function.[7] In a genetic female, a heterozygous SF-1 mutation has been associated with primary adrenal failure but normal ovarian development.[8] Thus, SF-1 mutations exist within a broad clinical spectrum that will undoubtedly continue to expand.

DAX-1 is an orphan nuclear receptor that is involved in steroidogenesis and functions as a repressor of SF-1 mediated transcription. Mutations have been identified in *NROB1*, the gene that encodes DAX1, on the Xp21 locus. Males with DAX1 mutations typically present with early-onset adrenal insufficiency and subsequent delayed puberty secondary to hypogonadotropic hypogonadism.[9] However, a delayed presentation of primary adrenal insufficiency has also been reported.[10] DAX1 mutations can lead to both hypothalamic and pituitary dysfunction with decreased GnRH and gonadotropin secretion.[11] DAX1 mutations can also cause defects in spermatogenesis, and in one study affected males also had evidence of azospermia.[12] Therefore, mutations in DAX-1, as in SF-1, can lead to the development of hypogonadism in a multitude of ways.

Kallman syndrome Impairment of GnRH secretion can also occur from defects in migration of GnRH producing neurons. Kallman syndrome (KS) refers to the combination of hypogonadotropic hypogonadism and anosmia. The X-linked form results from

Table 1
Molecular genetic causes of hypogonadotropic hypogonadism

Gene	Product	Inheritance	Target Sites	Additional Clinical Manifestations
SF-1	Orphan nuclear receptor	Autosomal recessive	Steroidogenesis in males Hypothalamus Pituitary Adrenals	XY sex reversal, adrenal failure In females: adrenal failure, normal ovarian function
DAX-1	Orphan nuclear receptor	X-linked recessive	Steroidogenesis Hypothalamus Pituitary Adrenals	In males: spectrum of hypogonadotropic hypogonadism and adrenal insufficiency
KAL-1	Anosmin	X-linked recessive	Hypothalamic neuronal migration	Anosmia
FGFR1	FGF receptor	Autosomal dominant	FGF receptor in hypothalamus Pituitary	Cleft palate Agenesis of corpus callosum
GPR54	G protein coupled receptor	Autosomal recessive	GnRH-secreting neurons Pituitary	Isolated hypogonadotropic hypogonadism
Prop-1	Transcription factor	Sporadic autosomal recessive	Pituitary gonadotrope development	Growth hormone deficiency Central hypothyroidism
Hesx1	Transcription factor	Sporadic	Prop-1 Pituitary gonadotrope development	Septo-optic dysplasia Central hypothyroidism Central hypocortisolism Diabetes insipidus
LEP	Leptin	Autosomal dominant	Hypothalamus	Obesity Hyperphagia T-cell immune dysfunction
LEPR	Leptin receptor	Autosomal dominant	Hypothalamus	Obesity Hyperphagia T-cell immune dysfunction

a defect in the migration of GnRH and olfactory neurons due to a mutation in the *KAL1* gene. This gene encodes for anosmin-1, a glycoprotein essential for neuronal migration and growth.[13] Individuals with KS also have aplasia of the olfactory bulb as noted on magnetic resonance imaging (MRI).[14] Although *KAL1* gene defects have been the prototype of KS, there is emerging evidence that autosomal forms may be more prevalent than previously thought. In one study, *KAL1* gene defects accounted for only 14% of cases with familial KS. Mutations in unidentified autosomal genes were postulated to cause the remainder. Subjects with presumed autosomal gene defects had some response to GnRH pulses, indicating partial preservation of hypothalamic GnRH-secreting neurons, though still with phenotypic similarity to the X-linked version of the syndrome.[15] Fibroblast growth receptor 1 (FGFR1) mutations may account for as many as 10% of cases,[16] and mutations in the prokineticin 2 (PROK2) gene have also been identified in individuals with KS and normosmic hypogonadotropic hypogonadism.[17] No matter what the underlying molecular genetic cause, lack of adequate GnRH secretion leads to decreased circulating gonadotropins in both autosomal and X-linked cases.

Isolated hypogonadotropic hypogonadism Isolated hypogonadotropic hypogonadism (IHH) refers to cases in which anosmia is absent. One potential cause is loss of function mutations of the GnRHR, a G-protein coupled receptor. At least 8 mutations of the GnRHR in 7 families have been identified. Notable genotype-phenotype variation exists even within members of the same kindred due to incomplete activation of GnRHR function.[18] Males with these mutations display signs of hypogonadism and small testes. Females typically present with primary amenorrhea.[19] Another important cause of IHH has been traced to mutations in GPR54, which has a critical role in hypothalamic GnRH signaling and release.[20] Of note, both KS and IHH may be found in the same kindred. IHH has also been noted to be reversible in some patients.[21]

Transcription factor mutations Even with intact GnRH production and signal transduction, pituitary gonadotropin synthesis may still be deficient due to mutations in a variety of transcription factors. An important transcription factor involved in the developmental cascade of pituitary gonadotrope cells is Prop-1. Prop-1 is the prophet of the pituitary transcription factor Pit 1, a paired-like homeodomain transcription factor that is responsible for early embryonic pituitary development. Prop-1 gene mutations can result in familial combined pituitary hormone deficiency including growth hormone deficiency, central hypothyroidism, and hypogonadotropic hypogonadism.[22] In one analysis of 8 members of a consanguineous family with Prop-1 gene mutations, all 8 family members had gonadotropin deficiency and failure of spontaneous sexual maturation.[23] There is also a variable pattern of phenotypic expressivity associated with Prop-1 mutations, with different deficiencies appearing at different time periods within the same family.

Like Prop-1, the transcription factor HESX1 is needed for normal pituitary development.[24] Deficiencies in HESX1, initially identified in 1998, are a rare cause of septo-optic dysplasia[25] which may be associated with hypogonadotropic hypogonadism.[26] Other transcription factors implicated in rare cases of hypogonadotropic hypogonadism include LHX4[27] and SOX 2.[28] All patients with hypopituitarism, including idiopathic forms, are at risk for hypogonadotropic hypogonadism.

Leptin and leptin receptor defects Congenital leptin deficiency results from loss of function mutations of the *LEP* gene, which encodes for the leptin protein. Leptin interacts with the leptin receptor, a member of the interleukin-6 family of receptors. This interaction stimulates the Jak-Stat pathway and leads to activation of downstream target genes. Leptin deficiency acts as a sign of nutritional deprivation and results in the suppression of the reproductive axis. Classic findings in individuals with leptin deficiency include hyperphagia, obesity, and hypogonadotropic hypogonadism. Administration of leptin seemingly rectifies these abnormalities.[29] Leptin receptor (LEPR) abnormalities have a similar phenotype to congenital leptin deficiency. Females with this mutation have hypogonadotropic hypogonadism. These girls present with delayed puberty, lack of a pubertal growth spurt, and reduced expression of secondary sexual characteristics. Some may have irregular menses due to aromatization of subcutaneous fat to estrogen, which then stimulates uterine hyperplasia. Males with leptin receptor mutations have hypogonadotropic hypogonadism and diminished testosterone production.[30]

Syndromes

Numerous syndromes include neuroendocrine dysfunction as a potential feature. Perhaps the best known is Prader-Willi syndrome (PWS), which is caused by a genetic defect involving paternal chromosome 15, usually in the form of a microdeletion within the long arm or maternal unipaternal disomy.[31] Hypothalamic dysfunction is marked in these patients as evidenced by their hypotonia, hyperphagia, and intermittent temperature instability. The hypothalamic dysfunction also leads to hypogonadism and may be attributed to an absence of or abnormal location of GnRH neurons. Early studies in individuals with PWS revealed low circulating serum gonadotropins and in males, attenuated testosterone response to human chorionic gonadotropin.[32] Physical findings in boys include micropenis, scrotal hypoplasia, cryptorchidism, and small testes. Either absent or delayed puberty may ensue. In girls, findings may be less remarkable and include hypoplasia of the clitoris or labia minora, primary amenorrhea, and delayed puberty.[33] However, a wide spectrum of hypogonadism exists in PWS, with some women achieving fertility without hormone replacement therapy.[34,35]

Acquired Origins

Any significant CNS insult can result in acquired hypogonadotropic hypogonadism. Two of the most common causes in children are traumatic brain injury and CNS tumors.

Traumatic brain injury

Traumatic brain injury (TBI) is an insult to the brain that results in neurologic dysfunction. TBI can have significant neurocognitive, neuropsychological, and neuroendocrine sequelae.[36,37] Anterior pituitary insufficiency resulting from TBI has been noted in the past, but is garnering more attention as a high prevalence of pituitary hormone insufficiency has been demonstrated.[38] Some retrospective studies indicate that gonadotropin deficiency may be found in 90% to 95% of those with history of TBI,[39] although prospective studies in adults have noted the prevalence to be far less. In one study, hormonal evaluation was conducted on TBI patients at baseline (acute phase) and at 12 months. In the acute phase, approximately 42% of those evaluated had gonadotropin deficiency. At the 12-month follow-up, many of these patients spontaneously recovered reproductive function. The final prevalence of hypogonadism was 7.7%.[40] It is clear that all patients with a history of TBI require ongoing surveillance for pituitary problems, including hypogonadotropic hypogonadism.

Central nervous system tumors

Intracranial injury can also occur as a result of CNS tumors. In children, resultant hypogonadotropic hypogonadism can exist as a result of the primary tumor or due to the therapeutic regimen needed to treat the lesion. In a prospective study of 75 children with various CNS tumors, 13% had an abnormality in gonadotropin secretion before initiation of therapy.[41] In a retrospective study focusing on craniopharyngioma, only 1 out of 64 patients had evidence of hypogonadism before treatment. However, after surgical resection and adjuvant radiotherapy, 80% of those evaluated at a pubertal age had evidence of hypogonadism.[42] Gonadotropin deficiency and delayed puberty are most likely in those who receive 40 Gy or more of radiation.[43] Gonadotropin deficiency may continue to evolve for many years after irradiation, with rates of total incidence ranging from 20% to 50%.[44,45] Therefore, all children who have CNS lesions should be monitored for gonadotropin deficiency and signs of pubertal delay.[46]

Hypothalamic amenorrhea

Hypothalamic amenorrhea is commonly associated with eating disorders such as anorexia nervosa, and also occurs in elite female athletes. Clinical manifestations include absence of menstrual cycles, increased exercise, and weight loss. In these girls, suppression of GnRH secretion results in attenuation of LH and FSH release, and decreased estrogen production.[47] Several theories have been postulated for this hypothalamic dysfunction, including low circulating energy levels due to high energy expenditure and relative deficiency of nutritional intake.[47] Girls with hypothalamic amenorrhea also have low circulating leptin levels. Administration of recombinant leptin to some women with hypothalamic amenorrhea leads to elevated LH and estradiol, resulting in follicular growth and ovulation.[48]

HYPERGONADOTROPIC HYPOGONADISM

Primary hypogonadism can be due to congenital origins such as chromosomal abnormalities, syndromes, or genetic mutations. Primary hypogonadism can also be acquired later in childhood or adolescence due to autoimmunity or exposure to chemotherapy or radiation. Alterations in gonadotropins, the gonadotropin receptors, or within the gonads themselves can lead to hypogonadism with decreased testosterone and estradiol secretion. The decreased sex steroid secretion causes increased production of gonadotropins manifesting as hypergonadotropic hypogonadism. Congenital causes of primary hypogonadism are outlined in **Table 2**.

Congenital Origins

The most common cause of congenital primary hypogonadism is sex chromosome aneuploidy as is present in Turner syndrome and Klinefelter syndrome. Isolated abnormalities of the X chromosome are also associated with primary ovarian failure.

Turner syndrome

Turner syndrome (TS) occurs in 1 in 2500 live born females.[49] Diagnosis of the syndrome requires the combination of characteristic physical features, including short stature as well as partial or complete absence of an X chromosome.[50] More than half of girls with TS have chromosomal mosaicism. Approximately 30% will begin puberty spontaneously, but only a small minority will progress to menarche.[51] Spontaneous pregnancy has been reported but is extremely rare in this population.[52] Although initially intrinsically normal, the ovaries in girls with TS undergo accelerated atresia such that ovarian failure is often already present and may be detected at birth. Precisely which genes on the X chromosome are necessary for ovarian maintenance is unknown. FSH levels during early life have been found to be significantly lower in girls with mosaic TS as compared with those who are monosomic.[53]

Table 2
Causes and clinical manifestations of congenital hypergonadotropic hypogonadism

Abnormality	Clinical Manifestations	
Turner syndrome	Short stature, webbed neck, cubitus valgus Streak ovaries	
Klinefelter syndrome	Tall stature Eunuchoid body habitus Small, firm testes	
X chromosome abnormality	Xq-premature ovarian failure XXX-tall stature GU abnormalities	
FSH and LH β subunit mutations	*Males* Delayed puberty Azospermia Infertility	*Females* Primary amenorrhea Menstrual irregularity Polycystic ovary syndrome
FSH and LH receptor mutations	*Males* Micropenis Ambiguous genitalia XY sex reversal Infertility	*Females* Primary amenorrhea Gonadal dysgenesis
Swyer syndrome (46, XY)	Tall stature Primary amenorrhea Delayed puberty Gonadal tumors	
CAIS (46, XY)	Primary amenorrhea Normal breast development Sparse body hair Absent mullerian and wolffian structures	
CAH (depending on deficiency)	Hypertension Hypokalemia XY sex reversal Adrenal crisis	
Galactosemia	Ovarian failure	
Testicular regression sequence	Normal external genitalia	

Klinefelter syndrome

Klinefelter syndrome is the most common congenital cause of primary hypogonadism and occurs in 1 in 1000 live male births.[54] The most common genotype is XXY, although variants exist with different numbers of X chromosomes. Tall stature, a eunuchoid body habitus, gynecomastia, and small, firm testes are cardinal features. Seminiferous tubule dysgenesis is a classic histologic feature of the testes. Individuals with Klinefelter syndrome exhibit a spectrum of gonadal failure, with many men going undiagnosed until they present with infertility in adulthood. However, a significant number come to attention during adolescence due to delayed puberty or lack of appropriate pubertal progression.

X chromosome abnormalities

Other X chromosome abnormalities, including Xq deletion and Triple X, can cause varying degrees of hypogonadism. Xq deletion can cause a phenotype similar to TS as well as isolated premature ovarian failure.[55] Deletions in the critical region, Xq13-q26, can also lead to premature ovarian failure.[56] Triple X, 47 XXX, is estimated to exist in 1 in 1000 girls and is marked by significant phenotypic variability.[57] Women with this condition can be tall and have normal external genitalia, with preservation of ovarian function.[57] These women can also have ovarian failure as well as significant genitourinary tract anomalies, including cloacal exstrophy and mullerian abnormalities.[58,59]

Abnormalities in gonadotropin production or action

Mutations within the β subunit of the gonadotropins, the gonadotropin receptors, or forms of resistance to gonadotropins can all result in hypergonadotropic hypogonadism. Females with mutations in the β subunit of FSH present with primary amenorrhea, delayed puberty, and poorly developed secondary sexual characteristics; they have low FSH levels, low estradiol levels, and high LH levels due to lack of feedback inhibition by estradiol.[60,61] Males with the same mutation have normal to delayed puberty and azospermia.[62]

A homozygous mutation within the LH β subunit has resulted in total functional loss in one male.[63] The individual in this case presented with delayed puberty, low serum testosterone, and high LH levels. It was discovered later that several male members in his family were infertile. In further studies, it was noted that females with this defect present with ovarian dysfunction, infertility, menstrual irregularity, or polycystic ovary syndrome.[64]

Inactivating mutations of the G-protein coupled FSH and LH receptors result in a phenotype similar to those with abnormalities in the LH and FSH β subunits. Complete LH resistance results from a loss of function mutation in the LH receptor gene. In males, this causes a phenotype that ranges from micropenis, to ambiguous genitalia, to completely female external genitalia.[65,66] In females, LH resistance results in normal puberty but subsequent amenorrhea, infertility, and elevated LH levels, demonstrating that ovulation requires LH as well as FSH.[67] FSH resistance due to FSH receptor mutations has also been reported, particularly in the Finnish population. Women who are homozygous for this defect have gonadal dysgenesis and primary amenorrhea.[68] In contrast, men from the same kindreds have variable degrees of infertility.

A rare congenital condition associated with gonadotropin resistance is carbohydrate-deficient glycoprotein syndrome, which causes defects in gonadotropin glycosylation. In females with this defect, FSH seems to have less bioactivity and leads to decreased serum estradiol levels. However, exogenous FSH results in an increase in estradiol. Males with this disease advance through puberty but have decreased testicular volume.[69]

Resistance syndromes can also be due to variations in the signal transduction pathway after gonadotropin binding. Pseudohypoparathyroidism is a disease in which the signal transduction pathway of many hormones is altered due to inactivating mutations of the G_s α subunit. The mutation leads to multiple hormone resistance. In a study of 12 patients with pseudohypoparathyroidism, 25% of the pubertal patients had evidence of gonadotropin resistance.[70]

Disorders of sex development

Disorders of sex development (DSDs) are congenital conditions in which development of chromosomal, gonadal, or anatomic sex is atypical.[71] This broad category includes common entities such as TS and Klinefelter Syndrome, as well as rare disorders such as cloacal exstrophy, mixed gonadal dysgenesis, and congenital aphallia. Many DSDs are associated with ambiguous genitalia, which is beyond the scope of this review. However, a few may present with delayed puberty or primary amenorrhea, and are important to consider in the differential diagnosis of an adolescent with apparent hypogonadism. These DSDs include Swyer syndrome, complete androgen insensitivity syndrome (CAIS), and rare forms of congenital adrenal hyperplasia (CAH), all of which result in female external genitalia.

Swyer syndrome Swyer syndrome, also known as XY pure gonadal dysgenesis, is characterized by tall stature, primary amenorrhea, and delayed puberty in a phenotypic female. Laboratory studies reveal elevated gonadotropins, and ultrasonographic examination reveals bilateral streak gonads and a hypoplastic uterus.[72] Fifteen to thirty percent of these individuals have mutations in SRY (sex-determining region of the Y chromosome) or alterations in the Y chromosome.[73] There is also a high risk of gonadal tumors such as dysgerminoma or gonadoblastoma.[73] Therefore, gonadectomy is routinely recommended when this diagnosis is made.

Complete androgen insensitivity syndrome CAIS is caused by mutations of the androgen receptor that result in loss of testosterone and dihydrotestosterone mediated action. Androgen receptor mutations are X-linked recessive in 70% of cases, and are found in 1 in 20,000 to 1 in 90,000 genetic males.[74] The most common phenotype is that of an adolescent girl who has normal breast development, but absent or scant body hair and primary amenorrhea. Examination of the external genitalia reveals a normal female phenotype with a blind ending vagina. Eighty percent to 90% of girls with CAIS will also eventually develop inguinal hernias,[75] with some presenting in infancy with this diagnosis.

Congenital adrenal hyperplasia Rare forms of CAH can present with hypogonadism due to lack of production of testosterone and estrogen. These conditions include deficiencies of 17α-hydroxylase, side chain cleavage enzyme (SCC), and steroid acute regulatory protein (StAR). Girls with 17α-hydroxylase deficiency can present with primary amenorrhea and absent secondary sexual characteristics. Boys have female external genitalia, a blind vagina, and intra-abdominal testes.[76] Hypertension and hypokalemia may also be present.[77] SCC is the first step in the steroidogenic pathway and converts cholesterol to pregnenolone. SCC deficiency leads to deficiencies in all steroid hormones. SCC deficiency in genetic males leads to XY sex reversal and adrenal insufficiency.[78] StAR, a protein expressed in the adrenal cortex and gonads, increases cholesterol transport in response to steroidogenic stimuli. Affected genetic males present in early infancy with adrenal crisis, and appear phenotypically female.[79] Affected genetic females are normally developed at birth and may have intact ovarian function.[80]

Galactosemia Another congenital cause of primary hypogonadism is galactosemia. Galactosemia results from a deficiency in galactose-1-phosphate uridyltransferase (GALT) and presents with clinical manifestations of cataracts, *Escherichia coli* sepsis, poor growth, and feeding dysfunction if undiagnosed in the newborn. In an initial study conducted in 1981, gonadal function was evaluated in 12 women and 8 men with galactosemia. Although gonadal function was normal in men with the disease, the women in this study had evidence of hypergonadotropic hypogonadism, with varying degrees of primary and secondary amenorrhea and oligomenorrhea.[81] Ultrasound studies of the ovaries in those affected demonstrated streak gonads in several women.[81] The cause of the hypogonadism is most likely premature ovarian failure, although the exact pathophysiology is not well understood. Numerous theories exist, including the hypothesis that galactose-1-phosphate is toxic and perhaps competitively inhibits UDP-Galactose transferase and alters FSH and FSH receptors, with subsequent failure of ovarian follicles to develop.[82] This process manifests as an elevated FSH in 85% of girls younger than 10 years who have galactosemia and premature ovarian failure.[82]

Testicular regression sequence Testicular regression sequence (TRS), or vanishing testis syndrome, occurs when an initially normal testicle that existed in fetal life subsequently atrophies. Most individuals with TRS have normal male external genitalia, reflecting that normal testicular function existed during prenatal life. The most likely cause of this syndrome is fetal or antenatal testicular torsion, or trauma to scrotal contents in utero.[83] This view is supported by the finding of hemosiderin laden macrophages and dystrophic calcifications under histopatholgic examination.[84] There has also been an association noted between testicular regression and persistence of mullerian duct structures.[85] Thus far, a search for a molecular genetic cause of TRS has been negative.[86]

Acquired Origins

The acquired forms of primary hypogonadism are as varied as the congenital forms. Important acquired origins include treatment for pediatric cancer (radiation and chemotherapy) and autoimmune conditions.

Chemotherapy and radiation

Both chemotherapy and radiation have been noted to cause primary hypogonadism. In girls, the dose of intra-abdominal radiation needed to destroy more than 50% of developing oocytes is less than 2 Gy.[87] In the 70% of patients who survive pediatric cancer, 1 in 6 female survivors develops primary ovarian failure. Those who do undergo spontaneous menarche have decreased ovarian reserve.[88] In boys, depressed spermatogenesis can be seen after a testicular radiation dose as low as 0.15 Gy, with temporary azoospermia occurring after doses of 0.3 Gy.[89] The effect of radiation on testicular function is age dependent, with prepubertal radiation exposure causing significantly more damage to Leydig cells than postpubertal radiation.[90] Cumulative doses of alkylating agents are also correlated with altered function.[89]

A high prevalence of hypogonadism was noted in young adult survivors of childhood cancer who participated in a study comparing 3 treatment arms for non-Hodgkin lymphoma (NHL) and acute lymphoblastic leukemia (ALL). The study compared treatment with chemotherapy alone (vincristine, prednisolone, l-asparaginase, methotrexate, 6-mercaptopurine), combined chemotherapy and prophylactic cranial radiation, and chemotherapy with total body radiation and bone marrow transplant. All women in the third category had premature ovarian failure. Women in the other 2 categories, however, had intact ovarian function. Among men in the third category, 83% had primary hypogonadism, with a low serum testosterone and elevated FSH and LH. Forty percent of men in all 3 treatment arms had alterations in spermatogenesis, with the greatest dysfunction appearing in those who had received total body radiation.[91]

Despite these findings, there have been reports of spontaneous recovery of testicular or ovarian function in childhood cancer survivors. Although more common in older children and adults, recovery of ovarian function has occurred as long as 12 years post exposure to radiation and alkylating chemotherapy in a young girl.[92] Due to the increased risk of gonadal dysfunction in pediatric cancer patients and also due to the chance of spontaneous recovery, recommendations for surveillance include yearly monitoring of pubertal status with Tanner staging and assessment of growth velocity. Laboratory measurements of FSH and LH as well as estradiol or testosterone are recommended for those with signs of pubertal delay.[93]

Autoimmune gonadal failure

Autoimmunity can lead to both testicular and ovarian failure, specifically in those who have other types of autoimmune endocrinopathies. Several autoimmune polyglandular syndromes (APS) have been identified. Of these, APS I and APS II have been associated with premature ovarian failure at prevalence rates of 30% to 50%.[94] APS I consists of a triad of hypoparathyroidism, mucocutaneous candidiasis, and adrenal insufficiency. The mutation is within the *AIRE* gene, the autoimmune regulator. In a Finnish cohort, approximately 50% of the females identified with APS I had premature ovarian failure. Two-thirds of these individuals had autoantibodies to side-chain cleavage enzyme (anti-SCC),[95] one of the enzymes identified in steroid production that is specific to the ovary and is noted in autoimmune ovarian failure. In those who have been diagnosed with APS I and who initially have signs of ovarian failure, the presence of steroid cell antibodies may signal progression of the disease process.[96] APS II consists of autoimmune adrenocortical failure along with thyroid disease or diabetes. Positive antibodies to the P450 enzymes, specifically ovary-specific antibodies, in the steroid production pathway are thought to mediate autoimmune ovarian failure in this syndrome as well.[97] Autoimmunity can also cause isolated premature ovarian failure,[98] and has also been reported in conditions such as systemic lupus erythematous and myasthenia gravis.

Testicular failure occurs at a lower rate than ovarian failure in APS.[99] Autoimmunity to the Leydig cells in APS may be mediated by P450 autoantibodies that are testis specific.[100] Antisperm antibodies have also been noted in prepubertal boys treated with chemotherapy and in those with urogenital tract abnormalities such as cryptorchidism, testicular torsion, or hypospadias.[101]

EVALUATION

Evaluation of a child with delayed puberty begins with a careful history and physical examination. Important elements on history include the parents' pubertal timing, because late menarche in the mother or delayed completion of adult height in the father is strongly suggestive of CDGP. Eliciting a family history of hypogonadism, autoimmune syndromes, DSDs, or consanguinity is also essential. History in the child should include attention to any CNS insult or symptoms of chronic disease. In the review of systems, lack of sense of smell can be an important clue to the presence of KS.

Physical examination should include height and weight measurements. Neurologic assessment should include evaluation of visual fields. Assessment of secondary sexual characteristics includes Tanner staging and recognition of evidence of androgen exposure. Testicular enlargement, which can sometimes go unnoticed by boys, indicates the onset of central puberty. Stigmata of TS or Klinefelter Syndrome should be noted. The external genitalia should be visually inspected for any signs of anatomic abnormality.

Laboratory evaluation including plasma gonadotropin levels, estradiol, or testosterone may be helpful. Low gonadotropin levels suggest CDGP or pathologic hypogonadotropic hypogonadism, and can be further evaluated with a GnRH stimulation test.[102] In contrast, elevated gonadotropins indicate primary gonadal failure. A bone age radiograph is an essential component of the evaluation. Other tests that may be indicated, depending on the individual situation, include a head MRI, karyotype, autoimmune panel, or molecular genetic analysis. In patients with suspected CDGP, a "wait and see" approach is typically employed to determine whether spontaneous puberty will ensue.

TREATMENT

Although there are many causes of hypogonadism in children, the treatment is primarily focused on hormone replacement with sex steroids. The overarching goal is to simulate a normal progression of pubertal development that also allows for the attainment of genetic potential for height.

Estrogen Replacement

Estrogen therapy is initially started for pubertal induction and breast development in girls with hypogonadism. Studies regarding estrogen therapy in children have focused primarily on girls with TS. Recommended starting doses of estrogen therapy in this population are one-eighth to one-tenth the doses used for adult replacement, and vary depending on the formulation used. Very low doses have been reported to have a salutary effect on linear growth in TS.[103] Multiple different formulations of estrogen are available, and include oral estradiol, oral conjugated estrogen, transdermal estrogen patches, and estrogen gel. The age at which estrogen therapy is initiated is individualized and incorporates factors such as chronologic age, bone age, absolute height, and psychosocial issues. The starting dose is low and is gradually increased over several years. Equivalent adult doses of oral therapy are micronized estradiol, 2 mg, esterified estrogen, 1.25 mg, ethinyl estradiol, 8 to 10 µg, and conjugated estrogens, 1.25 mg.[104] Addition of progesterone 1 week per month, usually in the form of medroxyprogesterone, after 1 to 2 years of estrogen therapy or post breakthrough bleeding, allows for adequate breast and uterine development. Formulations and available does of estrogen preparations are shown in **Table 3**.

Limitations of oral estrogen therapy include variable bioavailability due to first-pass metabolism within the liver, which subsequently affects liver function and clotting factors.[105,106] As a result, transdermal estrogen formulations are gaining in popularity. Estrogen patches are widely used in adult women, and doses of 0.625 and 1.25 mg of oral conjugated estrogens have been reported to be similar those of 50 and 100 µg of transdermal estradiol per 24 hours.[107] Pubertal induction can be accomplished with transdermal estradiol at a dose as low as 3.1 to 6.2 µg/24 hours.[106] Puberty can then be mimicked with subsequent doubling of the dose after a median duration of 8 months and addition of progesterone 2 years after estrogen initiation. A transdermal estrogen dose of 0.1 mg/d is equivalent to an adult regimen. When comparing transdermal estrogen to oral estrogen, significantly higher levels of 17β-estradiol were noted with oral estrogen. However, no differences in metabolic effects including

Table 3 Estrogen formulations		
Type of Estrogen	**Trade Name**	**Available Doses**
Oral estradiol	Estrace	0.5, 1, 2 mg
	Gynodiol	0.5, 1, 2 mg
Oral esterified estrogen	Menest	0.3, 0.625, 1.25, 2.5 mg
	Ogen	Equivalent to 0.625 mg and above
	Ortho-Est	Equivalent to 0.625 mg and above
Oral conjugated equine estrogen	Premarin	0.3, 0.45, 0.625, 0.9, 1.25 mg
Estradiol patches	Vivelle	0.025, 0.0375, 0.05, 0.075, 0.1 mg/d
	Menostar	0.014 mg/d
Estradiol gel	Divigel	0.5 mg estradiol/5 g gel

lipolysis, lipid, and carbohydrate oxidation, and resting energy expenditure from short-term transdermal versus oral estrogen therapy have been noted.[105] In contrast, a pilot study of transdermal versus oral conjugated estrogen in girls with TS found better bone mineral accrual and uterine development in the transdermal group.[108]

Percutaneous estradiol gel has also been investigated for pubertal induction in girls with TS at a starting dose of 0.1 mg nightly with increases of 0.1 mg for each additional year up to 5 years. Side effects of percutaneous gel therapy include local skin irritation, and this modality is not currently in use in the clinical setting.[109] For hypogonadal women, estrogen replacement is needed throughout reproductive life.

Testosterone Replacement

In boys, studies involving testosterone for pubertal induction have primarily focused on CDGP and KS. Testosterone therapy is usually initiated at 15% to 25% of adult doses. Approximately 50 to 100 mg of a testosterone ester formulation is given intramuscularly every 2 to 4 weeks for 4 to 6 months with gradual increases to adult doses.[110,111] In boys with CDGP, a 4- to 6-month course of 50 to 100 mg testosterone per month may be offered to bring about initial secondary sexual characteristics and boost linear growth.[110] In boys who have permanent hypogonadism, the need for therapy is lifelong. Even at the initial doses used for pubertal induction, there is a decrease in total fat mass, percent body fat, and whole body proteolysis once testosterone is initiated.[112]

Intramuscular, transdermal, and oral formulations of testosterone exist. The preparations testosterone enanthate and testosterone cypionate are the most often used formulations in children, due to the difficulty in delivering the small doses needed initially for pubertal induction with alternate forms.[113] Intramuscular injections of testosterone, however, can be painful for the adolescent patient population, and studies investigating other formulations are ongoing.

Formal guidelines regarding the use of oral preparations have yet to be delineated, and experience with this form of testosterone is far less than with the intramuscular form. Transdermal testosterone, in the form of testosterone gel, at doses of 50 mg/m^2/d has been used in children short-term to treat poor growth secondary to renal failure.[114] In a study of transdermal testosterone delivered via a 5-mg patch, overnight use in boys with delayed puberty resulted in pubertal testosterone concentrations as well short-term growth.[115] Side effects of transdermal testosterone include local skin

Table 4
Testosterone formulations

Formulation	Trade Name	Dose (Adult)
IM testosterone enanthate	Delatestryl	250 mg every 2–4 wk
IM testosterone cypionate	Depo-Testosterone	250 mg every 2–4 wk
Oral testosterone undecanoate	Andriol (40 mg capsules)	2 capsules (2–3 times per day)
Testosterone patch	Androderm	5 mg/patch changed twice weekly
Testosterone gel	Androgel (25 mg testosterone/2.5 g gel) (50 mg testosterone/5 g gel)	50–100 mg/d
Buccal testosterone	Striant 30 mg tablet	1 tablet twice a day
Testosterone implants	Testopel 75 mg per pellet	3–4 pellets every 4–6 mo

irritation. As in oral testosterone therapy, there are limited studies regarding the use of transdermal preparations of testosterone, and intramuscular testosterone therapy remains the mainstay of therapy for pediatric patients. Testosterone preparations and adult doses are shown in **Table 4**.

Adjunctive treatment in the form of human chorionic gonadotropin has been suggested in boys with PWS in whom beneficial effects on body composition and endogenous testosterone secretion have been observed.[116]

SUMMARY

In conclusion, causes of hypogonadism are heterogeneous and may involve any level of the reproductive system. Whereas some conditions are clearly delineated, the exact etiology and underlying pathogenesis of many disorders is unknown. Regardless of the form of hypogonadism, the crux of therapy in children revolves around sex steroid replacement. Continued molecular genetic investigation and prospective clinical trials will enhance knowledge and improve management of hypogonadism in pediatric patients.

REFERENCES

1. Boyar R, Finkelstein J, Roffwarg H, et al. Synchronization of augmented luteinizing hormone secretion with sleep during puberty. N Engl J Med 1972;287(12): 582–6.
2. Apter D, Butzow TL, Laughlin GA, et al. Gonadotropin-releasing hormone pulse generator activity during pubertal transition in girls: pulsatile and diurnal patterns of circulating gonadotropins. J Clin Endocrinol Metab 1993;76(4): 940–9.
3. Sedlmeyer IL, Palmert MR. Delayed puberty: analysis of a large case series from an academic center. J Clin Endocrinol Metab 2002;87(4):1613–20.
4. von Kalckreuth G, Haverkamp F, Kessler M, et al. Constitutional delay of growth and puberty: do they really reach their target height? Horm Res 1991;35(6): 222–5.
5. Bergada I, Bergada C. Long term treatment with low dose testosterone in constitutional delay of growth and puberty: effect on bone age maturation and pubertal progression. J Pediatr Endocrinol Metab 1995;8(2):117–22.
6. Achermann JC, Weiss J, Lee EJ, et al. Inherited disorders of the gonadotropin hormones. Mol Cell Endocrinol 2001;179(1–2):89–96.
7. Kohler B, Lin L, Ferraz-de-Souza B, et al. Five novel mutations in steroidogenic factor 1 (SF1, NR5A1) in 46, XY patients with severe underandrogenization but without adrenal insufficiency. Hum Mutat 2008;29(1):59–64.
8. Biason-Lauber A, Schoenle EJ. Apparently normal ovarian differentiation in a prepubertal girl with transcriptionally inactive steroidogenic factor 1 (NR5A1/ SF-1) and adrenocortical insufficiency. Am J Hum Genet 2000;67(6):1563–8.
9. Muscatelli F, Strom TM, Walker AP, et al. Mutations in the DAX-1 gene give rise to both X-linked adrenal hypoplasia congenita and hypogonadotropic hypogonadism. Nature 1994;372(6507):672–6.
10. Yang F, Hanaki K, Kinoshita T, et al. Late-onset adrenal hypoplasia congenita caused by a novel mutation of the DAX-1 gene. Eur J Pediatr 2009;168:329–31.
11. Habiby RL, Boepple P, Nachtigall L, et al. Adrenal hypoplasia congenita with hypogonadotropic hypogonadism: evidence that DAX-1 mutations lead to combined hypothalamic and pituitary defects in gonadotropin production. J Clin Invest 1996;98(4):1055–62.

12. Mantovani G, De Menis E, Borretta G, et al. DAX1 and X-linked adrenal hypoplasia congenita: clinical and molecular analysis in five patients. Eur J Endocrinol 2006;154(5):685–9.
13. Franco B, Guioli S, Pragliola A, et al. A gene deleted in Kallmann's syndrome shares homology with neural cell adhesion and axonal path-finding molecules. Nature 1991;353(6344):529–36.
14. Vogl TJ, Stemmler J, Heye B, et al. Kallman syndrome versus idiopathic hypogonadotropic hypogonadism at MR imaging. Radiology 1994;191(1):53–7.
15. Oliveira LM, Seminara SB, Beranova M, et al. The importance of autosomal genes in Kallmann syndrome: genotype-phenotype correlations and neuroendocrine characteristics. J Clin Endocrinol Metab 2001;86(4):1532–8.
16. Sato N, Katsumata N, Kagami M, et al. Clinical assessment and mutation analysis of Kallmann syndrome 1 (KAL1) and fibroblast growth factor receptor 1 (FGFR1, or KAL2) in five families and 18 sporadic patients. J Clin Endocrinol Metab 2004;89(3):1079–88.
17. Pitteloud N, Zhang C, Pignatelli D, et al. Loss-of-function mutation in the prokineticin 2 gene causes Kallmann syndrome and normosmic idiopathic hypogonadotropic hypogonadism. Proc Natl Acad Sci U S A 2007;104(44):17447–52.
18. de Roux N, Young J, Misrahi M, et al. A family with hypogonadotropic hypogonadism and mutations in the gonadotropin-releasing hormone receptor. N Engl J Med 1997;337(22):1597–602.
19. de Roux N, Milgrom E. Inherited disorders of GnRH and gonadotropin receptors. Mol Cell Endocrinol 2001;179(1–2):83–7.
20. de Roux N, Genin E, Carel JC, et al. Hypogonadotropic hypogonadism due to loss of function of the KiSS1-derived peptide receptor GPR54. Proc Natl Acad Sci U S A 2003;100(19):10972–6.
21. Raivio T, Falardeau J, Dwyer A, et al. Reversal of idiopathic hypogonadotropic hypogonadism. N Engl J Med 2007;357(9):863–73.
22. Pfaffle RW, Blankenstein O, Wuller S, et al. Combined pituitary hormone deficiency: role of Pit-1 and Prop-1. Acta Paediatr Suppl 1999;88(433):33–41.
23. Lazar L, Gat-Yablonski G, Kornreich L, et al. PROP-1 gene mutation (R120C) causing combined pituitary hormone deficiencies with variable clinical course in eight siblings of one Jewish Moroccan family. Horm Res 2003;60(5):227–31.
24. Dasen JS, Barbera JP, Herman TS, et al. Temporal regulation of a paired-like homeodomain repressor/TLE corepressor complex and a related activator is required for pituitary organogenesis. Genes Dev 2001;15(23):3193–207.
25. Dattani MT, Martinez-Barbera JP, Thomas PQ, et al. Mutations in the homeobox gene HESX1/Hesx1 associated with septo-optic dysplasia in human and mouse. Nat Genet 1998;19(2):125–33.
26. Haddad NG, Eugster EA. Hypopituitarism and neurodevelopmental abnormalities in relation to central nervous system structural defects in children with optic nerve hypoplasia. J Pediatr Endocrinol Metab 2005;18(9):853–8.
27. Pfaeffle RW, Hunter CS, Savage JJ, et al. Three novel missense mutations within the LHX4 gene are associated with variable pituitary hormone deficiencies. J Clin Endocrinol Metab 2008;93(3):1062–71.
28. Kelberman D, Rizzoti K, Avilion A, et al. Mutations within Sox2/SOX2 are associated with abnormalities in the hypothalamo-pituitary-gonadal axis in mice and humans. J Clin Invest 2006;116(9):2442–55.
29. Farooqi IS, Matarese G, Lord GM, et al. Beneficial effects of leptin on obesity, T cell hyporesponsiveness, and neuroendocrine/metabolic dysfunction of human congenital leptin deficiency. J Clin Invest 2002;110(8):1093–103.

30. Farooqi IS, Wangensteen T, Collins S, et al. Clinical and molecular genetic spectrum of congenital deficiency of the leptin receptor. N Engl J Med 2007;356(3): 237–47.
31. Wharton RH, Loechner KJ. Genetic and clinical advances in Prader-Willi syndrome. Curr Opin Pediatr 1996;8(6):618–24.
32. Jeffcoate WJ, Laurance BM, Edwards CR, et al. Endocrine function in the Prader-Willi syndrome. Clin Endocrinol (Oxf) 1980;12(1):81–9.
33. Crino A, Schiaffini R, Ciampalini P, et al. Hypogonadism and pubertal development in Prader-Willi syndrome. Eur J Pediatr 2003;162(5):327–33.
34. Schulze A, Mogensen H, Hamborg-Petersen B, et al. Fertility in Prader-Willi syndrome: a case report with Angelman syndrome in the offspring. Acta Paediatr 2001;90(4):455–9.
35. Akefeldt A, Tornhage CJ, Gillberg C. A woman with Prader-Willi syndrome gives birth to a healthy baby girl. Dev Med Child Neurol 1999;41(11):789–90.
36. Morton MV, Wehman P. Psychosocial and emotional sequelae of individuals with traumatic brain injury: a literature review and recommendations. Brain Inj 1995; 9(1):81–92.
37. Kelly DF, Gonzalo IT, Cohan P, et al. Hypopituitarism following traumatic brain injury and aneurysmal subarachnoid hemorrhage: a preliminary report. J Neurosurg 2000;93(5):743–52.
38. Lieberman SA, Oberoi AL, Gilkison CR, et al. Prevalence of neuroendocrine dysfunction in patients recovering from traumatic brain injury. J Clin Endocrinol Metab 2001;86(6):2752–6.
39. Benvenga S, Campenni A, Ruggeri RM, et al. Clinical review 113: hypopituitarism secondary to head trauma. J Clin Endocrinol Metab 2000;85(4): 1353–61.
40. Tanriverdi F, Senyurek H, Unluhizarci K, et al. High risk of hypopituitarism after traumatic brain injury: a prospective investigation of anterior pituitary function in the acute phase and 12 months after trauma. J Clin Endocrinol Metab 2006;91(6):2105–11.
41. Merchant TE, Williams T, Smith JM, et al. Preirradiation endocrinopathies in pediatric brain tumor patients determined by dynamic tests of endocrine function. Int J Radiat Oncol Biol Phys 2002;54(1):45–50.
42. Gonc EN, Yordam N, Ozon A, et al. Endocrinological outcome of different treatment options in children with craniopharyngioma: a retrospective analysis of 66 cases. Pediatr Neurosurg 2004;40(3):112–9.
43. Mills JL, Fears TR, Robison LL, et al. Menarche in a cohort of 188 long-term survivors of acute lymphoblastic leukemia. J Pediatr 1997;131(4):598–602.
44. Constine LS, Woolf PD, Cann D, et al. Hypothalamic-pituitary dysfunction after radiation for brain tumors. N Engl J Med 1993;328(2):87–94.
45. Rappaport R, Brauner R, Czernichow P, et al. Effect of hypothalamic and pituitary irradiation on pubertal development in children with cranial tumors. J Clin Endocrinol Metab 1982;54(6):1164–8.
46. Nandagopal R, Laverdiere C, Mulrooney D, et al. Endocrine late effects of childhood cancer therapy: a report from the Children's Oncology Group. Horm Res 2008;69(2):65–74.
47. Chan JL, Mantzoros CS. Role of leptin in energy-deprivation states: normal human physiology and clinical implications for hypothalamic amenorrhoea and anorexia nervosa. Lancet 2005;366(9479):74–85.
48. Welt CK, Chan JL, Bullen J, et al. Recombinant human leptin in women with hypothalamic amenorrhea. N Engl J Med 2004;351(10):987–97.

49. Nielsen J, Wohlert M. Chromosome abnormalities found among 34,910 newborn children: results from a 13-year incidence study in Arhus, Denmark. Hum Genet 1991;87(1):81–3.
50. Bondy CA. Care of girls and women with Turner syndrome: a guideline of the Turner Syndrome Study Group. J Clin Endocrinol Metab 2007;92(1):10–25.
51. Pasquino AM, Passeri F, Pucarelli I, et al. Spontaneous pubertal development in Turner's syndrome. Italian Study Group for Turner's Syndrome. J Clin Endocrinol Metab 1997;82(6):1810–3.
52. Hovatta O. Pregnancies in women with Turner's syndrome. Ann Med 1999;31(2):106–10.
53. Fechner PY, Davenport ML, Qualy RL, et al. Differences in follicle-stimulating hormone secretion between 45, X monosomy Turner syndrome and 45, X/46, XX mosaicism are evident at an early age. J Clin Endocrinol Metab 2006; 91(12):4896–902.
54. Bojesen A, Juul S, Gravholt CH. Prenatal and postnatal prevalence of Klinefelter syndrome: a national registry study. J Clin Endocrinol Metab 2003;88(2):622–6.
55. Abulhasan SJ, Tayel SM, al-Awadi SA. Mosaic Turner syndrome: cytogenetics versus FISH. Ann Hum Genet 1999;63(Pt 3):199–206.
56. Rizzolio F, Bione S, Sala C, et al. Chromosomal rearrangements in Xq and premature ovarian failure: mapping of 25 new cases and review of the literature. Hum Reprod 2006;21(6):1477–83.
57. Linden MG, Bender BG, Harmon RJ, et al. 47, XXX: what is the prognosis? Pediatrics 1988;82(4):619–30.
58. Lin HJ, Ndiforchu F, Patell S. Exstrophy of the cloaca in a 47, XXX child: review of genitourinary malformations in triple-X patients. Am J Med Genet 1993;45(6):761–3.
59. Holland CM. 47, XXX in an adolescent with premature ovarian failure and autoimmune disease. J Pediatr Adolesc Gynecol 2001;14(2):77–80.
60. Matthews CH, Borgato S, Beck-Peccoz P, et al. Primary amenorrhoea and infertility due to a mutation in the beta-subunit of follicle-stimulating hormone. Nat Genet 1993;5(1):83–6.
61. Layman LC, Lee EJ, Peak DB, et al. Delayed puberty and hypogonadism caused by mutations in the follicle-stimulating hormone beta-subunit gene. N Engl J Med 1997;337(9):607–11.
62. Lindstedt G, Nystrom E, Matthews C, et al. Follitropin (FSH) deficiency in an infertile male due to FSHbeta gene mutation. A syndrome of normal puberty and virilization but underdeveloped testicles with azoospermia, low FSH but high lutropin and normal serum testosterone concentrations. Clin Chem Lab Med 1998;36(8):663–5.
63. Weiss J, Axelrod L, Whitcomb RW, et al. Hypogonadism caused by a single amino acid substitution in the beta subunit of luteinizing hormone. N Engl J Med 1992;326(3):179–83.
64. Furui K, Suganuma N, Tsukahara S, et al. Identification of two point mutations in the gene coding luteinizing hormone (LH) beta-subunit, associated with immunologically anomalous LH variants. J Clin Endocrinol Metab 1994;78(1):107–13.
65. Kremer H, Kraaij R, Toledo SP, et al. Male pseudohermaphroditism due to a homozygous missense mutation of the luteinizing hormone receptor gene. Nat Genet 1995;9(2):160–4.
66. Latronico AC, Anasti J, Arnhold IJ, et al. Brief report: testicular and ovarian resistance to luteinizing hormone caused by inactivating mutations of the luteinizing hormone-receptor gene. N Engl J Med 1996;334(8):507–12.

67. Arnhold IJ, Latronico AC, Batista MC, et al. Clinical features of women with resistance to luteinizing hormone. Clin Endocrinol (Oxf) 1999;51(6):701–7.
68. Aittomaki K. The genetics of XX gonadal dysgenesis. Am J Hum Genet 1994; 54(5):844–51.
69. de Zegher F, Jaeken J. Endocrinology of the carbohydrate-deficient glycoprotein syndrome type 1 from birth through adolescence. Pediatr Res 1995;37(4 Pt 1):395–401.
70. Gelfand IM, Eugster EA, DiMeglio LA. Presentation and clinical progression of pseudohypoparathyroidism with multi-hormone resistance and Albright hereditary osteodystrophy: a case series. J Pediatr 2006;149(6):877–80.
71. Lee PA, Houk CP, Ahmed SF, et al. Consensus statement on management of intersex disorders. International Consensus Conference on Intersex. Pediatrics 2006;118(2):e488–500.
72. Michala L, Goswami D, Creighton SM, et al. Swyer syndrome: presentation and outcomes. BJOG May 2008;115(6):737–41.
73. Zielinska D, Zajaczek S, Rzepka-Gorska I. Tumors of dysgenetic gonads in Swyer syndrome. J Pediatr Surg 2007;42(10):1721–4.
74. Oakes MB, Eyvazzadeh AD, Quint E, et al. Complete androgen insensitivity syndrome—a review. J Pediatr Adolesc Gynecol 2008;21(6):305–10.
75. Sarpel U, Palmer SK, Dolgin SE. The incidence of complete androgen insensitivity in girls with inguinal hernias and assessment of screening by vaginal length measurement. J Pediatr Surg 2005;40(1):133–6 [discussion: 136–7].
76. Costa-Santos M, Kater CE, Auchus RJ. Two prevalent CYP17 mutations and genotype-phenotype correlations in 24 Brazilian patients with 17-hydroxylase deficiency. J Clin Endocrinol Metab 2004;89(1):49–60.
77. Yang J, Cui B, Sun S, et al. Phenotype-genotype correlation in eight Chinese 17alpha-hydroxylase/17,20 lyase-deficiency patients with five novel mutations of CYP17A1 gene. J Clin Endocrinol Metab 2006;91(9):3619–25.
78. al Kandari H, Katsumata N, Alexander S, et al. Homozygous mutation of P450 side-chain cleavage enzyme gene (CYP11A1) in 46, XY patient with adrenal insufficiency, complete sex reversal, and agenesis of corpus callosum. J Clin Endocrinol Metab 2006;91(8):2821–6.
79. Baker BY, Lin L, Kim CJ, et al. Nonclassic congenital lipoid adrenal hyperplasia: a new disorder of the steroidogenic acute regulatory protein with very late presentation and normal male genitalia. J Clin Endocrinol Metab 2006;91(12): 4781–5.
80. Fujieda K, Tajima T, Nakae J, et al. Spontaneous puberty in 46, XX subjects with congenital lipoid adrenal hyperplasia. Ovarian steroidogenesis is spared to some extent despite inactivating mutations in the steroidogenic acute regulatory protein (StAR) gene. J Clin Invest 1997;99(6):1265–71.
81. Kaufman FR, Kogut MD, Donnell GN, et al. Hypergonadotropic hypogonadism in female patients with galactosemia. N Engl J Med 1981;304(17):994–8.
82. Prestoz LL, Couto AS, Shin YS, et al. Altered follicle stimulating hormone isoforms in female galactosaemia patients. Eur J Pediatr 1997;156(2):116–20.
83. Smith NM, Byard RW, Bourne AJ. Testicular regression syndrome—a pathological study of 77 cases. Histopathology 1991;19(3):269–72.
84. Law H, Mushtaq I, Wingrove K, et al. Histopathological features of testicular regression syndrome: relation to patient age and implications for management. Fetal Pediatr Pathol 2006;25(2):119–29.
85. Imbeaud S, Rey R, Berta P, et al. Testicular degeneration in three patients with the persistent mullerian duct syndrome. Eur J Pediatr 1995;154(3):187–90.

86. Vinci G, Anjot MN, Trivin C, et al. An analysis of the genetic factors involved in testicular descent in a cohort of 14 male patients with anorchia. J Clin Endocrinol Metab 2004;89(12):6282–5.

87. Wallace WH, Thomson AB, Kelsey TW. The radiosensitivity of the human oocyte. Hum Reprod 2003;18(1):117–21.

88. Larsen EC, Muller J, Schmiegelow K, et al. Reduced ovarian function in long-term survivors of radiation- and chemotherapy-treated childhood cancer. J Clin Endocrinol Metab 2003;88(11):5307–14.

89. Lopez Andreu JA, Fernandez PJ, Ferris I Tortajada J, et al. Persistent altered spermatogenesis in long-term childhood cancer survivors. Pediatr Hematol Oncol 2000;17(1):21–30.

90. Shalet SM, Tsatsoulis A, Whitehead E, et al. Vulnerability of the human Leydig cell to radiation damage is dependent upon age. J Endocrinol 1989;120(1): 161–5.

91. Steffens M, Beauloye V, Brichard B, et al. Endocrine and metabolic disorders in young adult survivors of childhood acute lymphoblastic leukaemia (ALL) or non-Hodgkin lymphoma (NHL). Clin Endocrinol (Oxf) 2008;69(5):819–27.

92. Rahhal SN, Eugster EA. Unexpected recovery of ovarian function many years after bone marrow transplantation. J Pediatr 2008;152(2):289–90.

93. Meacham LR, Ghim TT, Crocker IR, et al. Systematic approach for detection of endocrine disorders in children treated for brain tumors. Med Pediatr Oncol 1997;29(2):86–91.

94. Schatz DA, Winter WE. Autoimmune polyglandular syndrome. II: clinical syndrome and treatment. Endocrinol Metab Clin North Am 2002;31(2):339–52.

95. Wolff AS, Erichsen MM, Meager A, et al. Autoimmune polyendocrine syndrome type 1 in Norway: phenotypic variation, autoantibodies, and novel mutations in the autoimmune regulator gene. J Clin Endocrinol Metab 2007;92(2):595–603.

96. Ahonen P, Miettinen A, Perheentupa J. Adrenal and steroidal cell antibodies in patients with autoimmune polyglandular disease type I and risk of adrenocortical and ovarian failure. J Clin Endocrinol Metab 1987;64(3):494–500.

97. Uibo R, Aavik E, Peterson P, et al. Autoantibodies to cytochrome P450 enzymes P450scc, P450c17, and P450c21 in autoimmune polyglandular disease types I and II and in isolated Addison's disease. J Clin Endocrinol Metab 1994;78(2): 323–8.

98. Hoek A, Schoemaker J, Drexhage HA. Premature ovarian failure and ovarian autoimmunity. Endocr Rev 1997;18(1):107–34.

99. Buzi F, Badolato R, Mazza C, et al. Autoimmune polyendocrinopathy-candidiasis-ectodermal dystrophy syndrome: time to review diagnostic criteria? J Clin Endocrinol Metab 2003;88(7):3146–8.

100. Perniola R, Falorni A, Clemente MG, et al. Organ-specific and non-organ-specific autoantibodies in children and young adults with autoimmune polyendocrinopathy-candidiasis-ectodermal dystrophy (APECED). Eur J Endocrinol 2000; 143(4):497–503.

101. Sinisi AA, D'Apuzzo A, Pasquali D, et al. Antisperm antibodies in prepubertal boys treated with chemotherapy for malignant or non-malignant diseases and in boys with genital tract abnormalities. Int J Androl 1997;20(1):23–8.

102. Goodpasture JC, Ghai K, Cara JF, et al. Potential of gonadotropin-releasing hormone agonists in the diagnosis of pubertal disorders in girls. Clin Obstet Gynecol 1993;36(3):773–85.

103. Rosenfield RL, Perovic N, Devine N, et al. Optimizing estrogen replacement treatment in Turner syndrome. Pediatrics 1998;102(2 Pt 3):486–8.

104. Donaldson MD, Gault EJ, Tan KW, et al. Optimising management in Turner syndrome: from infancy to adult transfer. Arch Dis Child 2006;91(6):513–20.

105. Mauras N, Shulman D, Hsiang HY, et al. Metabolic effects of oral versus transdermal estrogen in growth hormone-treated girls with turner syndrome. J Clin Endocrinol Metab 2007;92(11):4154–60.

106. Ankarberg-Lindgren C, Elfving M, Wikland KA, et al. Nocturnal application of transdermal estradiol patches produces levels of estradiol that mimic those seen at the onset of spontaneous puberty in girls. J Clin Endocrinol Metab 2001;86(7):3039–44.

107. Chetkowski RJ, Meldrum DR, Steingold KA, et al. Biologic effects of transdermal estradiol. N Engl J Med 1986;314(25):1615–20.

108. Nabhan ZM, DiMeglio LA, Qi R, et al. Oral versus transdermal estrogen replacement in girls with Turner syndrome: a pilot comparative study. J Clin Endocrinol Metab 2009;94(6):2009–14.

109. Piippo S, Lenko H, Kainulainen P, et al. Use of percutaneous estrogen gel for induction of puberty in girls with Turner syndrome. J Clin Endocrinol Metab 2004;89(7):3241–7.

110. Richman RA, Kirsch LR. Testosterone treatment in adolescent boys with constitutional delay in growth and development. N Engl J Med 1988;319(24):1563–7.

111. Soliman AT, Khadir MM, Asfour M. Testosterone treatment in adolescent boys with constitutional delay of growth and development. Metabolism 1995;44(8):1013–5.

112. Arslanian S, Suprasongsin C. Testosterone treatment in adolescents with delayed puberty: changes in body composition, protein, fat, and glucose metabolism. J Clin Endocrinol Metab 1997;82(10):3213–20.

113. Rogol AD. Pubertal androgen therapy in boys. Pediatr Endocrinol Rev 2005;2(3):383–90.

114. Kassmann K, Rappaport R, Broyer M. The short-term effect of testosterone on growth in boys on hemodialysis. Clin Nephrol 1992;37(3):148–54.

115. Mayo A, Macintyre H, Wallace AM, et al. Transdermal testosterone application: pharmacokinetics and effects on pubertal status, short-term growth, and bone turnover. J Clin Endocrinol Metab 2004;89(2):681–7.

116. Eiholzer U, Grieser J, Schlumpf M, et al. Clinical effects of treatment for hypogonadism in male adolescents with Prader-Labhart-Willi syndrome. Horm Res 2007;68(4):178–84.

Optimizing Potential for Fertility: Fertility Considerations for the Pediatrician

Peter A. Lee, MD, PhD[a,b,*], Alan Rogol, MD[b,c], Christopher P. Houk, MD[d]

KEY WORDS

- Cryopreservation • Sperm retrieval • Oocyte retrieval
- Infertility • Assisted fertility • Fertility preservation

Modern medicine now offers hope for many patients who would have been infertile in the past. Fertility preservation and assisted reproduction in adults has received considerable attention. In women, discussion of fertility preservation typically arises in patients with malignancies or nononcologic conditions that either require treatment with gonadotoxic drugs, ovariectomy,[1] or pelvic radiation. Among adult men, fertility preservation should be considered whenever testicular damage may result from medical/surgical therapy or from trauma. Fertility preservation is a consideration that should be discussed in those undergoing treatment for malignancy as well as those with genetic or other congenital conditions.

The dramatic success noted in the treatment for childhood cancers has resulted in a marked increase in survival rates creating many long-term cancer survivors with unique medical challenges. Preservation of fertility is one such challenge that has mandated the need to assess future reproduction among these individuals.[2] Topics related to fertility preservation in pediatric and adolescent patients being treated for cancers, including ethical considerations, have recently been summarized.[3] Given the recent improvements in fertility preservation, this issue must now become part of an overall care plan for such children and adolescents.

Portions of this article were previously published in the *Endocrinology and Metabolism Clinics of North America*, 38:4.

[a] Department of Pediatrics, Penn State College of Medicine, MC-H085, The Milton S. Hershey Medical Center, PO Box 850, 500 University Drive, Hershey, PA 17033-0850, USA
[b] Department of Pediatrics, Indiana University School of Medicine, Riley Hospital for Children, Indianapolis, IN 46202, USA
[c] Department of Pediatrics, University of Virginia, Charlottesville, VA 22908, USA
[d] Department of Pediatrics, Medical College of Georgia, Augusta, GA 31403, USA
* Corresponding author. Department of Pediatrics, MC-H085, The Milton S. Hershey Medical Center, PO Box 850, 500 University Drive, Hershey, PA 17033-0850.
E-mail address: plee@psu.edu

Pediatr Clin N Am 58 (2011) 1201–1215
doi:10.1016/j.pcl.2011.07.011
0031-3955/11/$ – see front matter © 2011 Elsevier Inc. All rights reserved.

Awareness of current and developing techniques is appropriate for the pediatric endocrinologist because of the improved potential for fertility in children with malignancy who have undergone chemotherapy or radiation therapy as well as children and adolescents with other diagnoses, including endocrinopathy, who have long been considered to be infertile.

Efforts to address fertility preservation should be considered as soon as the risk is realized. This applies to those with gonadal failure previously considered to be incompatible with biologic parenthood such as Turner or Klinefelter syndromes. Parenthood may also be possible, albeit at considerable expense, for patients with hypogonadotropic hypogonadism, polycystic ovarian disease, or other ovulatory dysfunction. The potential for such therapies should be assessed at an early age.

ATTAINMENT OF FERTILITY POTENTIAL IN THE HUMAN

Although fertility potential is not normally attained until early or midpuberty, a low level of gonadal activity is present during childhood with limited follicular development and early stages of spermatogenesis. Even though mature sperm are not present until a mean age of 14 years, meiosis results in development of spermatids in the prepubertal testis.[4] Semen cryopreservation has been reported to be feasible in roughly two-thirds of boys aged 13.7 to 18.9 years.[5] Although sperm counts cannot accurately be predicted by hormone measurements, it is likely that an adequate sample for preservation could be obtained around midpuberty in those without chronic debilitating illness. Similar findings have also been noted in 14- to 17-year-old boys with malignancies.[6] Among females, there is no conclusive evidence of further oocyte production after birth and meiosis occurs during follicular maturation. There is potential for in vitro maturation of primordial oocytes into oogonia. Before ovarian failure, all females will produce mature follicles in response to gonadotropin stimulation. In fact most females are capable of ovulation by midpuberty.

ETHICAL CONSIDERATIONS FOR THE CHILD

Ethical and legal issues including risk-benefit determination, must be considered[7] before implementing fertility preservation procedures. These must be proposed to parents, and, in an age-appropriate way, to the patient. Investigational review boards require a pediatric counselor to discuss the proposed preservation with the child. Such discussion may be awkward for families who have recently been given a diagnosis of malignancy. In addition, the importance of future fertility may be difficult for the prepubertal child to assess; therefore, parents can and should play a role in decision making in this arena. Consent must be obtained from parents with appropriate assent from the child before attempting to obtain and cryopreserve germ cells or gonadal tissue. Any procedures should be presented to an appropriate ethical review board as experimental, as protocols to preserve fertility in children are only now being developed.

DIAGNOSES IN CHILDREN AND ADOLESCENTS FOR FERTILITY PRESERVATION CONSIDERATIONS

Procedures for adolescent women and prepubertal boys and girls being investigated[8] are listed in **Box 1**. Efficacy of these procedures must be verified in adults before they are used in children. Procedures applicable to children include oocyte banking, ovarian tissue cryopreservation, in vitro follicular maturation for females, and testicular tissue cryopreservation and spermatogonial stem cell transplantation in males.[9]

Fertility preservation in children (**Box 2**) who face therapy that may preclude fertility or have congenital or early-onset gonadal dysfunction will focus on preserving remaining

Box 1
Potential methods to preserve or stimulate fertility in children and adolescents

A. Among prepubertal individuals being treated with gonadotoxic agents or radiation or those with endocrinological diagnoses of primary hypogonadism

  a. Girls

    i. Cryopreservation of immature oocytes and in vitro follicular maturation

    ii. Ovarian tissue cryopreservation

    iii. Ovarian transposition out of radiation field

  b. Boys

    i. Testicular tissue cryopreservation

    ii. Spermatogonial stem cell transplantation

    iii. Shielding testes from radiation

B. Pubertal and postpubertal adolescents

  a. Girls

    i. Oocyte cryopreservation

    ii. GnRH analog

    iii. Ovarian tissue cryopreservation

  b. Boys

    i. Semen cryopreservation

C. Among those with hypogonadotropic hypogonadism

  a. Gonadotropin or gonadotropin-releasing hormone (intermittent stimulation)

germ cells. Examples of children and adolescents in this category include those whose gonads have been damaged as a result of therapy for malignant or autoimmune diseases, those with incomplete primary hypogonadism, including patients with Klinefelter syndrome, Turner syndrome, some types of DSD (disorders of sex development) such as ovotesticular DSD and those with gonadal damage following trauma, torsion,

Box 2
Fertility preservation or stimulation among children and adolescents

1. To preserve germ cells among those who

  ○ Face therapy for malignant or autoimmune diseases that may preclude fertility

  ○ Have congenital or early-onset gonadal dysfunction

    ■ Males with incomplete primary hypogonadism, including most boys with Klinefelter syndrome, those with gonadal damage after torsion, orchitis, or partial removal of the testes

    ■ Females with Turner syndrome whose ovaries contain follicles, and some patients with potentially functional ovaries having disorders of sex development (DSD), such as the female with ovotesticular DSD.

2. Stimulate germ cell maturation via pulsatile administration of GnRH or intermittent gonadotropin stimulation

  ○ Males and females have congenital or acquired hypogonadotropic hypogonadism

inflammatory process, or surgery. For those with congenital or acquired hypogonado-tropic hypogonadism, the focus of therapy involves the pulsatile administration of GnRH (currently unavailable in the United States), or intermittent gonadotropin stimulation.

FERTILITY PRESERVATION IN MALIGNANT DISEASES OF CHILDHOOD AND ADOLESCENCE

Consequences of therapy for childhood cancers may interfere with the ability to produce mature germ cells and achieve future fertilization. Accordingly, survivors of childhood cancer may have difficulty becoming pregnant, have increased sponta-neous abortions as a consequence of altered uterine anatomy, and suffer higher rates of neonatal death and low-birth-weight infants.[10] An increased risk of congenital mal-formations or childhood cancer in the offspring of patients who received cancer treat-ment in childhood has not been reported.

Fertility preservation techniques have progressed as survival rates of many cancers have improved, particularly in young adult men and women. These techniques apply to adolescents who have completed puberty who show adult-type spermatogenesis or ovulation. For adolescent males, sperm banking is relatively simple, well tested, and does not delay therapy for the underlying malignancy. In the postmenarchal adolescent female, delay of therapy for the malignancy is usually necessary to permit retrieval of ova.

Although the need for fertility preservation for children and adolescents is clear, there are few outcome studies that examine only those who have not had fertility pres-ervation. Therefore, fertility rates are unknown. A survey of adult cancer survivors indi-cates that 34 of 260 participants or partners achieved pregnancy, with 30 of these having one or more children[11]; the data do not report what percentage of these patients had attempted pregnancy. Also, the data did not account for the almost 25% of participants who indicated that they did not want children, in part because of a fear that the cancer would return or would develop in their child.

Damage to the gonad from chemotherapy is age-related, varies between the sexes, and is more likely with use of gonadotoxic drugs. Adolescents treated before puberty are at high risk for severe damage to spermatogenetic potential and ovarian follicular dysfunction.[12] Impaired fertility following chemotherapy for malignancy[13] is related to the age at therapy. The prepubertal testicle appears to be more vulnerable to cytotoxic effects of chemotherapy than is the adult testis[14]; in contrast, the prepubertal ovarian reserve is less susceptible to cytotoxic damage than the mature ovary. In fact, most prepubertal girls are expected to retain normal ovarian function. Seventy-five percent of 25 male cancer survivors diagnosed between ages 0.9 and 15.9 years[15] had normal sperm counts. Sperm concentrations correlated positively with testicular volume and inhibin B levels and negatively with follicle stimulating hormone (FSH) concentrations.

In a group of men who had gonadotoxic therapy before puberty,[16] such fertility markers have been found to be indicative of compromised fertility although the utility of these measures in individual patients was less helpful. Differences in inhibin B, testosterone, luteinizing hormone (LH) and FSH levels, testicular volume, and sperm counts were found when men who were long-term cancer survivors were compared with a control group (Table 1). Low inhibin B levels but near normal testosterone levels are consistent with the greater vulnerability of sperm-producing elements than the testosterone-producing Leydig cells, both hormone levels being significantly lower in survivors than in control men. Increased LH levels in survivors suggest a component of compensation whereby greater stimulation is required to achieve physiologic testosterone levels. Mean testicular volume did not differ between the two groups,

Table 1
Parameters of fertility among adult male survivors of childhood cancer and control men

	Range Survivors	Range Controls	P value	% Abnormal Survivors	% Abnormal Controls
Inhibin B, ng/L	0–393	60–556	<.0001	65	25
Testosterone, nmol/L	2.8–45.1	4.7–27.7	.05	8	10
FSH, U/L	0.3–65.8	0.6–18.0	.01	32	17
LH, U/L	0.1–16.3	0.3–19.2	<.0001	10	2
Sperm density, 1×10^6 mL	0.0–158.0	21.1–234.0	<.0001	76	0
Testis vol, mL	2–35	11–30	.391	17	14

Although the range is of limited usefulness for the individual patient, the overlap among the subjects with controls is pertinent.
Abbreviations: FSH, follicle-stimulating hormone; LH, luteinizing hormone.
Data from Van Casteren NJ, ver der Linden GHM, Hakvoort-Cammel FGAJ, et al. Effect of childhood cancer treatment on fertility markers in adult male long-term survivors. Pediatr Blood Cancer 2009;52:108–12.

although sperm concentrations were dramatically lower in the survivors where 67% showed oligospermia or azoospermia. Individual assessment of sperm parameters, both concentration and motility, is clearly the best determinant of subfertility or infertility.

FERTILITY PRESERVATION IN ENDOCRINE DISORDERS IN CHILDREN AND ADOLESCENTS
Hypothalamic-pituitary Dysfunction

Patients with hypothalamic-pituitary dysfunction may also be candidates if the gonads developed or are preserved sufficiently so that gonadotropin-responsive germ cells are present. These conditions may be acquired, such as following high-dosage cranial irradiation, or congenital.

Gonadal Dysfunction, Hypoplasia, or Dysplasia

In patients with gonadal dysgenesis who show arrested gonad development or early gonadal degeneration, there may be sufficient germ cells to permit harvesting. A small portion of Turner syndrome patients have normal puberty and normal gonadotropin secretion and are likely to be spontaneously fertile[17]; such patients do not require fertility preservation.

Conversely, most patients with Turner syndrome have very little peripubertal gonadal function and are therefore not candidates for fertility preservation; only the small portion of patients with persistent oocytes will benefit from fertility preservation. Such patients are likely to have some early, albeit usually limited, pubertal development. Their karyotype is likely mosaic or involves the loss of only a portion of the X chromosome. Moderate elevations of circulating gonadotropin levels may be present as evidence of follicular dysfunction. Because ultrasonography or MRI evaluations do not accurately assess ovarian structure or detect the presence of follicles, it is important to verify the presence of ovarian follicles with a definitive technique such as laparoscopic ovarian biopsy.

Evaluation of prognostic factors for follicular development have been reported for 57 patients with Turner syndrome.[18] The patients were categorized into three groups: (1)

15 found to have follicles after laparoscopic ovarian biopsy, (2) 32 with no follicles seen on biopsy, and (3) ovarian streaks identified and no biopsy done. Results are summarized in **Table 2** and **Fig. 1**. Baseline data are the most compelling in group one (those with follicles), which showed that 12 had mosaic karyotypes or structural abnormalities, 11 had spontaneous puberty, and 8 reached spontaneous menarche. The eight patients reaching menarche had Tanner stage 4 or 5 breast development at the time of evaluation.

In addition to spontaneous pubertal development and karyotype, positive predictive factors for detecting follicles in Turner syndrome patients were a normal serum FSH level (<11 mIU/mL) and a serum anti-Müllerian hormone (AMH) level higher than 2 pmol/L. Negative predictive values for lack of follicles (in order of importance) were: 45X karyotype, serum AMH less than 2 pmol/L, lack of spontaneous pubertal onset, an FSH value greater than 15 IU/L, and the presence of structural chromosomal abnormalities. These recent data confirm the overall impression that the presence of follicles in Turner syndrome patients will manifest itself in the data commonly obtained as part of clinical evaluation and care. These are the patients who should be considered for fertility preservation.

Although a normal FSH concentration is a positive predictive factor, the presence of an elevated FSH level does not preclude spontaneous ovulation, pregnancy, and successful birth. One such case with elevated FSH has been described in a patient with a mosaic karyotype, spontaneous puberty, and menarche who had a dominant follicle by ultrasonography.[19]

Fertility preservation has been attempted in a 16-year-old adolescent with mosaic Turner syndrome.[20] After laparoscopic wedge resection, visible follicles were

Table 2
Findings among three groups of Turner patients: those having (1) follicles on ovarian biopsy,(2) no follicles on biopsy, and (3) streak ovaries on laparoscopy and not biopsy

Group	1	2	3
N	15	32	10
Age range	11.8–18.3 y	8–18.8 y	8.4–17.8 y
LH			
Range, IU/L	0.1–62.8 (13)	0.1–96.2 (24)	1.0–49.6
Median	3.4	7.1	14.6
FSH			
Range, IU/L	1–122 (13)	3.3–96.2 (24)	10.4–123
Median	6.1	19	110
AMH			
Range, pM	0.75–12.27	0.55–5.96	0.7–3.66
Median	2.25	1.1	1.25
Spontaneous puberty	11/15	8/32	0/10
Spontaneous menarche	8/11	0/32	0/10
Tanner stage-range	2–5	1	1
Median	5		
Biopsied	15/15	32/32	0-streaks

N in parentheses if less than total group.
Abbreviations: AMH, anti-Müllerian hormone; FSH, follicle-stimulating hormone; LH, luteinizing hormone.
Data from Birgit B, Julius H, Carsten R, et al. Fertility preservation in girls with Turner syndrome—prognostic signs of the presence of ovarian follicles. J Clin Endocrinol Metab 2009;94:74–80.

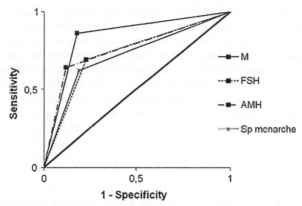

Fig. 1. ROC curves showing that there is higher sensitivity than specificity for the following variables: presence of a mosaic karyotype (M), normal FSH for age and stage of development (FSH), normal AMH for age (AMH) and spontaneous menarche (Sp menarche) (*From* Birgit B, Julius H, Carsten R, et al. Fertility preservation in girls with Turner syndrome—Prognostic signs of the presence of ovarian follicles. J Clin Endocrinol Metab 2009;94:74–80; with permission.)

aspirated. Eight of the 11 immature oocytes were permitted to mature in vitro and were cryopreserved. However, it is unclear whether this type of a patient is more likely to achieve pregnancy using cryopreservation than she would be without any intervention.

Testicular Damage, Including Those with Klinefelter Syndrome

Boys with the Klinefelter syndrome progressively lose spermatogenic capacity. From early to midpuberty, there is clear histologic change from a testicle showing relatively normal seminiferous tubules, reduced germ cells, and normal Sertoli/Leydig-cell appearance to the adult condition showing extensive fibrosis and hyalinization of the seminiferous tubules.[21,22] As a result of Sertoli cell dysfunction, virtually all men with Klinefelter syndrome are azoospermic or markedly oligospermic by late adolescence or early adulthood. This progressive gonadal failure is correlated with increasing FSH and decreasing inhibin B and AMH levels over time.[21]

In addition to Klinefelter syndrome, if compromised spermatogenesis is found in males with a history of varicocele, cryptorchidism, testicular torsion, or orchitis, procedures of sperm retrieval and cryopreservation may be a worthwhile consideration. Because progression of testicular damage and dysfunction may occur during adolescence, early consideration of fertility preservation is paramount.

TREATMENTS AND PROCEDURES TO PRESERVE FERTILITY

Efforts to preserve fertility depend on the sex and sexual maturation of the patient. Strategies involve two phases[23]: the first involves removal of gonadal tissue and germ cells, possible in vitro maturation, and cryopreservation, which occurs during childhood; the second phase involves using this previously obtained material in the adult who desires fertility. This may involve auto retransplantation of ovarian or testicular tissue or in vitro fertilization (IVF) using mature oocytes or spermatogonia. Autologous ovarian grafting in an oophorectomized female has resulted in a return of "ovarian" cycling.[24] Successful pregnancies have also been reported using immature spermatozoa and spermatids.[25] These techniques may also be successful in the patient with limited and progressively diminishing fertility, including the pubertal adolescent (**Figs. 2** and **3**). Procedures remain limited for the prepubertal child.

The status of fertility preservation for adult men and women has been reviewed by an expert advisory panel.[26] Techniques may be attempted in patients receiving chemotherapy or radiation therapy for malignancies, autoimmune diseases such as lupus erythematosis, and hematologic conditions such as sickle cell anemia, thalassemia major, and aplastic anemia as well as those who are undergoing gonadectomy. The lack of complete and accurate data concerning the gonadal effects of chemotherapy makes selection of at-risk patients, in which fertility preservation should be strongly considered, difficult.[27] Because of evolving chemotherapeutic regimens, the precise extent of gonadal damage remains difficult to predict. During puberty and thereafter, gonadotropin levels (LH and FSH) as well as AMH and inhibin B levels can be used as indices of gonadal integrity. Because damage may be only transient following chemotherapy or radiation therapy, these hormone measurements should be followed over time to identify trends of recovery or progressive damage.

Procedures for Females

Ovulation induction in anovulatory women has been well documented[28] in those with ovarian pathology. These induction strategies can also be used in those with hypothalamic-pituitary deficiencies (hypogonadotropic or secondary gonadal failure).

Among the technical procedures, embryo cryopreservation remains the most successful and widely available modality for storing germ cells for future pregnancy. This process requires availability of both ova and sperm. For females, this procedure involves ovulation induction, harvesting ova, and storage as ova or fertilized gametes. Obtaining and cryopreserving oocytes involves a complex and time-consuming ovarian stimulation called superovulation. Egg fertilization to permit cryopreservation of embryos is appropriate only when the sperm donor has been identified.

In addition to embryo cryopreservation, there have also been recent attempts to cryopreserve ova or sections of ovary. This procedure is done in anticipation of future

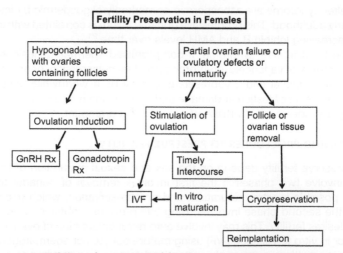

Fig. 2. Schematic possibilities for attempted fertility preservation among females, including children and adolescents. GnRH, gonadotropin-releasing hormone (currently unavailable in the United States; IVF, in vitro fertilization).

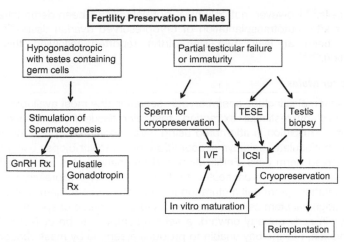

Fig. 3. Schematic algorithm for fertility preservation among prepubertal, pubertal and adult males. TESE, testicular sperm extraction; IVF, in vitro fertilization; ICSI, intracytoplasmic sperm injection.

ovarian tissue autotransplantation[29] and is dependent on type of malignancy, timing of chemotherapy, partner status, and patient's age.

Because both oocyte and embryo freezing require ovarian stimulation, novel stimulation regimens using aromatase inhibitors have been developed for women with estrogen-sensitive cancers that may be exacerbated by estrogen stimulation.[30] In vitro maturation has also been assessed in the unstimulated ovary, which avoids the issues of high cost and potential side effects of ovarian stimulation protocols.[31]

Ovarian tissue cryopreservation, a novel technology, is the only fertility preservation option for prepubertal children and the only treatment strategy allowing restoration of ovarian function. In vitro maturation, if successful, could be used in combination with ovarian tissue cryopreservation to improve fertility rates. Although fertilization of oocytes from unstimulated ovaries has been successful after in vitro maturation,[32] this process may be difficult to use in the prepubertal child, as the factors used to predict success and therefore candidacy for this technique include estradiol and FSH levels and antral follicular count[31]— measurements that would be appropriately low in the prepubertal child.

Although most prepubertal girls receiving therapy for malignancy retain some ovarian function, ovarian tissue harvesting may be appropriate for those patients judged to be at highest risk. Currently, fertilization of the egg and cryopreserving embryos would not be considered appropriate for most adolescent females, because only rarely would a sperm source be identified. The freezing of oocytes remains an option for an adolescent girl; however, the chance of retrieving an oocyte that will result in a live birth is currently very low (3%–5%).[33]

The harvesting and cryopreservation of ovarian cortex tissue for reimplantation is another option; however, limited experience with this technique precludes any meaningful estimation of its success rate. Oocytes retrieved from ovarian tissue excised before chemotherapy or radiotherapy, mature in vitro, and may then be cryopreserved.[34,35] In one report of five women who had ovarian tissue cryopreserved before chemotherapy and who later had this tissue reimplanted showed a restoration of ovarian function, albeit with elevated FSH levels, 4 to 6 months afterward.[36] Unsolved issues include cortical ischemia and follicle loss[37] and the risk of the seeding of malignant cells.[38] However, not only have normal follicles been demonstrated more than a year after autotransplantation of cryopreserved ovarian tissue,[39] but there have also been at least two live births reported following this type of reimplantation.[40,41]

Procedures for Males

Techniques for males include sperm cryopreservation (the most available technique), sperm retrieval by testicular extraction, testicular tissue freezing, and hormonal suppression. Fertilization is attempted using intracytoplamsic sperm injection (ICSI) obtained from ejaculate, epididymal aspiration, or testicular biopsy using both fresh or cryopreserved germ cells. Fertilization and pregnancy rates using epididymal or testicular spermatozoa are unaffected by the duration of cryopreservation.[42] Germ cell transplantation, germ cell maturation in vitro, stem-cell-to-germ-cell maturation, and spermatogonial stem cells can also be used as a source of sperm.

In the boy in early puberty onward, a semen sample can be collected for sperm cryopreservation. For the boy unable to produce a sample by masturbation, alternative procedures can be used. While these methods are not well developed for prepubertal boys, the goal is to establish procedures to obtain stem cells for storage and potential reimplantation or testicular tissue for storage and culture for in vitro spermatogenesis. Although the retrieval of spermatogonial stem cells, precursors of spermatozoa, have not been attempted in prepubertal boys, studies of animal models[13,43] may form the basis for in vitro maturation of sperm or reimplantation of testicular tissue. Currently, testicular sperm extraction and testicular tissue freezing in the prepubertal child is experimental.

For pubertal or adult men with incomplete primary testicular failure who show rare sperm in the ejaculate, ICSI, a well-established treatment for men with almost any form of infertility[44] can be attempted[45] and a detailed ICSI procedure has been published.[46] The preferred technique in azoospermic men is microdissection testicular sperm extraction (TESE) from which sperm are obtained slightly more than 50% of the time. Using an operating microscope, tubules containing sperm are identified, opened, and biopsied for sperm extraction.[47] Cryopreserved testicular biopsies may also be helpful in men with congenital or acquired reproductive obstruction.

Comparisons between sperm exposed to the maturation process of passing through the reproductive tract and those obtained by TESE show that transit through the male genital tract is unnecessary. In fact, the use of testicular extracted sperm resulted in more conceptions than did ejaculated sperm from severely oligospermic men.[45]

Pretherapy planning is critical for males with malignancy. Depending on patient age and status, procedures include (1) collection and cryopreservation of ejaculated sperm for possible cryopreservation and ICSI,(2) TESE in azoospermic males or early pubertal males to obtain sperm for cryopreservation, and (3) in the future, banking testicular *stem* cells, a technique successful in laboratory animals.[48] TESE and spermatogonial stem cell retrieval[49–51] should be considered for boys with Klinefelter syndrome and other forms of gonadal failure. In a man with nonmosaic Klinefelter syndrome, testicular sperm extraction, cryopreservation, oocyte recovery, and ICSI has been reported.[52]

In men with congenital or acquired hypogonadotropic hypogonadism, pulsatile GnRH administration or intermittent gonadotropin therapy may be used for hypothalamic (GnRH) or pituitary (LH and FSH) deficiency. Both techniques effectively induce spermatogenesis and have resulted in paternity in men with responsive germ cells.[53,54]

GONADAL PROTECTION DURING AT-RISK THERAPY

Gonad shielding during radiation therapy is a common practice and lead shielding of the testes is used when possible. In females, oophoropexy, a procedure where the ovaries are moved to a different position in the abdomen, out of the radiation field, may be used.

Hormonal suppression techniques, such as gonadotropin-releasing hormone agonist analogs (GnRHa) therapy, can be used to create a hypogonadotropic or prepubertal state and decrease the metabolic activity of the gonad, to attempt to reduce damage to germ cells.[55] Desensitizing the pituitary and indirectly and directly the ovary or testis with GnRHa therapy is a theoretical, but as yet not well demonstrated mechanism to preserve the fertility potential of a pubertal or postpubertal patient. Suggested mechanisms of action for GnRHa in females include decreasing the number of primordial follicles, decreasing vascular supply to the ovary to reduce the exposure to chemotherapeutic agents, and stimulation of antiapoptotic activity within the ovary,[56] and consequent to directly binding to the ovarian follicle, independent of gonadotropin levels.

Amelioration of the gonadotoxic effect of chemotherapy may reduce the incidence of premature ovarian failure.[57] Early data suggest that GnRHa therapy decreases rates of primary ovarian failure and is followed by a higher rate of spontaneous ovulation and menses in women treated for malignant and nonmalignant diseases.[55] A recent randomized, prospective, controlled study in adult women younger than 40 with breast cancer[58] found that 8 months after therapy, in those who received GnRH therapy, 89.6% resumed menses, 69.2% had spontaneous ovulation, and 11.4% developed ovarian failure. In the non-GnRH–treated control group, only 33.3% resumed menses and 25.6% had spontaneous ovulation.

Use of GnRHa involves a delay of 7 to 10 days before therapy for the underlying condition; although the use of a GnRH antagonist used alone, or in combination with GnRHa, would reduce that interval. Because antagonists immediately block GnRH receptors and gonadotropin release, the delay in therapy could be reduced to 3 or 4 days. GnRHa therapy as adjunctive therapy at the time of chemotherapy resulted in a larger number having resumption of cyclic ovarian function and fewer having premature ovarian failure than in the group receiving chemotherapy alone.[59]

It has been suggested that GnRHa be used for fertility preservation in conjunction with other methods, such as embryo cryopreservation after IVF.[56] There are no data that suggest the utility of GnRHa for gonadal protection in the prepubertal individual. Overall, results are encouraging that GnRHa therapy may play a role in fertility preservation in the peripubertal patient. A large, multicentered, well-defined, age-stratified randomized trial should be considered.

SUMMARY

Significant advances are being made in optimizing potential for fertility for children and adolescents. Although among adolescents at risk for impaired fertility adult techniques can be used, strong consideration should be given pediatric-aged patients, including prepubertal children, to removal of gonadal tissue for cryopreservation. Success with technique is summarized among adult women.[60] Ovarian cortical slices or primordial follicles obtained in childhood could be reimplanted at a later date, allowing for the possibility of successful pregnancy. In males, isolation of germ cells, either from ejaculate of TESE for future autotransplantation or in vitro maturation and cryopreservation in anticipation of ICSI should be considered. Because the duration of ovarian function following reimplantation may be short lived, transplantation should be done only when fertility is desired. For parents of patients, the parents section in the Web site www. myoncofertility.org may be helpful.

ACKNOWLEDGMENTS

The comments and suggestions of William C. Dodson, MD, Penn State College of Medicine are sincerely appreciated.

REFERENCES

1. Tulandi T, Huang JY, Tan SL. Preservation of female fertility. An essential progress. Obstet Gynecol 2008;112:1160–72.
2. Wallace WHB, Thomson AB. Preservation of fertility in children treated for cancer. Arch Dis Child 2003;88:493–6.
3. Fallat ME, Hutter J, The Committee on Bioethics, Section on Hematology/ Oncology, and Section on Surgery, American Academy of Pediatrics. Preservation of fertility in pediatric and adolescent patients with cancer. Pediatrics 2008; 121:e1461–9.
4. Gerris J. Methods of semen collection not based on masturbation or surgical sperm retrieval. Hum Reprod Update 1999;5:211–5.
5. Van Casteren NJ, Dohle GR, Romijn MSC, et al. Semen cryopreservation in puberty; boys before gonadotoxic treatment and the role of endocrinologic evaluation in predicting sperm yield. Fertil Steril 2008;90:1119–25.
6. Müller J, Sønksen J, Sommer P, et al. Cryopreservation of semen from pubertal boys with cancer. Med Pediatr Oncol 2000;34:191–4.
7. Hart R. Preservation of fertility in adults and children diagnosed with cancer. BMJ 2008;337:1045–8.
8. Anderson RA. Fertility preservation techniques: laboratory and clinical progress and current issues. Reproduction 2008;136:667–9.
9. Deepinder F, Agarwal A. Technical and ethical challenges of fertility preservation in young cancer patients. Reprod Biomed Online 2008;16:784–91.
10. Blatt J. Pregnancy outcome in long-term survivors of childhood cancer. Med Pediatr Oncol 1999;33:29–33.
11. Reinmuth S, Lieeskind AK, Wickmann L, et al. Having children after surviving cancer in childhood or adolescence—results of a Berlin survey. Kiln Paediatr 2008;220:159–65.
12. Mackie EJ, Radford M, Shalet SM. Gonadal failure following chemotherapy for childhood Hodgkin's disease. Med Pediatr Oncol 1996;27:74–8.
13. Revel A, Revel-Vilk S. Pediatric fertility preservation: is it time to offer testicular tissue cryopreservation? Mol Cell Endocrinol 2008;66:784–9.
14. Edgar AB, Wallace WHB. Pregnancy in women who had cancer in childhood. Eur J Cancer 2007;43:1890–4.
15. Lahteenmäki PM, Arola M, Suominen J, et al. Male reproductive health after childhood cancer. Acta Paediatr 2008;97:935–42.
16. Van Casteren NJ, ver der Linden GHM, Hakvoort-Cammel FGAJ, et al. Effect of childhood cancer treatment on fertility markers in adult male long-term survivors. Pediatr Blood Cancer 2009;52:108–12.
17. Cools M, Rooman RPA, Wauters J, et al. A nonmosaic 45, X karyotype in a mother with Turner's syndrome and in her daughter. Fertil Steril 2004;82:923–5.
18. Birgit B, Julius H, Carsten R, et al. Fertility preservation in girls with Turner syndrome—prognostic signs of the presence of ovarian follicles. J Clin Endocrinol Metab 2009;94:74–80.

19. Livadas S, Xekouki P, Kafiri G, et al. Spontaneous pregnancy and birth of a normal female from a woman with Turner syndrome and elevated gonadotropins. Fertil Steril 2005;83:769–72.
20. Huang JYJ, Tulandi T, Holzer H, et al. Cryopreservation of ovarian tissue and in vitro matured oocytes in a female with mosaic Turner syndrome: case report. Humanit Rep 2008;23:336–9.
21. Bastida MG, Rey RA, Bergada I, et al. Establishment of testicular endocrine function impairment during childhood and puberty in boys with Klinefelter syndrome. Clin Endocrinol 2007;67:863–70.
22. Alsglaede L, Wikstrom AM, Rajpert-De Meyts, et al. Natural history of seminiferous tubule degeneration in Klinefelter syndrome. Hum Reprod Update 2006; 12:39–48.
23. Nidker J, Baylis K, McLeod C. Choice of fertility preservation in girls and adolescent women with cancer. Cancer 2006;107(Suppl):1686–9.
24. Oktay K, Karlikaya G. Ovarian function after transplantation of frozen, banked, autologous ovarian tissue. N Engl J Med 2000;342:1919.
25. Tesarik J. Fertilization of oocytes by injecting spermatozoa, spermtids, and spermatocytes. Rev Reprod 1996;1:149–52.
26. Lamar CA, DeCherney AH. Fertility preservation: state of the science and future research directions. Fertil Steril 2009;91:316–9.
27. Anderson RA, Wallace WHB, Baird DT. Ovarian cryopreservation for fertility preservation: indications and outcomes. Reproduction 2008;136:681–9.
28. The Practice Committee of the American Society for Reproductive Medicine. Use of exogenous gonadotropins in anovulatory women: a technical bulletin. Fertil Steril 2008;90(Suppl 3):S7–12.
29. Donnez J, Martinez-Madrid B, Jadoul P, et al. Ovarian tissue cryopreservation and transplantation: a review. Hum Reprod Update 2006;12:519–35.
30. Sonmezer M, Oktay K. Assisted reproduction and fertility preservation techniques in cancer patients. Curr Opin Endocrinol Diabetes Obes 2008;15:514–22.
31. Fadini R, Dal Canto MB, Renzini MM, et al. Predictive factors in in-vitro maturation in unstimulated women with normal ovaries. Reprod Biomed Online 2009;18:251–61.
32. Zhao JZ, Zhou W, Zhang W, et al. In vitro maturation and fertilization of oocytes from unstimulated ovaries in infertile women with polcystic ovary syndrome. Fertil Steril 2009;91:2568–71.
33. Gook DA, Edgar DH. Human oocyte cryopreservation. Hum Reprod Update 2007;20:591–605.
34. Huang JYJ, Tulandi T, Holzer H, et al. Combining ovarian tissue cryobanking with retrieval of immature oocytes followed by in vitro maturation and vitrification: an additional strategy of fertility preservation. Fertil Steril 2008;89:567–72.
35. Huang JYJ, Buckett WM, Gilbert L, et al. Retrieval of immature oocytes followed by in vitro maturation and vitrification: a case report on a new strategy of fertility preservation in women with borderline ovarian malignancy. Gynecol Oncol 2007; 105:542–4.
36. Donnez J, Squifflet J, Van Eyck AS, et al. Restoration of ovarian function in orthotopically transplanted cryopreserved ovarian tissue: a pilot experience. Reprod Biomed Online 2008;16:694–704.
37. Newton H, Aubard Y, Rutherford A, et al. Low temperature storage and grafting of human ovarian tissue. Humanit Rep 1996;11:1487–91.
38. Meirow D, Hardan I, Dor J, et al. Searching for evidence of disease and malignant cell contamination in ovarian tissue stored from hematologic cancer patients. Humanit Rep 2008;23:1007–13.

39. Camboni A, Martinez-Madrid B, Dolmans MM, et al. Autotransplantation of frozen-thawed ovarian tissue in a young woman: ultrastructure and viability of grafted tissue. Fertil Steril 2007;90:1215–8.
40. Donnez J, Dolmans MM, Demyalle D, et al. Live birth after orthotopic transplantation of cryopreserved ovarian tissue. Lancet 2004;364:1405–10.
41. Demeestere I, Simon P, Emiliani S, et al. Fertility preservation: successful transplantation of cryopreserved ovarian tissue in a young patient previously treated for Hodgkin's disease. Oncologist 2007;12:1437–42.
42. Wood S, Sephton V, Searle T, et al. Effect on clinical outcome of the interval between collection of epididymal and testicular spermatozoa and intracytoplamsic sperm injection in obstructive azoopsermia. J Androl 2003;24: 67–72.
43. Ehmcke J, Schlatt S. Animal models for fertility preservation in the male. Reproduction 2008;136:717–23.
44. Silber SJ, Van Steirtegehem A, Liu J, et al. Normal pregnancies resulting from testicular sperm extraction and intracytoplasmic sperm injection for azoospermia due to maturation arrest. Fertil Steril 1996;66:110–7.
45. Bendikson BA, Neri QV, Takeuchi T, et al. The outcome of intracytoplasmic sperm injection using occasional spermatozoa in the ejaculate of men with spermatogenic failure. J Urol 2008;180:1060–4.
46. Palermo GD, Schlegel PN, Colombero LT, et al. Aggressive sperm immobilization prior to intracytoplasmic sperm injection with immature spermatozoa improves fertilization and pregnancy rates. Humanit Rep 1999;15:1023–9.
47. Schlegel PN. Male infertility: evaluation and sperm retrieval. Clin Obstet Gynecol 2006;49:55–72.
48. Zhang Z, Renfree MB, Short RV. Successful intra- and interspecific male germ cell transplantation in the rat. Biol Reprod 2003;68:961–7.
49. Paduch DA, Fine RG, Bolyakov A, et al. New concepts in Klinefelter syndrome. Curr Opin Urol 2008;18:621–7.
50. Krausz C, Forti G. Sperm cryopreservation in male infertility due to genetic disorders. Cell Tissue Bank 2006;7:105–12.
51. Tournaye H, Goosens E, Verheven G, et al. Preserving the reproductive potential of men and boys with cancer: current concepts and future prospects. Hum Reprod Update 2004;10:525–32.
52. Greco E, Iacobelli M, Rienzi L, et al. Birth of a healthy boy after fertilization if cryopreserved oocytes with cryopreserved testicular spermatozoa from a man with nonmosaic Klinefelter syndrome. Fertil Steril 2008;89:e5–7.
53. Büchter D, Behre HM, Kliesch S, et al. Pulsatile GnRH or human chorionic gonadotropin/human menopausal gonadotropin as effective treatment for men with hypogonadotropic hypogonadism: a review of 42 cases. Eur J Endocrinol 1998;139: 298–303.
54. Zitzmann M, Nieschlag E. Hormone substitution in male hypogonadism. Mol Cell Endocrinol 2000;161:73–88.
55. Lee PA, Houk CP. Recommendation on the use of GnRH in pediatrics. In: Lunenfeld B, editor. GnRH analogs in human reproduction. London: Taylor & Francis; 2005. p. 89–100. Chapter 6.
56. Blumenfeld Z. How to preserve fertility in young women exposed to chemotherapy? The role of GnRH agonist cotreatment in addition to cryopreservation of embryos, oocytes, or ovaries. Oncologist 2007;12:1044–54.
57. Blumenfeld Z. GnRH-agonist in fertility preservation. Curr Opin Endocrinol Diabetes Obes 2008;15:523–8.

58. Badawy A, Elnashar A, El-Ashry M, et al. Gonadotropin-releasing hormone agonists for prevention of chemotherapy-induced ovarian damage: prospective randomized study. Fertil Steril 2008;91:694–7.
59. Blumenfeld Z, Avivi I, Eckman A, et al. Gonadotropin-releasing hormone agonist decreases chemotherapy-induced gonadotoxicity and premature ovarian failure in young female patients with Hodgkin lymphoma. Fertil Steril 2008;89:166–73.
60. Meirow D. Fertility preservation in cancer patients using stored ovarian tissue: clinical aspects. Curr Opin Endocrinol Diabetes Obes 2008;15:536–47.

Pediatric Obesity: Etiology and Treatment

Melissa K. Crocker, MBA, MD, Jack A. Yanovski, MD, PhD*

KEYWORDS

- Overweight • Differential diagnosis • Pharmacotherapy
- Bariatric surgery • Adiposity • Leptin

In the United States, the prevalence of pediatric overweight, defined by the Centers for Disease Control as a body mass index (BMI) ≥95th percentile for age and sex, has more than tripled during the past 4 decades.[1–3] Of children and adolescents, 16.3% are now obese, and an additional 15.6% are classified as overweight (BMI in the 85th–95th percentile).[3] Of all children, 11.3% have a BMI that exceeds the 97th percentile for age and sex,[3] a degree of excess weight that some believe may be a reasonable cut-point for pediatric obesity.[4] Some racial and ethnic minority populations, especially African American, Hispanic, and American Indian groups, are at particular risk for the development of overweight and obesity.[3] The increase in obesity prevalence among children is particularly alarming because obesity-related diseases rarely seen in children in the past, including obesity-associated sleep apnea,[5] non-alcoholic fatty liver disease[6] with resultant cirrhosis,[7] and type 2 diabetes,[8,9] are increasingly diagnosed in pediatric patients. The earlier onset of chronic health conditions such as type 2 diabetes in childhood has been shown to lead to an earlier onset of related medical complications such as end-stage renal disease.[10] Pediatric obesity has been shown to have a tremendous impact on later health,[11] even independent of adult weight.[12] In the absence of effective strategies to prevent and treat childhood obesity, millions of children will enter adulthood with the physical and psychologic consequences of excess adiposity. The current childhood obesity epidemic in the United States also has the potential to reverse the improvements in life expectancy that have been seen during the twentieth century[13] and to result in more functional disability and decreased quality of life for those who survive to old age.[14]

Portions of this article were previously published in the Endocrinology and Metabolism Clinics of North America, 38:3.

This research was supported by the Intramural Research Program of the Eunice Kennedy Shriver National Institute of Child Health and Human Development. Dr Yanovski is a Commissioned Officer in the United States Public Health Service, Department of Health and Human Services.

Unit on Growth and Obesity, Program in Developmental Endocrinology and Genetics, Eunice Kennedy Shriver National Institute of Child Health and Human Development, National Institutes of Health, Department of Health and Human Services, 9000 Rockville Pike, Hatfield Clinical Research Center, Room 1-3330, MSC 1103, Bethesda, MD, 20892-1103, USA

* Corresponding author.

E-mail address: jy15i@nih.gov

This article reviews factors that contribute to excessive weight gain in children and outlines current knowledge regarding approaches for treating pediatric obesity.

ETIOLOGY

Obesity is a genetic disease, because all available data suggest that 60% to 80% of the observed variance in human body weight can be accounted for by inherited factors.[15] Obesity is also just as clearly an environmentally caused disorder; our genetic endowments have changed minimally during the last 40 years, yet the prevalence of abnormally high BMI in US children has tripled, an observation that can only be explained by changes in external factors affecting children's energy economy (**Fig. 1**).

Some theorists hypothesize that in the past it was evolutionarily advantageous for proto-humans to have to the capacity to consume energy in excess of the quantity now needed to maintain normal body composition. One version of this theory proposes that overeating enough to store calories in adipose tissue would augment the human's ability to survive periods of relative starvation. Another version makes the assumption that normal daily human energy expenditure was frequently significantly greater than commonly found today, such that most humans had body weight below that considered ideal in terms of reproductive fitness. All versions of this hypothesis lead to an expectation that natural selection would favor polymorphisms in perhaps many genes that would predispose children and adults to overeat whenever excessive energy was available. More than 300 genetic loci that are potentially

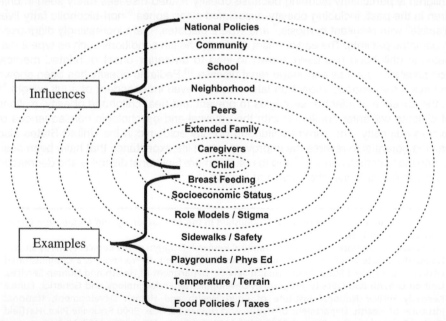

Fig. 1. A social-ecological model of influences on pediatric obesity and its treatment. Levels of environmental influence begin with the family environment and extend to larger spheres of influence, including peers as well as neighborhoods, schools, community, and national factors. Some of the influences within each of these spheres are also given. For instance, the neighborhood environment may influence children's activity if there are no sidewalks or if safe areas for play are not available. (*Courtesy of* Denise E. Wilfley, PhD, St Louis, MO.)

involved in human body weight regulation have been identified through analyses in humans, rodents, and *Caenorhabditis elegans*.[16,17] Some exceedingly rare gene variants affect gene function and behavior to such an extent that obesity results even without a particularly "obesogenic" environment (**Fig. 2**), but the vast majority of genetic factors are presumed to affect body weight enough to cause obesity only when specific environmental conditions pertain. Factors known to influence body weight are described in the following sections.

Classical Endocrine Disorders Associated with Weight Gain

Children with identifiable endocrinopathies are believed to comprise only a small minority of children referred for the evaluation of overweight, ranging from 2% to 3%[18]; however, because treatment of these conditions generally resolves obesity, they are frequently considered.

Hypothyroidism

Hypothyroidism is associated with modest weight gain and may cause a BMI increase in children of approximately 1 to 2 BMI units (ie, only a few kilograms).[19] Hypothyroidism leads to increased permeability of capillary walls,[20] which creates extravascular leakage and retention of water[21] causing excess weight gain; consequently, most of the weight gained in patients who have hypothyroidism appears to be fluid rather than triglyceride. Resting energy expenditure may also decrease, potentially

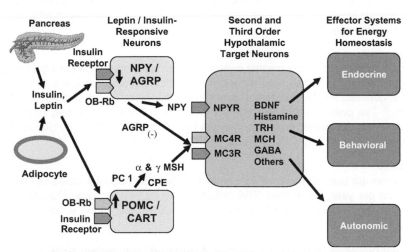

Fig. 2. A simplified model of the leptin-signaling pathway. Central insulin can bind to the same neurons as leptin and is an anorexigenic signal. The ligands leptin, POMC, CART, and BDNF, the receptors for leptin, melanocortins, and BDNF, and the enzyme PC1 have been found to have function-altering mutations associated with obesity in children. Mutations in the ligands and receptors for NPY, AGRP, CPE, and MCH have been found to cause excessive weight gain when mutated in rodents but have not been as convincingly shown to be associated with human obesity. AGRP, agouti-related protein; BDNF, brain-derived neurotrophic factor; CART, cocaine-amphetamine related transcript; CPE, carboxypeptidase E; GABA, gamma amino butyric acid; MCH, melanin-concentrating hormone; MC3R, melanocortin 3 receptor; MC4R, melanocortin 4 receptor; MSH, melanocyte-stimulating hormone; NPY, neuropeptide Y; NPYR, neuropeptide Y receptor; OB-Rb, signal-transducing form of the leptin receptor; PC1, prohormone convertase 1; POMC, pro-opiomelanocortin; TRH, thyrotropin-releasing hormone.

biasing energy balance toward storage of ingested calories.[22] Because children with hypothyroidism usually have diminished linear growth, their BMI may be high even though weight does not exceed the 95th percentile.[23] Any overweight child with a diminution of linear growth should be evaluated for the possibility of hypothyroidism with measurement of both serum thyroid-stimulating hormone and free T4 concentrations. Few data are available regarding the weight response in children treated for hypothyroidism, but the accelerated linear growth during treatment of these children appears to lead to a reduction in BMI.[24]

Growth hormone deficiency

In obese children who have no true endocrinopathy, the 24-hour secretion of growth hormone (GH), the GH peak during the night,[25] and the GH response to various pharmacologic stimuli are invariably diminished.[26–29] Interpretation of the results of provocative testing in obese children may be difficult. Growth velocity is either normal or supranormal, and the concentration of insulin-like growth factor 1 (IGF-1) is generally normal or only modestly decreased in obesity,[30,31] whereas both growth velocity and IGF-1 are diminished in true GH deficiency. Diminished linear growth that is accompanied by continued increase in body weight should lead to consideration of GH deficiency.

In addition to its ability to stimulate protein synthesis and increase fat-free mass, GH also stimulates adipocyte lipolysis.[32] GH deficiency leads to increased fat mass, especially in a central distribution, along with decreased lean mass. Adults with GH deficiency are more likely to develop metabolic syndrome.[33] In GH-deficient children, improvements in body composition can be detected as early as 6 weeks after the initiation of GH therapy.[34]

Cushing syndrome

Cushing syndrome in adults causes central obesity, although the weight gain may be more generalized in children. The excess glucocorticoid production leads to increased gluconeogenesis, insulin resistance, inhibition of lipolysis,[35] and stimulation of lipogenesis.[36] The prevalence of Cushing syndrome in children is low; only one child in every million is diagnosed with endogenous hypercortisolism. Obesity due to hypercortisolism is associated with markedly diminished height velocity.[37,38]

Insulinoma

Insulinomas are even rarer in children, with an incidence rate of 4 cases per 5 million population per year; fewer than 10% occur before 20 years of age. Elevated insulin production leads to increased food intake to counter lower blood sugars and leads to obesity.[39,40]

Structural Disorders of the Hypothalamus Associated with Weight Gain

Hypothalamic obesity may arise after injury to, or congenital malformation of, the hypothalamus. The ventromedial hypothalamic nucleus, arcuate nucleus, paraventricular nucleus, dorsomedial nucleus, and the lateral hypothalamic area are all involved in control of appetite and energy expenditure. These areas produce several neuropeptides involved in appetite regulation, including orexigenic peptides such as neuropeptide Y and anorexigenic peptides such as the melanocortins (see **Fig. 2**).[41] Injury or malformation may also affect binding of peripheral intake-related signals, including cholecystokinin, glucagon-like peptide, ghrelin, insulin, and leptin. These peptides cross the blood-brain barrier and bind to their receptors in the hypothalamus to regulate appetite. Loss of function of the hypothalamic developmental factor Sim1 leads to obesity in mice. Chromosomal deletions inactivating one copy of Sim1 have also been found to be associated with obesity in humans,[42] although point mutations in Sim1 associated with obesity are not common.[43] Many congenital disorders associated with hypothalamic neuroanatomical disruption are associated with obesity. Obesity occurs in approximately 50% of children treated surgically for craniopharyngioma.[33,44,45]

Leptin Signaling Pathway Genes

One of the major advances in obesity science over the last 15 years has been elucidation of the leptin signaling pathway (see **Fig. 2**). Inactivating mutations affecting these genes may account for as much as 3% or 4% of severe, early-onset obesity.

Leptin

Leptin is produced by adipose tissues and binds to leptin receptors in the arcuate nucleus and elsewhere in the brain. Leptin concentrations rise with increasing fat mass; individuals with low fat mass, such as those with lipodystrophy syndromes and anorexia nervosa, have low circulating leptin concentrations.[46–49] Fasting acutely lowers leptin, and absence of sufficient leptin is a potent signal that stimulates food seeking and consummatory behaviors and promotes reduced energy use. Restoration of normal leptin concentration leads to reductions in food intake[50,51] and changes in activation of brain regions involved in appetitive control.[52] Inactivating mutations affecting both alleles of the leptin gene result in excessive food intake and severe, early-onset obesity in the context of very low (<5 ng/mL) serum leptin concentrations.[53,54] These features are successfully reversed with leptin therapy.[50] Heterozygous leptin deficiency may present with no findings other than somewhat lower leptin concentrations out of proportion to fat mass.[55] Individuals with inactivating mutations of both alleles of the leptin receptor gene may also have central hypothyroidism and excess cortisol along with delay in sexual development[56]; heterozygotes appear to have a normal phenotype.[57] Leptin receptor mutations were first described in the context of markedly supraphysiologic serum leptin; however, more recent studies suggest substantial overlap in serum leptin among those with and without function-altering leptin receptor mutations.[58] Leptin concentrations have not been successfully used to identify patients bearing leptin receptor abnormalities.

Pro-opiomelanocortin

In some leptin-responsive hypothalamic neurons, leptin stimulates the production of pro-opiomelanocortin (POMC), which is the precursor for corticotropin (ACTH), alpha, beta, and gamma melanocyte-stimulating hormone (MSH), beta-lipoprotein, and beta-endorphin. Alpha-MSH binds to the melanocortin receptors MC3R and MC4R in the arcuate nucleus to regulate appetite and energy expenditure. A handful of patients have been described who have inactivating mutations of POMC that prevent its cleavage into alpha-MSH or ACTH. Such patients have hyperphagia (presumed secondary to absent signaling at MC3R and MC4R), red hair (lack of peripheral alpha-MSH to bind at melanocortin 1 receptors), and adrenal insufficiency (insufficient ACTH to bind at adrenal melanocortin 2 receptors).[59–64]

Pro-opiomelanocortin processing

Mutations in prohormone convertase 1 (PC1), an enzyme that cleaves POMC, have also been found in a few pediatric patients. PC1 is involved in the processing of numerous hormones. PC1 deficiency presents not only with obesity and ACTH deficiency but also with postprandial hypoglycemia (insufficient cleavage of pro-insulin), hypogonadotropic hypogonadism, and small bowel malabsorption.[65–67]

Melanocortin receptors

Alpha-MSH exerts it effects on weight regulation by binding to MC3R and MC4R.[68] MC3R appears to act by affecting feeding efficiency,[69–71] whereas MC4R seems mostly involved in appetite regulation in mouse models. In humans, heterozygous and homozygous MC4R mutations cause obesity, hyperphagia, hyperinsulinism, and increased linear growth during childhood.[72] MC4R inactivating mutations are the most common known cause of severe, early-onset obesity; in some series, as many as 3% of patients may have heterozygous or homozygous inactivating MC4R mutations.[73] Recent data suggest that MC4R is important not only for body weight but also for blood pressure regulation via effects on the sympathetic nervous system.[74] Some data also support a role for polymorphisms in the MC3R for regulation of body weight, particularly in African American children.[75]

Brain-derived neurotrophic factor

Brain-derived neurotrophic factor (BDNF) is believed to function downstream from MC4R in the leptin signaling pathway. In mice, haploinsufficiency for BDNF or its receptor TrkB leads to obesity. Haploinsufficiency for BDNF has been suggested to be the cause of pediatric-onset obesity in patients with WAGR syndrome (Wilms' tumor, aniridia, genitourinary malformations, and mental retardation), which results from heterozygous contiguous 11p gene deletions.[76] In one recent case series, 100% of patients with WAGR syndrome whose deletions included BDNF were obese by age 10 years; serum BDNF concentrations in such patients were found to be reduced by 50% when compared with serum BDNF in patients with WAGR syndrome retaining two copies of the BDNF gene. A heterozygous inactivating mutation in the gene coding for the BDNF receptor TrkB has also been found in a single patient with obesity, seizures, and developmental delay.[77]

Albright's hereditary osteodystrophy

Albright's hereditary osteodystrophy describes a phenotype of short stature and obesity found in pseudohypoparathyroidism 1a (PHP1a) and in pseudopseudohypoparathyroidism (PPHP), both of which are the result of inactivating defects in the Gs alpha protein complex. PHP1a is the result of maternally derived mutations, whereas PPHP is caused by paternally derived gene abnormalities. PHP1a is also associated with endocrinopathies resulting from insufficient signal transduction through the Gs alpha subunit in tissues where expression of Gs alpha is affected by paternal imprinting. PPHP does not have such associated endocrine disorders but presents with the Albright's hereditary osteodystrophy phenotype, although the obesity is less severe.[78] The etiology of the obesity in PHP1a may be related, in part, to diminished signaling via the Gs alpha subunit in the many Gs alpha-coupled receptors found in the leptin pathway.[79]

Common Allelic Variation in Genes that May Affect Energy Balance

Single nucleotide polymorphisms (SNPs) of many genes and chromosomal regions have been found to be associated with body weight or body composition.[80–82] The mechanisms explaining how such SNPs might change energy balance are often not fully understood. Even in studies including thousands of genotyped people, such SNPs can be linked to body weight only when they are relatively common in the population.

Fat mass and obesity associated gene locus

Recent genome-wide association studies have found that common SNPs in the fat mass and obesity associated (FTO) gene locus are consistently associated with higher

BMI and adiposity in children and adults.[83–87] Rodent studies indicate that *FTO* mRNA is highly expressed in brain areas important for regulation of energy- and reward-driven consumption.[88] Food deprivation alters *FTO* expression in the hypothalamus in rats and mice.[88–90] When compared with children with the more common *FTO* T allele at rs9939609, children with two copies of the A allele variant have greater BMI and fat mass. Some limited data also suggest such children may have greater food intake[91,92] and reduced satiety[93] but show no differences in energy expenditure.[91]

Peroxisome proliferator-activated receptors

Peroxisome proliferator-activated receptors (PPAR-γ) help regulate metabolism and storage of fat and are involved in differentiation of adipocytes from precursors. A rare gain-of-function mutation is associated with extreme obesity.[94] Heterozygous Pro12Ala substitution is associated with a differential response to dietary fats; a high saturated fat intake compared with polyunsaturated fats leads to higher fasting insulin levels in patients with this allelic variation.[95]

Beta adrenergic receptor

Activation of the beta-2 adrenergic receptor stimulates lipolysis in adipocytes. Polymorphisms rs1042713 (Arg16) and rs1042714 (Glu27) have shown associations with obesity, although the data show some inconsistencies among studies. A recent meta-analysis described increased risk for obesity among Asians, Pacific Islanders, and American Indians with the Glu27 variation. No other populations reached statistical significance for obesity risk factors with either of these polymorphisms.[96]

Perilipin

Perilipin proteins protect lipid droplets in adipocytes from unregulated lipolysis. Studies of the perilipin A gene have suggested that carriers of some perilipin SNPs may be more resistant to weight loss when compared with controls.[97]

Syndromic Obesity

Multiple genetic syndromes involve obesity as part of their presentation, although patients with these syndromes usually come to medical attention for reasons other than obesity. Even when grouped together, these etiologies (**Box 1**) account for only a small percentage of overweight children. All of these syndromes involve multiple other medical problems or dysmorphic features. The root of obesity in these disorders is often poorly understood.

Particularly notable for hyperphagia are the Prader-Willi, Bardet-Biedl, and Alström syndromes. Patients with Prader-Willi syndrome display high circulating concentrations of ghrelin,[98] a factor that is primarily stomach-derived and is a peripheral orexigen, at least in short-term studies in humans.[99] The role of hyperghrelinemia in the obesity of Prader-Willi syndrome remains in dispute. The Bardet-Biedl and Alström syndromes appear to be associated with disruption of ciliary function. Cilia have been demonstrated to be necessary for body weight regulation in mice, in which inducible disruption of primary cilia by inactivating the ciliogenic genes Tg737 and Kif3a specifically in POMC-expressing neurons leads to hyperphagia and obesity.[100] Some recent data also suggest that the proteins affected by several of the Bardet-Biedl syndromes may interact with the leptin receptor and alter its trafficking.[101]

Acquired Obesity

Medications associated with weight gain

Multiple medications may lead to weight gain. Iatrogenic obesity can result from administration of insulin or insulin secretagogues, glucocorticoids, psychotropic drugs

---

Box 1
Genetic syndromes associated with obesity

Achondroplasia

Alström syndrome

Bannayan-Riley-Ruvalcaba syndrome

Bardet-Biedl syndrome

Beckwith-Wiedemann syndrome

Borjeson-Forssman-Lehmann syndrome

Carpenter syndrome

CDG 1a

Cohen syndrome

Fragile X

Mehmo syndrome

Meningomyelocoele

Prader-Willi syndrome

Pseudohypoparathyroidism 1a

Simpson-Golabi-Behmel syndrome

Smith-Magenis syndrome

Sotos syndrome

Turner syndrome

Ulnar-Mammary Schinzel syndrome

Weaver syndrome

Wilson-Turner syndrome

---

including antipsychotics such as olanzapine and clozapine, mood stabilizers such as lithium, antidepressants including the tricyclics, anticonvulsants such as valproate and carbamazepine, antihypertensives including propranolol, nifedipine, and clonidine, antihistamines, and chemotherapeutic agents.[102]

AD36: the "obesity virus"

An avian form of adenovirus has been found to cause increased adiposity in infected chickens, both from spontaneous infection and inoculation.[103] After the publication of that observation, the consequence of infection with human adenovirus strain AD36 on body weight was studied in rhesus monkeys, marmosets,[104] chickens, and mice.[105] All species showed increased adipose tissue but paradoxically decreased serum cholesterol in those infected with the virus. In vitro studies of human adipose-derived stem/stromal cells infected with AD36 demonstrate increased accumulation of lipids and induction of pre-adipocytes to become lipid-accumulating adipocytes.[106] Prevalence studies suggest that humans with antibodies to AD36 (indicating past infection) also tend to have higher rates of obesity and lower serum cholesterol and triglycerides[107]; twin pair studies have also demonstrated associations between sero-positivity for AD36 and higher BMI and body fat.[108] Such evidence suggests this virus may potentially have a role in acquired obesity.

Environment and behavior

As outlined in **Fig. 1**, the sociocultural environment has a major role in determining who becomes obese. This observation is demonstrated by comparing human samples that share the same genetic background but are raised in different cultures. Arizona Pima Indians who live on a reservation have much higher rates of obesity and diabetes than their counterparts in an isolated Mexican village,[109] and Asian and Hispanic adolescents born in the United States have a higher prevalence of obesity than immigrant members of the same community.[110] A full discussion of social and environmental factors is beyond the scope of this article but has been elegantly summarized elsewhere.[111,112]

Epigenetics

The differential response of some people to environmental conditions may be the result of genetic variation alone, but there is increasing recognition that genetic expression related to disease risk may be modified by the environment during development. These so-called "epigenetic changes" include methylation and alterations to histone proteins that alter the likelihood that specific genes are transcribed. Epigenetic changes usually occur during prenatal development or the early postnatal period. Strong evidence suggests that maternal nutrition is a key factor leading to epigenetic changes. Maternal nutrition includes levels of vitamins consumed in pregnancy, such as folate, methionine, and vitamin B_{12}, which affect methylation.[113] Undernutrition during prenatal development has been suggested to lead to postnatal consumption of a fatty diet.[114] The most convincingly shown factor is glycemic status during pregnancy. Hyperglycemia clearly affects infants' birth weight but, beyond its effects on body weight, may increase the risk for subsequent development of insulin resistance and obesity. Nutritional signals reaching the developing hypothalamus during pregnancy may influence the sensitivity of these neurons to respond to similar signals postnatally.[113] Infant nutrition in the neonatal period may also potentially affect future risk for obesity and its complications. Although some studies have shown protection against obesity after extended breastfeeding, others have not confirmed these findings.[113]

Evaluation

Most genetic and hormonal causes of obesity are rare. The decision to test for these abnormalities should depend upon the presence of clinical features suggesting the possibility of a diagnosable disorder. **Fig. 3** provides an algorithm for this evaluation.

THERAPY
Indications

The Maternal and Child Health Bureau of the Department of Health and Human Services recommended in 1998 that children aged 7 years and older with a BMI greater than the 95th percentile for age should be offered obesity interventions.[115] For adolescents, a cut-off BMI of 30 kg/m² should be used when the 95th percentile standard is above 30 kg/m².[116] Some practitioners refer to these patients as obese, whereas others avoid the terminology in pediatrics given the associated stigma and instead describe these patients as "at risk for obesity" or "overweight." "Overweight" is the word choice that children with a BMI ≥95th percentile greatly prefer.[117] Consensus statements from the American Academy of Pediatrics as well as from the Endocrine Society recommend use of the term obesity to denote elevated adipose tissue.[116,118] Some suggest a BMI above the 99th percentile should be called severe obesity.[116] Regardless of the title, the prevalence of comorbidities rises as BMI increases, such that half of those persons with a BMI exceeding the 99th percentile

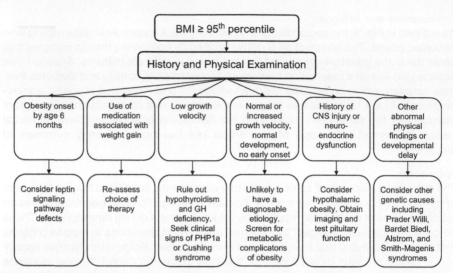

Fig. 3. An algorithm for the evaluation of an obese child. Physical examination, growth patterns, and the child's age should narrow the scope of the differential diagnosis and dictate appropriate testing.

meet criteria for the metabolic syndrome.[119] Those with a BMI in the 85th to 95th percentiles, referred to as overweight in both sets of guidelines[116,118] and by the Centers for Disease Control, should also be considered for dietary counseling if they have overfatness but should probably not be involved with medical or surgical treatments unless they already sustain medical complications secondary to obesity. The American Academy of Pediatrics expert panel has recommended assessing risk factors for these patients, including family history, trends in the patient's weight gain, their fitness level, and the distribution of adipose tissue versus lean mass to determine the need for intervention.[116] Additionally, the American Academy of Pediatrics expert panel, noting that younger patients have the benefit of significant future vertical growth, has suggested such growth can compensate for weight already gained; therefore, the goal for young patients (particularly those aged <5 years) is weight maintenance to allow the height to attain the same percentile as the weight. Nevertheless, there are few data demonstrating that approaches aiming for weight maintenance, rather than weight reduction, are successful in reducing adiposity. For older children, weight loss is needed, because for most height gain alone will not correct the obesity; for these children, a goal of 0.5 to 1 kg loss per month is appropriate, although adolescents may tolerate 1 to 2 kg of weight loss per month.[116]

Interventions for obesity in pediatric patients range from basic diets and lifestyle interventions to more intensive very low energy diets, medications, and surgery. Each of these methods has varying levels of success, both short and long term, as well as side effects that must be considered. None of these interventions will be successful if the patient and family lack motivation and education. The participation and cooperation of the entire family is critical regardless of the mode of therapy employed.

Diets

Several dietary approaches are available, including low fat, low carbohydrate, low calorie, Mediterranean (based on diets of that region which are high in olive oil and nuts), and others. Despite many studies in adults comparing and contrasting these diets, few have been performed on adolescents and fewer still in younger children. A meta-analysis through February 2006 has examined trials using diet alone as a weight loss intervention in pediatrics. Six such articles were found using a comprehensive literature review, including studies that employed a reduced glycemic load diet, a protein-sparing modified diet, a low carbohydrate diet, a high protein diet, and a hypocaloric diet. Overall pooled benefit showed an effect size of only 0.22 points in the treatment arms.[120] Although dietary therapy in the context of behavioral management is recommended for all obese children because some children experience long-lasting weight reductions and do not require other therapy,[121] diets by themselves are considered relatively ineffective for those with severe obesity.

Very low energy diets are based on restricting energy intake to 600 to 800 kilocalories per day. In the past, these diets were frequently liquid based but may be food based and are usually designed to be "protein-sparing modified fasts" intended to maximize fat loss while minimizing loss of lean body mass. These diets are reviewed in detail elsewhere.[122] To avoid nutritional deficiencies, such diets must contain 1.5 to 2.5 g of high quality protein per kilogram of ideal body weight. Typically, such diets limit carbohydrates to 20 to 40 g per day. A multivitamin should be included in the daily regimen given the lack of sources for many critical elements. A total of 1500 mL of free water is also recommended to avoid dehydration. These diets are rapid in their weight loss among teens (up to 11 kg in 10 weeks has been noted); most published data limit the length of the diet to 12 weeks. These diets are generally prescribed only in patients who need to lose substantial amounts of weight (ie, adolescents usually above the 99th percentile for body weight). Risks associated with the rapid weight loss include cholelithiasis, hyperuricemia, decreased serum proteins, orthostatic hypotension, halitosis, and diarrhea.[122] Unfortunately, the short-term improvement in weight is often reversed in the long term when regular dietary habits are resumed.[123] Most clinicians refrain from using such diets in children unless rapid weight loss is needed for medical purposes.

Exercise

Most recommendations for weight loss rarely endorse exercise without additional dietary intervention. A few pediatric studies have analyzed weight loss from exercise alone. A meta-analysis examining 17 of these trials in pediatric patients demonstrated inconsistent results across studies. Studies that considered adiposity as the outcome found a moderate decrease in the treatment arm, but those using BMI as the outcome saw little or no effect. When the effect of a combination of exercise and diet was analyzed among 23 trials, there was a small-to-moderate effect of intervention. The largest change in weight was found in the trials that involved parents in the therapy. Although not statistically significant, there was a trend toward improved outcomes in younger children, primarily those aged 8 years or less.[120]

Behavior Modification

Behavior modification as an approach to weight loss may include encouragement to reduce screen time and increase physical activity, psychologic training to motivate a change in eating behaviors or exercise, family counseling to support weight loss goals, and school-based changes to promote physical activity and healthy eating. Often, these interventions involve frequent meetings with a counselor individually or in group sessions. Studies employing these techniques have recently been reviewed elsewhere.[124] A Cochrane review[125] compared four studies of children aged less than 12 years and three studies of adolescents enrolled in behavioral intervention versus conventional treatment. Among the children under 12 years, there was a 0.06 point change in BMI standard deviation score (SDS) in the parent-focused behavioral interventions. Among the older patients, a 0.14 point decrease in BMI SDS and a 3.04 point decrease in BMI were seen with behavioral therapy.[125] A meta-analysis of 14 studies using behavioral interventions compared with no intervention or standard weight loss counseling interventions found significant but small effect sizes ranging from 0.48 to 0.91.[126] Although short-term success has primarily been the endpoint of behavior modification, one group has shown long-term improvement in weight control over 10-year periods when the family was also involved in counseling and behavior changes.[121,127,128] Some data support better maintenance of weight loss using continued behavioral management strategies.[129]

Schools settings may serve as outlets for implementing behavior modification programs. One study of increased exercise during an after school program, which also served healthy snacks, showed a decrease in body fat throughout the school year but negative progress during the summer.[130] Another study provided education on nutrition and healthy behaviors during school along with physical activity sessions; results demonstrated decreases in obesity rates over several years, although only in females.[131]

Recommendations on Combined Treatment Approaches

The American Academy of Pediatrics recommends a four-step approach to obesity treatment, the first three of which are dietary and lifestyle interventions of escalating intensity.[116] If there is insufficient progress after 3 to 6 months, the guidelines recommend advancing to each successive stage and, finally, to referral to obesity management experts for specialized interventions such as medication or surgery.[116]

Medications

Although several forms of medications to treat obesity are on the market, only one is approved for children aged less than 16 years. Success has been limited with these medications, which usually only show promise in combination with exercise and dietary interventions. The Endocrine Society has suggested limiting pharmacotherapy to patients with a BMI over the 95th percentile who have failed diet and lifestyle intervention, or in limited cases with a BMI over the 85th percentile and severe comorbidities.[118] Others have suggested, given the limited efficacy of medications, that only pediatric-aged patients with a BMI over the 95th percentile who also have significant medical complications of their obesity should be exposed to the risks of obesity pharmacotherapy.[132]

Anorexigenic agents

A major class of medications used in weight treatment is appetite suppressants. Currently available agents affect the neurotransmitters norepinephrine, dopamine, and serotonin in the brain to regulate appetite.[133] In 1997, the appetite suppressant sibutramine was approved by the US Food and Drug Administration (FDA) for long-term use in adults. Sibutramine was removed from use in 2010, when a greater incidence of cardiovascular events were found among adults who took the drug. Sibutramine inhibited reuptake of all three of these anorexigenic neurotransmitters. The increased levels of these hypothalamic neurotransmitters promote satiety and decrease hunger.[134] Side effects included hypertension, tachycardia, premature ventricular contractions, prolonged QTc, insomnia, dizziness, dry mouth, cholelithiasis, and constipation.[122,134] Four randomized controlled trials examined the effect of sibutramine on weight in adolescents and on average found 7.7 kg of weight loss in the short term.[134] A meta-analysis of three of these trials showed a change in BMI by 2.4 units after 6 months of medication treatment.[120] The largest sibutramine trial enrolled 498 patients aged 12 to 16 years with a BMI 2 points above the 95th percentile for age and randomized them to sibutramine or placebo. After 12 months of therapy, 24% of the treatment group and 38% of the placebo group had left the study. Of those remaining, the sibutramine group had a decrease in BMI by 2.9 units more than the control arm; however, they also had a statistically significant increase in tachycardia.[135] There were no published reports of sibutramine treatment for adolescent obesity that have lasted longer than 1 year.[122] Another trial has examined the use of sibutramine in patients with syndromes or conditions that made behavioral interventions difficult. Of the 50 patients, 22 had hypothalamic obesity from central nervous system damage, Bardet-Biedl syndrome, MC4R mutations, or Prader-Willi syndrome. The other 28 patients had mental retardation, autism spectrum disorder, attention deficit hyperactivity disorder, or a myelomeningocele. During a cross-over period during which each group received sibutramine for 20 weeks and placebo for 20 weeks, the overall loss of BMI SDS was 0.7 units on sibutramine; however, the hypothalamic obesity group only lost 0.3 to 0.4 BMI SD units, whereas the remaining patients lost closer to 0.9 to 1 BMI SD units.[136]

Other neurotransmitter regulators that are marketed for weight loss include phentermine, chlorphentermine, mazindol, and diethylpropion, all of which have shown short-term weight loss of 2 to 5 kg in excess of placebo over 1 to 3 months in adults. There are no long-term follow-up data in pediatric samples for these medications. Ephedrine in combination with caffeine induced significant weight loss but was banned by the FDA after reported deaths from hypertensive crises and arrhythmias. Fenfluramine was also withdrawn after valvulopathies developed due to what appears to have been a serotonin excess syndrome.[137] Another appetite suppressant, rimonabant, which has never been FDA-approved in the United States and was recently withdrawn in Europe, works as an inhibitor of the central nervous system cannabinoid type 1 receptor, leading to decreased appetite; rimonabant probably also acts peripherally to increase thermogenesis.[138] No randomized controlled trials have been published in adolescents. In adults, side effects included anxiety, depression, insomnia, dizziness, nausea, and vomiting.

Gastrointestinal lipase inhibition

Blocking the absorption of fat from the gastrointestinal tract provides another medical approach to weight loss. Orlistat, an inhibitor of gastrointestinal lipases, prevents the breakdown of triglycerides into absorbable fatty acids and monoglycerols. When orlistat 120 mg capsules are taken three times a day with meals, approximately one third of dietary triglycerides are excreted intact rather than absorbed. Side effects of this medication include oily stools, flatulence, and uncontrolled leakage of oil from the rectum. In addition, gallbladder disease has been seen in greater frequency in trials of orlistat when compared with a control group. Diminished fat absorption also limits absorption of the fat-soluble vitamins A, D, E, and K; therefore, a multivitamin should be part of the diet regimen, with consumption of the vitamin more than 2 hours apart from administration of orlistat. Additionally, because orlistat must be consumed at each meal, pediatric patients will require therapy during school hours, which adds logistical complications to the regimen.[118] An analysis of three randomized control trials in adolescents found a net loss of 0.7 units in the BMI but with increased rates of abdominal pain and discomfort as well as oily stools when compared with placebo.[120] The largest adolescent orlistat study[139] enrolled 539 patients aged 12 to 16 years who were randomized to placebo or orlistat. After 1 year of therapy, approximately 35% of participants had dropped out. The BMI in the orlistat group fell by 0.55 and rose by 0.31 kg/m^2 in the placebo group, leading to a small but significant difference in BMI. Although adult patients have experienced improvement in glucose and insulin levels while taking orlistat, no similar effects have been observed in the pediatric studies conducted to date.[134]

Therapies altering insulin secretion or insulin resistance

Another medical approach to weight control involves metformin, which inhibits hepatic gluconeogenesis, diminishes insulin resistance and hyperinsulinemia, and may decrease lipogenesis in adipose tissues.[134] Currently, metformin is approved for treatment of type 2 diabetes mellitus in patients aged 10 years and older. Several randomized controlled trials have evaluated metformin as an obesity medication in adolescents, including one trial lasting 48 weeks[140] and one in children 6–12y.[141] An average loss of 3.15 kg was noted by one investigator,[134] although another meta-analysis described the pooled results as "a small nonsignificant change in obesity outcome at 6 months."[120] Additionally, a randomized controlled trial of 39 patients (of whom 30 completed the study) aged 10 to 17 years taking atypical antipsychotics showed a decrease of 0.13 kg and 0.43 BMI points in the metformin arm compared with a weight gain of 4.01 kg and BMI gain of 1.12 points in the placebo arm after 16 weeks of intervention.[142] Improvements in steatohepatitis have also been noted.[122] All studies thus far are 1 year or shorter; therefore, the degree of long-term improvement in body weight or its complications is unknown. Patients treated with metformin report abdominal discomfort, which improves when the medication is taken with food. There is also a risk of vitamin B$_{12}$ deficiency; therefore, a multivitamin is recommended.[122] There is a risk of lactic acidosis, which has been observed in adults but not seen in pediatric patients thus far.[134] Metformin is contraindicated in heart, kidney, and liver disease; however, because the clearance is renal, patients with liver function tests less than three times the upper limit of normal are considered appropriate to take the medication.

Octreotide has been investigated as a treatment for hypothalamic obesity. This somatostatin analogue binds receptors on the beta cells of the pancreas and inhibits insulin release. A randomized controlled trial comparing octreotide with placebo demonstrated reduced weight gain among those treated with octreotide given subcutaneously three times per day. Over 6 months, the placebo group experienced an average weight gain of 9.2 kg and a BMI change by 2.2 points, whereas the treatment group gained 1.6 kg and decreased their BMI by 0.2.[143] Because of its mode of action, octreotide use is associated with significant risks for cholelithiasis and abnormalities of glucose homeostasis.

Leptin

Leptin poses another possibility for obesity treatment. Thus far, clinical trials in obese subjects without leptin deficiency have shown only small effects on weight loss. Leptin must be delivered as frequent subcutaneous injections given its short half-life, and patients in these studies experienced painful injection site reactions, especially in the larger dosages needed to alter body weight.[144] Among those rare individuals with true leptin deficiency, leptin is effective at reducing BMI and fat mass over the long term.[50,145]

Bariatric Surgery

Bariatric surgery is by far the most definitive and longest lasting form of weight loss treatment. In adults, surgical intervention leads to significant weight loss and improvement or resolution of multiple other problems, including type 2 diabetes, hypertension, and obstructive sleep apnea. Similar effects have been noted in smaller studies of adolescents following bariatric surgery.[146] Surgical interventions are not without significant drawbacks. As with any surgery, immediate complications can include mild wound infections, more serious pneumonias and abscesses, and life-threatening pulmonary emboli and sepsis. Bowel obstructions and perforations are also described. The decision to perform bariatric surgery should not be taken lightly.

Adult patients are considered candidates for bariatric surgery if they have a BMI of 40 or higher, or a BMI of 35 or higher along with comorbid conditions directly as a result of their weight. For pediatric patients, most practitioners of bariatric surgery recommend a stricter guideline of a BMI greater than 50, or a BMI greater than 40 with comorbidities present along with insufficient weight loss from at least a 6-month trial of a nonsurgical weight loss program.[118,147–149] Given that nutritional insufficiencies after surgery could impact growth and development, guidelines recommend that adolescents have achieved Tanner IV staging in their pubertal development and a bone age that demonstrates 95% of their final height has been reached.[147] Extensive pre- and postoperative counseling and evaluation are required from a multidisciplinary team,[150] particularly to evaluate the family's capacity to support the patient and the patient's ability to maintain a healthy lifestyle postoperatively.

Three forms of bariatric surgery have been most commonly used in adolescent patients. The first, the Roux-en-Y gastric bypass, involves marked reduction of stomach size along with bypass of the proximal small bowel. This configuration restricts total food intake and creates a situation of malabsorption. Studies have also demonstrated decreased production of ghrelin[151] as well as increases in peptide YY and glucagon-like peptide 1.[152–154] Bariatric case series in adolescents show large degrees of weight loss, with many patients maintaining a lower weight several years after the surgery. Steatohepatitis also improves significantly.[122] A recent retrospective review[146] of Roux-en-Y procedures performed at five centers over a course of 2 years found that 11 adolescent patients (age <21 years) with type 2 diabetes lost an average of 34.4% of their body weight 1 year after the surgery. BMI changed by an average of 17 points. Weight loss ranged from 33 to 99 kg. All of the patients remained at least somewhat overweight; however, all but one had remission of their diabetes.[146]

The two other forms of bariatric surgery in adolescents involve decreasing the size of the stomach to impact satiety and food intake but do not produce malabsorption because no bypass is involved. One of these methods, vertical banded gastroplasty, involves stapling the stomach into a smaller pouch. One report of adolescents followed up 5 years postoperatively found an average of 55% of excess weight was lost, and only one of the 14 patients did not have a significant decrease of BMI.[122] The other approach is laparoscopic adjustable gastric banding (LAGB). Although not currently approved for adolescents by the FDA,[118] LAGB has been performed on several pediatric patients. In this procedure, a saline-filled band that is attached to an externally accessible port is placed around the exterior of the stomach. Using the port, the degree of outflow restriction from the small proximal pouch created by the procedure can be modified according to the amount of saline placed in the band. Problems have arisen when the band has slipped or leaked, and gastric perforation has occurred during initial surgery. There have also been reports of anemia despite placing patients on vitamin supplementation. Several studies that have observed patients during the first 4 years after LAGB have shown an average BMI change of 8 to 14.5 points and a loss of 40% to 70% of excess weight. Based on adult data, LAGB is expected to be somewhat less efficacious than malabsorptive procedures but potentially safer. Currently, more long-term data are available for the Roux-en-Y gastric bypass procedure.[148]

One review of surgeries registered in the Health Care Cost and Use Nationwide Inpatient Sample from 1996 to 2003 found 566 cases of either gastric bypass or gastroplasty involving adolescents (aged 10–19 years) with a diagnosis of obesity.[155] The overall complication rate of any kind was 4.2%, and 84.4% of these complications were respiratory in nature. In the same surgeries in adults, the complication rate was 6.6%. No in-hospital deaths were observed among adolescents.[155] The context in which these encouraging results have been obtained must be understood before surgical procedures are promulgated more widely for adolescent obesity. In general, the adolescents selected for surgery in the past have had significant obesity-related health problems that were considered likely to lead to an early death and supportive families expected to be able to care for them successfully after the operation; therefore, the cost-benefit ratio for adolescent bariatric surgery may have been maximized. Given the high frequency with which adolescents choose to undertreat their chronic diseases,[156] there is great concern that the risks from procedures that induce nutritional deficiencies might outweigh the benefits of weight reduction. In one study of adolescents treated with Roux-en-Y gastric bypass, only 14% were regularly taking nutritional supplements as prescribed.[157] Neurologic complications of bariatric procedures, believed largely to be due to vitamin B_{12}, folate, and thiamine deficiencies, are common, reported in 5% to 16% of patients,[158,159] and not always reversible, even after prompt nutritional repletion.[160] Bariatric surgery should continue to be offered only to adolescents who have life-threatening complications of their obesity.

SUMMARY

Treating obesity in children and adolescents is critical to prevent adult obesity-related complications, decrease health care costs, and provide patients with higher qualities of life. Despite the rapidly rising rates of obesity in the United States, few successful approaches have emerged. Clearly, given the large impact of environmental factors, behavioral changes are critical to include in any weight loss program. School systems may seem to be optimal targets for reaching large numbers of children and providing health education; however, results of prevention and intervention programs in schools have generally been modest. The genetic predisposition to obesity is also a large element of the picture but is incompletely understood. Research in the future needs to address these predispositions in the hope of dictating which weight loss approaches will be successful in individual patients.

REFERENCES

1. Ogden CL, Flegal KM, Carroll MD, et al. Prevalence and trends in overweight among US children and adolescents, 1999–2000. JAMA 2002;288(14):1728–32.
2. Ogden CL, Carroll MD, Curtin LR, et al. Prevalence of overweight and obesity in the United States, 1999–2004. JAMA 2006;295(13):1549–55.
3. Ogden CL, Carroll MD, Flegal KM. High body mass index for age among US children and adolescents, 2003–2006. JAMA 2008;299(20):2401–5.
4. l'Allemand D, Wiegand S, Reinehr T, et al. Cardiovascular risk in 26,008 European overweight children as established by a multicenter database. Obesity (Silver Spring) 2008;16(7):1672–9.
5. Muzumdar H, Rao M. Pulmonary dysfunction and sleep apnea in morbid obesity. Pediatr Endocrinol Rev 2006;3(Suppl 4):579–83.
6. Ogden CL, Yanovski SZ, Carroll MD, et al. The epidemiology of obesity. Gastroenterology 2007;132(6):2087–102.

7. Molleston JP, White F, Teckman J, et al. Obese children with steatohepatitis can develop cirrhosis in childhood. Am J Gastroenterol 2002;97(9):2460–2.
8. Dabelea D, Bell RA, D'Agostino RB Jr, et al. Incidence of diabetes in youth in the United States. JAMA 2007;297(24):2716–24.
9. Liese AD, D'Agostino RB Jr, Hamman RF, et al. The burden of diabetes mellitus among US youth: prevalence estimates from the SEARCH for Diabetes in Youth Study. Pediatrics 2006;118(4):1510–8.
10. Pavkov ME, Bennett PH, Knowler WC, et al. Effect of youth-onset type 2 diabetes mellitus on incidence of end-stage renal disease and mortality in young and middle-aged Pima Indians. JAMA 2006;296(4):421–6.
11. Baker JL, Olsen LW, Sorensen TI. Childhood body-mass index and the risk of coronary heart disease in adulthood. N Engl J Med 2007;357(23):2329–37.
12. Must A, Jacques PF, Dallal GE, et al. Long-term morbidity and mortality of overweight adolescents: a follow-up of the Harvard Growth Study of 1922 to 1935. N Engl J Med 1992;327(19):1350–5.
13. Olshansky SJ, Passaro DJ, Hershow RC, et al. A potential decline in life expectancy in the United States in the 21st century. N Engl J Med 2005;352(11): 1138–45.
14. Alley DE, Chang VW. The changing relationship of obesity and disability, 1988–2004. JAMA 2007;298(17):2020–7.
15. Wardle J, Carnell S, Haworth CMA, et al. Evidence for a strong genetic influence on childhood adiposity despite the force of the obesogenic environment. Am J Clin Nutr 2008;87:398–404.
16. Ashrafi K, Chang FY, Watts JL, et al. Genome-wide RNAi analysis of Caenorhabditis elegans fat regulatory genes. Nature 2003;421(6920):268–72.
17. Rankinen T, Zuberi A, Chagnon YC, et al. The human obesity gene map: the 2005 update. Obesity (Silver Spring) 2006;14(4):529–644.
18. Crino A, Greggio NA, Beccaria L, et al. Diagnosis and differential diagnosis of obesity in childhood. Minerva Pediatr 2003;55(5):461–70.
19. Ning C, Yanovski JA. Endocrine disorders associated with pediatric obesity. In: Goran M, Sothern M, editors. Handbook of pediatric obesity. Boca Raton (FL): CRC Press; 2006. p. 135–55.
20. Wheatley T, Edwards OM. Mild hypothyroidism and oedema: evidence for increased capillary permeability to protein. Clin Endocrinol (Oxf) 1983;18(6): 627–35.
21. Villabona C, Sahun M, Roca M, et al. Blood volumes and renal function in overt and subclinical primary hypothyroidism. Am J Med Sci 1999;318(4):277–80.
22. AL-Adsani H, Hoffer LJ, Silva JE. Resting energy expenditure is sensitive to small dose changes in patients on chronic thyroid hormone replacement. J Clin Endocrinol Metab 1997;82(4):1118–25.
23. Abbassi V, Rigterink E, Cancellieri RP. Clinical recognition of juvenile hypothyroidism in the early stage. Clin Pediatr (Phila) 1980;19(12):782–6.
24. Teng L, Bui H, Bachrach L, et al. Catch-up growth in severe juvenile hypothyroidism: treatment with a GnRH analog. J Pediatr Endocrinol Metab 2004; 17(3):345–54.
25. Meistas MT, Foster GV, Margolis S, et al. Integrated concentrations of growth hormone, insulin, C-peptide and prolactin in human obesity. Metabolism 1982; 31(12):1224–8.
26. Bell JP, Donald RA, Espiner EA. Pituitary response to insulin-induced hypoglycemia in obese subjects before and after fasting. J Clin Endocrinol Metab 1970;31(5):546.

27. Copinschi G, Wegienka LC, Hane S, et al. Effect of arginine on serum levels of insulin and growth hormone in obese subjects. Metabolism 1967;16(6):485–91.
28. Mims RB, Stein RB, Bethune JE. The effect of a single dose of L-dopa on pituitary hormones in acromegaly, obesity, and in normal subjects. J Clin Endocrinol Metab 1973;37(1):34–9.
29. Topper E, Gil-Ad I, Bauman B, et al. Plasma growth hormone response to oral clonidine as compared to insulin hypoglycemia in obese children and adolescents. Horm Metab Res 1984;16(Suppl 1):127–30.
30. Attia N, Tamborlane WV, Heptulla R, et al. The metabolic syndrome and insulin-like growth factor I regulation in adolescent obesity. J Clin Endocrinol Metab 1998;83(5):1467–71.
31. Kamoda T, Saitoh H, Inudoh M, et al. The serum levels of proinsulin and their relationship with IGFBP-1 in obese children. Diabetes Obes Metab 2006;8(2):192–6.
32. Dietz J, Schwartz J. Growth hormone alters lipolysis and hormone-sensitive lipase activity in 3T3-F442A adipocytes. Metabolism 1991;40(8):800–6.
33. Srinivasan S, Ogle GD, Garnett SP, et al. Features of the metabolic syndrome after childhood craniopharyngioma. J Clin Endocrinol Metab 2004;89(1):81–6.
34. Hoos MB, Westerterp KR, Gerver WJ. Short-term effects of growth hormone on body composition as a predictor of growth. J Clin Endocrinol Metab 2003;88(6):2569–72.
35. Ottosson M, Lonnroth P, Bjorntorp P, et al. Effects of cortisol and growth hormone on lipolysis in human adipose tissue. J Clin Endocrinol Metab 2000;85(2):799–803.
36. Berdanier CD. Role of glucocorticoids in the regulation of lipogenesis. FASEB J 1989;3(10):2179–83.
37. Greening JE, Storr HL, McKenzie SA, et al. Linear growth and body mass index in pediatric patients with Cushing's disease or simple obesity. J Endocrinol Invest 2006;29(10):885–7.
38. Magiakou MA, Mastorakos G, Oldfield EH, et al. Cushing's syndrome in children and adolescents: presentation, diagnosis, and therapy. N Engl J Med 1994;331(10):629–36.
39. Bonfig W, Kann P, Rothmund M, et al. Recurrent hypoglycemic seizures and obesity: delayed diagnosis of an insulinoma in a 15-year-old boy. Final diagnostic localization with endosonography. J Pediatr Endocrinol Metab 2007;20(9):1035–8.
40. Dizon AM, Kowalyk S, Hoogwerf BJ. Neuroglycopenic and other symptoms in patients with insulinomas. Am J Med 1999;106(3):307–10.
41. Woods SC, D'Alessio DA. Central control of body weight and appetite. J Clin Endocrinol Metab 2008;93(11 Suppl 1):S37–50.
42. Holder JL Jr, Butte NF, Zinn AR. Profound obesity associated with a balanced translocation that disrupts the SIM1 gene. Hum Mol Genet 2000;9(1):101–8.
43. Hung CC, Luan J, Sims M, et al. Studies of the SIM1 gene in relation to human obesity and obesity-related traits. Int J Obes (Lond) 2007;31(3):429–34.
44. Hoffman HJ, De Silva M, Humphreys RP, et al. Aggressive surgical management of craniopharyngiomas in children. J Neurosurg 1992;76(1):47–52.
45. Muller HL, Bueb K, Bartels U, et al. Obesity after childhood craniopharyngioma: German multicenter study on preoperative risk factors and quality of life. Klin Padiatr 2001;213(4):244–9.
46. Considine RV, Sinha MK, Heiman ML, et al. Serum immunoreactive-leptin concentrations in normal-weight and obese humans. N Engl J Med 1996;334(5):292–5.

47. Havel PJ, Kasim-Karakas S, Mueller W, et al. Relationship of plasma leptin to plasma insulin and adiposity in normal weight and overweight women: effects of dietary fat content and sustained weight loss. J Clin Endocrinol Metab 1996;81(12):4406–13.
48. Maffei M, Halaas J, Ravussin E, et al. Leptin levels in human and rodent: measurement of plasma leptin and ob RNA in obese and weight-reduced subjects. Nat Med 1995;1(11):1155–61.
49. Oral EA, Simha V, Ruiz E, et al. Leptin-replacement therapy for lipodystrophy. N Engl J Med 2002;346(8):570–8.
50. Farooqi IS, Matarese G, Lord GM, et al. Beneficial effects of leptin on obesity, T cell hyporesponsiveness, and neuroendocrine/metabolic dysfunction of human congenital leptin deficiency. J Clin Invest 2002;110(8):1093–103.
51. McDuffie JR, Riggs PA, Calis KA, et al. Effects of exogenous leptin on satiety and satiation in patients with lipodystrophy and leptin insufficiency. J Clin Endocrinol Metab 2004;89(9):4258–63.
52. Farooqi IS, Bullmore E, Keogh J, et al. Leptin regulates striatal regions and human eating behavior. Science 2007;317(5843):1355.
53. Montague CT, Farooqi IS, Whitehead JP, et al. Congenital leptin deficiency is associated with severe early-onset obesity in humans. Nature 1997;387(6636):903–8.
54. Strobel A, Issad T, Camoin L, et al. A leptin missense mutation associated with hypogonadism and morbid obesity. Nat Genet 1998;18(3):213–5.
55. Farooqi IS, Keogh JM, Kamath S, et al. Partial leptin deficiency and human adiposity. Nature 2001;414(6859):34–5.
56. Tanofsky-Kraff M, Yanovski SZ, Wilfley DE, et al. Eating-disordered behaviors, body fat, and psychopathology in overweight and normal-weight children. J Consult Clin Psychol 2004;72(1):53–61.
57. Lahlou N, Issad T, Lebouc Y, et al. Mutations in the human leptin and leptin receptor genes as models of serum leptin receptor regulation. Diabetes 2002; 51(6):1980–5.
58. Farooqi IS, Wangensteen T, Collins S, et al. Clinical and molecular genetic spectrum of congenital deficiency of the leptin receptor. N Engl J Med 2007;356(3): 237–47.
59. Krude H, Biebermann H, Luck W, et al. Severe early-onset obesity, adrenal insufficiency and red hair pigmentation caused by POMC mutations in humans. Nat Genet 1998;19(2):155–7.
60. Krude H, Biebermann H, Schnabel D, et al. Obesity due to proopiomelanocortin deficiency: three new cases and treatment trials with thyroid hormone and ACTH4-10. J Clin Endocrinol Metab 2003;88(10):4633–40.
61. Challis BG, Pritchard LE, Creemers JW, et al. A missense mutation disrupting a dibasic prohormone processing site in pro-opiomelanocortin (POMC) increases susceptibility to early-onset obesity through a novel molecular mechanism. Hum Mol Genet 2002;11(17):1997–2004.
62. Creemers JW, Lee YS, Oliver RL, et al. Mutations in the amino-terminal region of proopiomelanocortin (POMC) in patients with early-onset obesity impair POMC sorting to the regulated secretory pathway. J Clin Endocrinol Metab 2008; 93(11):4494–9.
63. Farooqi IS, Drop S, Clements A, et al. Heterozygosity for a POMC-null mutation and increased obesity risk in humans. Diabetes 2006;55(9):2549–53.
64. Lee YS, Challis BG, Thompson DA, et al. A POMC variant implicates beta-melanocyte-stimulating hormone in the control of human energy balance. Cell Metab 2006;3(2):135–40.

65. Jackson RS, Creemers JW, Ohagi S, et al. Obesity and impaired prohormone processing associated with mutations in the human prohormone convertase 1 gene. Nat Genet 1997;16(3):303–6.

66. Jackson RS, Creemers JW, Farooqi IS, et al. Small-intestinal dysfunction accompanies the complex endocrinopathy of human proprotein convertase 1 deficiency. J Clin Invest 2003;112(10):1550–60.

67. Farooqi IS, Volders K, Stanhope R, et al. Hyperphagia and early-onset obesity due to a novel homozygous missense mutation in prohormone convertase 1/3. J Clin Endocrinol Metab 2007;92(9):3369–73.

68. Cone RD. Anatomy and regulation of the central melanocortin system. Nat Neurosci 2005;8(5):571–8.

69. Butler AA, Cone RD. Knockout studies defining different roles for melanocortin receptors in energy homeostasis. Ann N Y Acad Sci 2003;994:240–5.

70. Chen AS, Marsh DJ, Trumbauer ME, et al. Inactivation of the mouse melanocortin-3 receptor results in increased fat mass and reduced lean body mass. Nat Genet 2000;26(1):97–102.

71. Butler AA. The melanocortin system and energy balance. Peptides 2006;27(2): 281–90.

72. Farooqi IS, Keogh JM, Yeo GS, et al. Clinical spectrum of obesity and mutations in the melanocortin 4 receptor gene. N Engl J Med 2003;348(12): 1085–95.

73. Farooqi IS, Yeo GS, Keogh JM, et al. Dominant and recessive inheritance of morbid obesity associated with melanocortin 4 receptor deficiency [see comments]. J Clin Invest 2000;106(2):271–9.

74. Greenfield JR, Miller JW, Keogh JM, et al. Modulation of blood pressure by central melanocortinergic pathways. N Engl J Med 2009;360(1):44–52.

75. Feng N, Young SF, Aguilera G, et al. Co-occurrence of two partially inactivating polymorphisms of MC3R is associated with pediatric-onset obesity. Diabetes 2005;54(9):2663–7.

76. Han JC, Liu QR, Jones M, et al. Brain-derived neurotrophic factor and obesity in the WAGR syndrome. N Engl J Med 2008;359(9):918–27.

77. Yeo GS, Connie Hung CC, Rochford J, et al. A de novo mutation affecting human TrkB associated with severe obesity and developmental delay. Nat Neurosci 2004;7(11):1187–9.

78. Long DN, McGuire S, Levine MA, et al. Body mass index differences in pseudohypoparathyroidism type 1a versus pseudopseudohypoparathyroidism may implicate paternal imprinting of G alpha(s) in the development of human obesity. J Clin Endocrinol Metab 2007;92(3):1073–9.

79. Xie T, Chen M, Gavrilova O, et al. Severe obesity and insulin resistance due to deletion of the maternal Gs alpha allele is reversed by paternal deletion of the Gs alpha imprint control region. Endocrinology 2008; 149(5):2443–50.

80. Meyre D, Delplanque J, Chevre JC, et al. Genome-wide association study for early-onset and morbid adult obesity identifies three new risk loci in European populations. Nat Genet 2009;41(2):157–9.

81. Thorleifsson G, Walters GB, Gudbjartsson DF, et al. Genome-wide association yields new sequence variants at seven loci that associate with measures of obesity. Nat Genet 2009;41(1):18–24.

82. Willer CJ, Speliotes EK, Loos RJ, et al. Six new loci associated with body mass index highlight a neuronal influence on body weight regulation. Nat Genet 2009; 41(1):25–34.

83. Frayling TM, Timpson NJ, Weedon MN, et al. A common variant in the FTO gene is associated with body mass index and predisposes to childhood and adult obesity. Science 2007;316(5826):889–94.

84. Dina C, Meyre D, Gallina S, et al. Variation in FTO contributes to childhood obesity and severe adult obesity. Nat Genet 2007;39(6):724–6.

85. Hinney A, Nguyen TT, Scherag A, et al. Genome wide association (GWA) study for early onset extreme obesity supports the role of fat mass and obesity associated gene (FTO) variants. PLoS One 2007;2(12):e1361.

86. Hunt SC, Stone S, Xin Y, et al. Association of the FTO gene with BMI. Obesity (Silver Spring) 2008;16(4):902–4.

87. Scuteri A, Sanna S, Chen WM, et al. Genome-wide association scan shows genetic variants in the FTO gene are associated with obesity-related traits. PLoS Genet 2007;3(7):e115.

88. Fredriksson R, Hagglund M, Olszewski PK, et al. The obesity gene, FTO, is of ancient origin, up-regulated during food deprivation and expressed in neurons of feeding-related nuclei of the brain. Endocrinology 2008;149(5):2062–71.

89. Stratigopoulos G, Padilla SL, LeDuc CA, et al. Regulation of Fto/Ftm gene expression in mice and humans. Am J Physiol Regul Integr Comp Physiol 2008;294(4):R1185–96.

90. Gerken T, Girard CA, Tung YC, et al. The obesity-associated FTO gene encodes a 2-oxoglutarate-dependent nucleic acid demethylase. Science 2007; 318(5855):1469–72.

91. Cecil JE, Tavendale R, Watt P, et al. An obesity-associated FTO gene variant and increased energy intake in children. N Engl J Med 2008;359(24):2558–66.

92. Wardle J, Llewellyn C, Sanderson S, et al. The FTO gene and measured food intake in children. Int J Obes (Lond) 2008;33(1):42–5.

93. Wardle J, Carnell S, Haworth CM, et al. Obesity associated genetic variation in FTO is associated with diminished satiety. J Clin Endocrinol Metab 2008;93(9):3640–3.

94. Celi FS, Shuldiner AR. The role of peroxisome proliferator-activated receptor gamma in diabetes and obesity. Curr Diab Rep 2002;2(2):179–85.

95. Luan J, Browne PO, Harding AH, et al. Evidence for gene-nutrient interaction at the PPARgamma locus. Diabetes 2001;50(3):686–9.

96. Jalba MS, Rhoads GG, Demissie K. Association of codon 16 and codon 27 beta 2-adrenergic receptor gene polymorphisms with obesity: a meta-analysis. Obesity (Silver Spring) 2008;16(9):2096–106.

97. Corella D, Qi L, Sorli JV, et al. Obese subjects carrying the 11482G>A polymorphism at the perilipin locus are resistant to weight loss after dietary energy restriction. J Clin Endocrinol Metab 2005;90(9):5121–6.

98. Cummings DE, Clement K, Purnell JQ, et al. Elevated plasma ghrelin levels in Prader Willi syndrome. Nat Med 2002;8(7):643–4.

99. Wren AM, Seal LJ, Cohen MA, et al. Ghrelin enhances appetite and increases food intake in humans. J Clin Endocrinol Metab 2001;86(12):5992.

100. Davenport JR, Watts AJ, Roper VC, et al. Disruption of intraflagellar transport in adult mice leads to obesity and slow-onset cystic kidney disease. Curr Biol 2007;17(18):1586–94.

101. Seo S, Guo DF, Bugge K, et al. Requirement of Bardet-Biedl syndrome proteins for leptin receptor signaling. Hum Mol Genet 2009;18(7):1323–31.

102. Aronne LJ, Segal KR. Weight gain in the treatment of mood disorders. J Clin Psychiatry 2003;64(Suppl 8):22–9.

103. Dhurandhar NV, Kulkarni P, Ajinkya SM, et al. Effect of adenovirus infection on adiposity in chicken. Vet Microbiol 1992;31(2,3):101–7.

104. Dhurandhar NV, Whigham LD, Abbott DH, et al. Human adenovirus Ad-36 promotes weight gain in male rhesus and marmoset monkeys. J Nutr 2002; 132(10):3155–60.

105. Dhurandhar NV, Israel BA, Kolesar JM, et al. Increased adiposity in animals due to a human virus. Int J Obes Relat Metab Disord 2000;24(8):989–96.

106. Pasarica M, Mashtalir N, McAllister EJ, et al. Adipogenic human adenovirus Ad-36 induces commitment, differentiation, and lipid accumulation in human adipose-derived stem cells. Stem Cells 2008;26(4):969–78.

107. Dhurandhar NV, Kulkarni PR, Ajinkya SM, et al. Association of adenovirus infection with human obesity. Obes Res 1997;5(5):464–9.

108. Atkinson RL, Dhurandhar NV, Allison DB, et al. Human adenovirus-36 is associated with increased body weight and paradoxical reduction of serum lipids. Int J Obes (Lond) 2005;29(3):281–6.

109. Ravussin E, Valencia ME, Esparza J, et al. Effects of a traditional lifestyle on obesity in Pima Indians. Diabetes Care 1994;17(9):1067–74.

110. Popkin BM, Udry JR. Adolescent obesity increases significantly in second and third generation US immigrants: the National Longitudinal Study of Adolescent Health. J Nutr 1998;128(4):701–6.

111. Hawkins SS, Cole TJ, Law C. An ecological systems approach to examining risk factors for early childhood overweight: findings from the UK Millennium Cohort Study. J Epidemiol Community Health 2009;63(2):147–55.

112. Lang T, Rayner G. Overcoming policy cacophony on obesity: an ecological public health framework for policymakers. Obes Rev 2007;8(Suppl 1): 165–81.

113. Waterland RA. Does nutrition during infancy and early childhood contribute to later obesity via metabolic imprinting of epigenetic gene regulatory mechanisms? Nestle Nutr Workshop Ser Pediatr Program 2005;56:157–74.

114. Wu Q, Suzuki M. Parental obesity and overweight affect the body-fat accumulation in the offspring: the possible effect of a high-fat diet through epigenetic inheritance. Obesity Reviews 2006;7:201–8.

115. Barlow SE, Dietz WH. Obesity evaluation and treatment: Expert Committee recommendations. The Maternal and Child Health Bureau, Health Resources and Services Administration and the Department of Health and Human Services. Pediatrics 1998;102(3):E29.

116. Barlow SE. Expert committee recommendations regarding the prevention, assessment, and treatment of child and adolescent overweight and obesity: summary report. Pediatrics 2007;120(Suppl 4):S164–92.

117. Cohen ML, Tanofsky-Kraff M, Young-Hyman D, et al. Weight and its relationship to adolescent perceptions of their providers (WRAP): a qualitative and quantitative assessment of teen weight-related preferences and concerns. J Adolesc Health 2005;37(2):163–578.

118. August GP, Caprio S, Fennoy I, et al. Prevention and treatment of pediatric obesity: an Endocrine Society clinical practice guideline based on expert opinion. J Clin Endocrinol Metab 2008;93(12):4576–99.

119. Weiss R, Dziura J, Burgert TS, et al. Obesity and the metabolic syndrome in children and adolescents. N Engl J Med 2004;350(23):2362–74.

120. McGovern L, Johnson JN, Paulo R, et al. Clinical review: treatment of pediatric obesity: a systematic review and meta-analysis of randomized trials. J Clin Endocrinol Metab 2008;93(12):4600–5.

121. Epstein LH, Valoski A, Wing RR, et al. Ten-year follow-up of behavioral, family-based treatment for obese children. JAMA 1990;264(19):2519–23.

122. Han JC, Yanovski JA. Intensive therapies for the treatment of pediatric obesity. In: Jelalian E, Steele RC, editors. Handbook of child and adolescent obesity. New York: Springer; 2008. p. 241–60.

123. Figueroa-Colon R, von Almen TK, Franklin FA, et al. Comparison of two hypocaloric diets in obese children. Am J Dis Child 1993;147(2):160–6.

124. Epstein LH, Myers MD, Raynor HA, et al. Treatment of pediatric obesity. Pediatrics 1998;101(3 Pt 2):554–70.

125. Oude Luttikhuis H, Baur L, Jansen H, et al. Interventions for treating obesity in children. Cochrane Database Syst Rev 2009;(1):1–189.

126. Wilfley DE, Tibbs TL, Van Buren DJ, et al. Lifestyle interventions in the treatment of childhood overweight: a meta-analytic review of randomized controlled trials. Health Psychol 2007;26(5):521–32.

127. Epstein LH. Family-based behavioural intervention for obese children. Int J Obes Relat Metab Disord 1996;20(1):S14–21.

128. Epstein LH, Valoski A, Wing RR, et al. Ten-year outcomes of behavioral family-based treatment for childhood obesity. Health Psychol 1994;13(5):373–83.

129. Wilfley DE, Stein RI, Saelens BE, et al. Efficacy of maintenance treatment approaches for childhood overweight: a randomized controlled trial. JAMA 2007;298(14):1661–73.

130. Gutin B, Yin Z, Johnson M, et al. Preliminary findings of the effect of a 3-year after-school physical activity intervention on fitness and body fat: the Medical College of Georgia Fit kid Project. Int J Pediatr Obes 2008;3 (Suppl 1):3–9.

131. Gortmaker SL, Peterson K, Wiecha J, et al. Reducing obesity via a school-based interdisciplinary intervention among youth: planet health. Arch Pediatr Adolesc Med 1999;153(4):409–18.

132. Yanovski JA. Intensive therapies for pediatric obesity. Pediatr Clin North Am 2001;48(4):1041–53.

133. Samanin R, Garattini S. Neurochemical mechanism of action of anorectic drugs. Pharmacol Toxicol 1993;73(2):63–9.

134. Freemark M. Pharmacotherapy of childhood obesity: an evidence-based, conceptual approach. Diabetes Care 2007;30(2):395–402.

135. Berkowitz RI, Fujioka K, Daniels SR, et al. Effects of sibutramine treatment in obese adolescents: a randomized trial. Ann Intern Med 2006;145(2):81–90.

136. Danielsson P, Janson A, Norgren S, et al. Impact of sibutramine therapy in children with hypothalamic obesity or obesity with aggravating syndromes. J Clin Endocrinol Metab 2007;92(11):4101–6.

137. Connolly HM, Crary JL, McGoon MD, et al. Valvular heart disease associated with fenfluramine-phentermine. N Engl J Med 1997;337(9):581–8.

138. Akbas F, Gasteyger C, Sjodin A, et al. A critical review of the cannabinoid receptor as a drug target for obesity management. Obes Rev 2009;10(1): 58–67.

139. Chanoine JP, Hampl S, Jensen C, et al. Effect of orlistat on weight and body composition in obese adolescents: a randomized controlled trial. JAMA 2005; 293(23):2873–83.

140. Wilson DM, Abrams SH, Aye T, et al. Metformin extended release treatment of adolescent obesity: a 48-week randomized, double-blind, placebo-controlled trial with 48-week follow-up. Arch Pediatr Adolesc Med 2010;164:116–23.

141. Yanovski JA, Krakoff J, Salaita CG, et al. Effects of metformin on body weight and body composition in obese insulin-resistant children: a randomized clinical trial. Diabetes 2011;60(2):477–85.

142. Klein DJ, Cottingham EM, Sorter M, et al. A randomized, double-blind, placebo-controlled trial of metformin treatment of weight gain associated with initiation of atypical antipsychotic therapy in children and adolescents. Am J Psychiatry 2006;163(12):2072–9.

143. Lustig RH, Hinds PS, Ringwald-Smith K, et al. Octreotide therapy of pediatric hypothalamic obesity: a double-blind, placebo-controlled trial. J Clin Endocrinol Metab 2003;88(6):2586–92.

144. Heymsfield SB, Greenberg AS, Fujioka K, et al. Recombinant leptin for weight loss in obese and lean adults: a randomized, controlled, dose-escalation trial [see comments]. JAMA 1999;282(16):1568–75.

145. Farooqi IS, Jebb SA, Langmack G, et al. Effects of recombinant leptin therapy in a child with congenital leptin deficiency. N Engl J Med 1999;341(12):879–84.

146. Inge TH, Miyano G, Bean J, et al. Reversal of type 2 diabetes mellitus and improvements in cardiovascular risk factors after surgical weight loss in adolescents. Pediatrics 2009;123(1):214–22.

147. Inge TH, Krebs NF, Garcia VF, et al. Bariatric surgery for severely overweight adolescents: concerns and recommendations. Pediatrics 2004;114(1):217–23.

148. Apovian CM, Baker C, Ludwig DS, et al. Best practice guidelines in pediatric/adolescent weight loss surgery. Obes Res 2005;13(2):274–82.

149. Xanthakos SA, Inge TH. Extreme pediatric obesity: weighing the health dangers. J Pediatr 2007;150(1):3–5.

150. Inge TH, Garcia V, Daniels S, et al. A multidisciplinary approach to the adolescent bariatric surgical patient. J Pediatr Surg 2004;39(3):442–7.

151. Cummings DE, Weigle DS, Frayo RS, et al. Plasma ghrelin levels after diet-induced weight loss or gastric bypass surgery. N Engl J Med 2002;346(21):1623–30.

152. Korner J, Bessler M, Cirilo LJ, et al. Effects of Roux-en-Y gastric bypass surgery on fasting and postprandial concentrations of plasma ghrelin, peptide YY, and insulin. J Clin Endocrinol Metab 2005;90(1):359–65.

153. Morinigo R, Moize V, Musri M, et al. Glucagon-like peptide-1, peptide YY, hunger, and satiety after gastric bypass surgery in morbidly obese subjects. J Clin Endocrinol Metab 2006;91(5):1735–40.

154. Reinehr T, Roth CL, Schernthaner GH, et al. Peptide YY and glucagon-like peptide-1 in morbidly obese patients before and after surgically induced weight loss. Obes Surg 2007;17(12):1571–7.

155. Tsai WS, Inge TH, Burd RS. Bariatric surgery in adolescents: recent national trends in use and in-hospital outcome. Arch Pediatr Adolesc Med 2007;161(3):217–21.

156. Rianthavorn P, Ettenger RB. Medication non-adherence in the adolescent renal transplant recipient: a clinician's viewpoint. Pediatr Transplant 2005;9(3):398–407.

157. Sugerman HJ, Sugerman EL, DeMaria EJ, et al. Bariatric surgery for severely obese adolescents. J Gastrointest Surg 2003;7(1):102–7.

158. Berger JR. The neurological complications of bariatric surgery. Arch Neurol 2004;61(8):1185–9.

159. Thaisetthawatkul P, Collazo-Clavell ML, Sarr MG, et al. A controlled study of peripheral neuropathy after bariatric surgery. Neurology 2004;63(8):1462–70.

160. Xanthakos SA, Daniels SR, Inge TH. Bariatric surgery in adolescents: an update. Adolesc Med Clin 2006;17(3):589–612.

Metabolic Syndrome in Pediatrics: Old Concepts Revised, New Concepts Discussed

Ebe D'Adamo, MD[a,b], Nicola Santoro, MD, PhD[a], Sonia Caprio, MD[a,*]

KEYWORDS

- Obesity • Children • Metabolic syndrome
- Insulin resistance • Type 2 diabetes

The worldwide epidemic of childhood obesity in the last decades is responsible for the occurrence in pediatrics of disorders once mainly found in adults, such as the metabolic syndrome (MS). First described by Gerald Reaven, MS has been defined as "a link between insulin resistance, hypertension, dyslipidemia, impaired glucose tolerance and other metabolic abnormalities associated with an increased risk of atherosclerotic cardiovascular diseases in adults."[1] A key factor in the pathogenesis of MS is insulin resistance, a phenomenon occurring mainly in obese subjects with a general resistance to the insulin effect only on carbohydrates and lipid metabolism.[2] The pathogenesis of insulin resistance has been studied for many years and it is now known that free fatty acid (FFA) accumulation in the liver, fat cells, pancreas and, particularly, skeletal muscle of obese patients, interfering with the normal insulin signaling cascade, appears as the primary determinant of insulin resistance.[2] Moreover, FFA accumulation in the liver makes it resistant to insulin in terms of the ability of the hormone to suppress glucose production. Under these conditions, hyperinsulinemia turns the liver into a "fat-producing factory" with all of its negative downstream effects, including the genesis of hypertriglyceridemia.[2] On the other hand, the fat cells' resistance to insulin causes an increase in lipolisis, with a consequent increase in

Portions of this article were previously published in the *Endocrinology and Metabolism Clinics of North America*, 38:3.

This study was supported by grants from the National Institutes of Health: R01-HD40787, R01-HD28016 and K24-HD01464 to S. Caprio; M01-RR00125 to the Yale Clinical Research Center and R01-EB006494 to the Bioimage Suite.

[a] Department of Pediatrics, Yale University School of Medicine, PO Box 208064, New Haven, CT 6520, USA
[b] Department of Pediatrics, University of Chieti, Chieti, Italy
* Corresponding author. Department of Pediatrics, Yale University School of Medicine, PO Box 208064, New Haven, CT 6520.
E-mail address: sonia.caprio@yale.edu

dismissing lipids in the plasma.[2] As a consequence of insulin resistance, the pancreas needs to increase its insulin production to maintain normal value of glycemia, promoting, in this way, the FFA accumulation, further worsening insulin resistance and generating a vicious cycle.

In spite of the emerging difficulties in transposing the definition of MS from adults to children,[3] MS in children is commonly defined as the co-occurrence of three or more of the following features: severe obesity (usually with a waist circumference higher than the nintieth sex- and age-specific percentile), dyslipidemia (increase of triglycerides and decrease of high-density lipoprotein or HDL), hypertension and alterations of glucose metabolism, such as impaired glucose tolerance (IGT) and type 2 diabetes (T2D).[4–8]

Recently, to overcome conflicts arising from different definitions, the International Diabetes Federation consensus group proposed an easy-to-apply definition to begin using in clinical setting (Table 1).[3] In fact, the numerous definitions now used make it difficult to follow the epidemiology of MS in childhood. A study by Goodman and colleagues[9] has clearly shown how changes in MS definitions dramatically influence prevalence differences, ranging from 15% to 50% according to which definition is used. Moreover, given that MS is driven by obesity, the prevalence of the latter will strongly influence the prevalence of MS. One should also take into account that, because the known differences of insulin resistance between different ethnic groups (with African American and Hispanic children more insulin-resistant than Caucasians) it may be important to consider ethnicity in the evaluation of MS.[10–13] Difficulties in defining MS in children and adolescents also come by the lack—for some components of MS, such as HDL, triglycerides, waist circumference and blood pressure (BP)—of normative values that might find a worldwide application. This inevitably determines that the definition of MS in pediatrics is driven by that given for adults.

Table 1
International Diabetes Federation criteria for metabolic syndrome in children. Diagnosis requires the presence of central obesity plus any two of other criteria

Age Group	Obesity (WC)	Triglycerides (mg/dl)	HDL (mg/dl)	Blood Pressure (mmHg)	Glucose (mg/dl)
6 < 10	≥90th percentile				
10 < 16	≥90th percentile or adult cut-off if lower	≥150	< 40	Systolic BP >130 or diastolic BP > 85	FPG >100 or T2D
>16 Adult criteria	WC ≥94 cm for males and ≥80 for females	≥150	< 40 in males, < 50 in females	Systolic BP >130 or diastolic BP > 85	FPG >100 or T2D

According to these criteria, MS cannot be diagnosed under 6 years of age, but further measurement and a strict follow-up should be provided according to family history. Different thresholds for different ethnicity are also suggested.

Abbreviations: BP, blood pressure; FPG, fasting plasma glucose; T2D, type 2 diabetes; WC, waist circumference.

Data from Zimmet P, Alberti KG, Kaufman F, et al. IDF Consensus Group. The metabolic syndrome in children and adolescents—an IDF consensus report. Pediatr Diabetes 2007;8:299-306.

Beyond any definition, the precocious identification of the components of MS is of primary importance to address the treatment and the behavior of those children who will develop cardiovascular and metabolic issues in adulthood. That is why several studies have been focused on clinical and biochemical markers predicting MS, demonstrating in some cases a strong link between changes of the risk variables of MS, such as body mass index (BMI), HDL, triglycerides, glucose, and insulin from childhood to early adulthood and cardiovascular risk later in the life.[14]

IDENTIFYING CHILDREN WITH MS

Although there is no complete agreement on the fine definition of MS in youth, given the limitations described above, the cornerstones of its definition still remain and need to be identified by pediatricians.

BMI is a predictor of coronary artery disease (CAD) risk factors among children and adolescents,[15,16] and its utility has been endorsed by International Obesity Task Force and the Centers for Disease Control (CDC).[17–19] The cut-off points of the CDC, based on a distribution approach, identify children with a BMI higher than the eighty-fifth percentile as "at-risk of overweight" and children with a BMI higher than the ninety-fifth percentile as "overweight." Data from multiracial cohorts of obese children, in which obesity was defined according to the CDC cut-off, showed that the severity of obesity and the prevalence of MS are strongly associated.[5] However, obesity per se is not a marker sufficient for identifying children at-risk for MS and consequently for CAD. Fat distribution plays an important role in influencing the occurrence of metabolic complications consequent to obesity. Visceral fat accumulation, in fact, is strongly associated with MS in childhood[20] and CAD later in life,[21] and waist circumference has been recognized as the best clinical predictor of visceral fat accumulation.[22] Although reference values for waist circumference in children do exist for Canada,[23] Italy,[24] the United Kingdom,[25] and the United States,[20] and cut-off points beyond which there is an increase of the prevalence of CAD risk factors have been provided,[20] this measure is not commonly used in children, probably because no organization has endorsed a waist circumference cut-off for children.

The importance of measuring waist circumference is corroborated by multiracial cohort studies in children and adolescents showing that subjects with high waist-circumference values are more likely to have elevated CAD risk factors, compared with those with low waist circumference, within a given BMI category.[21] This means that waist circumference may be, for such an extent, considered a more reliable measure for predicting MS than BMI alone. In fact, as in adults,[26–30] in children an increased waist circumference has been correlated with abnormal systolic and diastolic blood pressure and elevated levels of serum cholesterol, low density lipoprotein (LDL), triglycerides, insulin, and lower HDL concentrations.[31–33] The association between the clustering of cardiovascular risk factors and waist circumference is not only a reflection of the obesity degree, but it has a psychopathologic background, given that visceral adiposity is one of the main risk factors for the development of insulin resistance, diabetes mellitus (DM), hypertension, and cardiovascular disease.[34,35] The mechanisms involved in these common clinical associations are not completely known, but include the impaired suppression of hepatic glucose production,[36] the increased portal release of FFAs,[37] the increased visceral production of glycerol,[38] and the abnormal production of adipose tissue-derived hormones and cytokines, such as tumor necrosis factor (TNF)-α, leptin, and adiponectin.[39,40] In fact, some studies have shown that the removal of visceral fat reverses insulin resistance in two models of obesity, and that the metabolic consequences of visceral fat removal were associated with improved hepatic insulin action[41,42] and with reduced adipose tissue expression of proinflammatory cytokines.[43]

Although the anthropometric measurements obtained during the physical examination, such as BMI and waist circumference, can be very helpful and rich in meaning,[44] family history needs to be deeply investigated as well, given that heritability of the single components of MS has been well demonstrated.[45,46] In fact, heritability for obesity ranges from 60% to 80% and heritability for blood pressure varies from 11% to 37%, while those for lipid levels varies from 43% to 54%.[45] Moreover, a recent study by Weiss and colleagues[47] shows that those children who do not show MS early in childhood are less prone to develop it later, further supporting, indirectly, a strong genetic component in the development of MS.

METABOLIC PHENOTYPE OF CHILDREN AND ADOLESCENTS WITH MS

Because insulin resistance represents one of the most important pathogenetic primers in the development of MS, all patients should be investigated for insulin resistance. Weiss and colleagues[5] have demonstrated how the increase of insulin resistance parallels the increase of the risk of MS in obese children and adolescents. In this latter study, a strong loading of insulin resistance to obesity and glucose metabolism factor and moderate loading to the dyslipidemia factor has been shown.[5] Some studies suggest a direct effect of hyperinsulinemia consequent to insulin resistance on the single components of the syndrome.[48]

Although it is difficult to dissect the effect of insulin resistance and obesity on blood pressure, it has been demonstrated that insulin resistance per se may determine hypertension. Insulin levels in children between 6 and 9 years of age have been shown to predict blood pressure levels in adolescence[49]; moreover, the Bogalusa Heart Study showed a strong correlation between the persistently high fasting insulin levels and the development of CAD in children and young adults.[50] Some studies showed not only a strong correlation between hyperinsulinemia and blood pressure in children, but also that fasting insulin predicted the levels of blood pressure 6 years later.[49] As has been suggested, the adverse direct effect of hyperinsulinemia on blood pressure may be ascribed to the effect of insulin on (i) sympathetic nervous system activity,[51] (ii) sodium retention by kidney,[52] and (iii) vascular smooth-muscle growth stimulation.[53]

A strong effect of hyperinsulinemia on lipid metabolism has also been demonstrated. In vivo studies showed that hyperinsulinemia stimulates the synthesis of tryglicerydes by increasing the transcription of genes for lipogenic enzymes in the liver.[54] Moreover, recent reports showed that the forkhead transcription factor FoxO1 acts in the liver to integrate hepatic insulin action to very low-density lipoprotein (VLDL) production. Augmented FoxO1 activity in insulin-resistant livers promotes hepatic VLDL overproduction and predisposes to the development of hypertriglyceridemia.[55]

Although obesity is the most important cause of insulin resistance among obese and adolescents, one should not forget that a transient insulin-resistant state occurs in children during puberty, possibly because of the increase in growth hormone and insulin-like growth factor 1,[56] and that this state may worsen the insulin resistance present in obese children, accelerating the progression to MS and T2D.

Along with insulin resistance, MS in children is associated with a proinflammatory state,[5] which in turn seems to be associated with a worsening in the risk of CAD. The relationship between inflammatory markers and individual components of MS is still unclear. In fact, it is not yet known if the proinflammatory state is a result of MS and insulin resistance or if, vice versa, the increase of inflammatory cytokines derived from adipocytes may be partly responsible for insulin resistance and MS.

It has been demonstrated that obese children show an elevation of C-reactive protein (CRP), which is a biomarker of the inflammation associated with adverse cardiovascular outcomes and altered glucose metabolism (**Fig. 1**).[5] However, most studies in children do not conclusively confirm that CRP levels are associated with insulin resistance or MS,[7,57–59] which is why some investigators suggest that an underlying inflammation may be an additional factor contributing to adverse long-term cardiovascular outcomes, independent of the insulin-resistance degree.[5] Because CRP is just an indirect marker of inflammation, several studies have been focused on the contribution of proinflammatory adipocytokines, such as TNF-α and interleukin (IL)-6 molecules produced by adipose tissue (or adipose resident macrophages). In a multiethnic cohort of obese and lean children, IL-6 levels have been shown to increase with the degree of obesity (see **Fig. 1**); results concerning the association between TNF-α, childhood obesity, and its metabolic complications are less clear.[60] In particular, studies dealing with TNF-α in obese children show contrasting results, with some of them showing a positive association with body fat and other

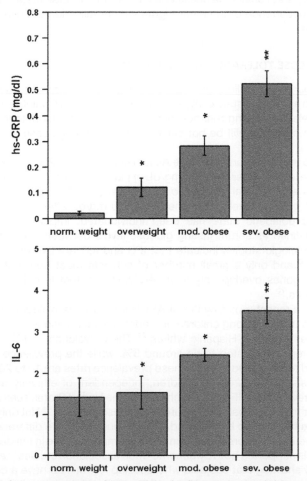

Fig. 1. Impact of severe obesity on biomarkers of inflammation in children and adolescents (*asterisks*).

showing a decrease of TNF-α in obese prepubertal children[61,62]; on the other hand, the effect of TNF-α on insulin resistance has been well demonstrated. In fact, this cytokine induces lipolysis in adipose tissue, inhibits insulin signaling, and affects the expression of some genes that are important for adipocyte function. TNF-α may also enhance the release of FFAs from adipose tissue, which affects whole-body energy homeostasis and overall insulin sensitivity.[63] Furthermore, a recent report demonstrated a positive correlation between IL-6, TNF-α, and adipocyte diameter studied by a needle biopsy of subcutaneous abdominal fat in obese children.[64]

Along with the increase of cytokines affecting insulin sensitivity and CAD risk, adipose tissue of obese children reduces the production of the adiponectin, which is a cytokine exclusively expressed by adipocytes and that can be found in high concentration in the human blood.[60] It exerts several beneficial actions, such as anti-atherogenetic, antidiabetogenic, and anti-inflammatory, hence protecting against the development of T2D and CAD.[65,66] Interestingly, adiponectin is decreased in obesity and the decreased adiponectin levels are associated with parameters of MS in obese children.[67,68] In summary, the co-occurrence of the insulin resistance and an adverse proinflammatory state drives the obese child to develop a worse metabolic asset, with a consequent occurrence of the most frightened complication of childhood obesity: type-2 diabetes.

IMPAIRED GLUCOSE TOLERANCE AND T2D IN YOUTH

The β-cell response to insulin resistance occurring in obese children and adolescents is by producing a vigorous state of hyperinsulinemia, which will maintain normal values of glucose levels. In the long run, however, β-cell function may deteriorate in some, and the insulin secretion will be not sufficient to maintain glucose levels within the normal range.

According to the American Diabetese Association criteria, T2D is defined as fasting plasma glucose levels higher than 126 mg/dL or plasma glucose levels higher than 200 mg/dL 2 hours after an oral glucose tolerance test (OGTT), while IGT is defined as having plasma glucose levels are higher than 140 mg/dL after OGTT.[69] Along with IGT, another prediabetic state has been individuated: impaired fasting glucose (IFG). IFG is defined as serum fasting glucose levels between 100 mg/dL and 125 mg/dL. Epidemiologic studies indicate that IFG and IGT are two distinct categories of individuals,[70] and only a small number of subjects meet both criteria, showing that these categories overlap only to a very limited extent in children, as already reported in adults.[70]

According to a recent report by the SEARCH for Diabetes in Youth Study Group,[71] incidence rates of T2D among children and adolescents are higher among racial and ethnic minorities than non-Hispanic whites.[71] The prevalence of T2D in the United States in children is estimated to be around 5%, while the prevalence of IGT it has been estimated to be around 15%.[72] These prevalence rates are 10 to 20 times higher than those observed in European children, independent of ethnicity and race.[73] In addition, the prevalence of IFG among children in the United States seems to be about 10 times higher than that observed in European obese children.[74] Not only the environment, but more the genetic background may account for these differences.

Surely, different genetic predisposition plays an important role in the development of T2D. This idea is supported both by genome-wide association studies[75] and by clinical studies, clearly showing that subjects who develop IGT or T2D have a compromising insulin secretion, even before developing IGT or T2D. When estimating insulin secretion in the context of the "resistant milieu" of IGT subjects, and thus using the disposition index (DI), it has been found that IGT subjects had a significantly lower DI than the normal glucose tolerance group. The lower DI indicates that the secretion of insulin is not able to compensate for the increased resistance, resulting in a marked decrease in insulin-stimulated glucose metabolism in the IGT subjects.[76] More recently, Cali and colleagues[77] showed that obese adolescents with normal glucose tolerance who successively progress to IGT manifest a primary defect in β-cell function. These data are in agreement with those reported by Lyssenko and colleagues[75] on mineral protein preparation and Botnia studies on adults showing that impaired insulin secretion and action, particularly insulin secretion adjusted for insulin resistance (DI), are strong predictors of future diabetes. Moreover, the progression of obese children with insulin resistance to T2D seems to be faster than in adults.[78] An accurate case report by Gungor and colleagues[78] suggested that, despite relatively robust initial insulin secretion, the deterioration in β-cell function in youth with T2DM may be much more accelerated (approximately 15% per year) than that observed in adults.

However, because T2D in youth is a recent phenomenon, longitudinal long-term follow-up data are lacking. Findings from the SEARCH study showed that youth with T2D and relatively short diabetes duration (1.5 years in mean) have a higher prevalence of CAD risk factors compared with nondiabetic of similar age, sex, and race.[79] In the same study, it has been also suggested that adiposity and glycemic control account for much of the association between T2D and an unfavorable CAD risk-factor profile in youth.[79]

ASSOCIATION BETWEEN FATTY LIVER AND MS

The intrahepatic fat accumulation induced by insulin resistance causes the development of nonalcoholic fatty liver disease (NAFLD), which is a clinic pathologic condition of emerging importance in obese children.[80] NAFLD encompasses the entire spectrum of liver conditions, ranging from asymptomatic steatosis with elevated or normal aminotransferases to steatohepatitis (nonalcoholic steatohepatitis or NASH) and advanced fibrosis with cirrhosis.[81,82] Concurrent with the worldwide epidemic increase in childhood obesity,[80,83] NAFLD is rapidly becoming one of the most important metabolic complications in the pediatric population. NAFLD affects 2.6% of normal children[84] and up to 77% in obese individuals.[85,86] Studies from autopsies of 742 children (ages 2–19 years) reported fatty liver prevalence at 9.6%, and in obese children this rate increased to an alarming 38%.[86] Moreover, in the United States, 3% of adolescents present abnormal serum aminotransferases values.[87]

The natural history of NAFLD is not entirely known; nevertheless, mortality among NASH patients is higher than in those with NAFLD without fibrosis or inflammation.[88] Alarming data have been shown in pediatric population. NASH is increasingly recognized in obese children[89,90] and it has been demonstrated that it may progress to cirrhosis in this age group.[89]

Although a multifactorial pathogenesis for the development of NAFLD has been demonstrated, a strong relationship between hepatic steatosis and insulin resistance has been clearly documented in large cohort-based studies of adults[91,92] and in obese adolescent populations.[80,93] To date, a widely accepted model for the pathogenesis of NAFLD is the "two-hit" hypothesis, where insulin resistance seems to be responsible for abnormalities in lipid storage and lipolysis in insulin-sensitive tissues, leading to an increased fatty acids flux from adipose tissue to the liver[94] and subsequent accumulation of triglycerides in the hepatocytes.[95]

The "second hit" is oxidative stress, which activates inflammatory cytokines like TNF-α and generates reactive oxygen species, such as hydroxyl radicals and superoxide anions, which can react with the excess lipid to form peroxides.[96,97] Lipids per oxidation products may injure cells directly by interfering with membrane function or stimulate fibrosis by hepatic stellate cells.[95,98]

It is becoming increasingly clear that NAFLD in obese youth is not only a marker of liver disease, but is also associated with important cardiovascular risk factors.[99] In fact, it has been suggested that, because of the high prevalence of fatty liver in association with obesity, insulin resistance, and alterations in glucose and lipid metabolism,[80,99] NAFLD may be considered the hepatic manifestation of MS.

The association between NAFLD and MS has been clearly demonstrated by Burgert and colleagues.[80] In this latest study, as surrogate of liver injury, alanine aminotransferase (ALT) levels were measured in 392 obese adolescents. Elevated ALT (>35 U/L) levels were found in 14% of participants, with a predominance of White/Hispanic. After adjusting for potential confounders, rising ALT levels were associated with deterioration in insulin sensitivity and glucose tolerance, as well as increasing FFA and triglyceride levels. Furthermore, increased hepatic fat accumulation (assessed using fast MRI) was found in 32% of obese adolescents and was associated with decreased insulin sensitivity and adiponectin levels, and with increased triglycerides and visceral fat (**Fig. 2**).[80] These results demonstrate that in obese children and adolescents, hepatic fat accumulation is associated with the components of MS, such as insulin resistance, dyslipidemia, and altered glucose metabolism.

The relationship between fatty liver and glucose dysregulation has been recently demonstrated in a multiethnic group of 118 obese adolescents.[100] The cohort was stratified according to tertiles of hepatic fat content, measured by fat gradient MRI. All children underwent an oral glucose tolerance test and insulin sensitivity was estimated by the Matsuda Index and HOMA-IR. Independently of obesity, the severity of fatty liver was associated with the presence of prediabetes (IGT and IFG/IGT). In fact, paralleling the severity of hepatic steatosis, there was a significant decrease in insulin sensitivity and impairment in β-cell function, as indicated by the fall in the DI. Given the association with prediabetic phenotype and fatty liver, NAFLD may be considered a strong risk factor for T2DM in youth.[80,100,101] Furthermore, paralleling the severity of fatty liver, there was a significant increase in the prevalence of MS, suggesting that hepatic steatosis may probably be a predictive factor of MS in children.[100]

Recent studies have shown that patterns of fat partitioning are probably one major link between insulin resistance, NAFLD, and MS in obese children.[102] In a multiethnic cohort study, 118 obese adolescents were stratified into tertiles based on the proportion of abdominal fat in the visceral depot. Abdominal fat and intramyocellular lipid were respectively measured by MRI and by proton magnetic resonance spectroscopy. A high proportion of visceral fat was associated with muscle and hepatic steatosis, insulin resistance, high triglycerides, and low HDL and adiponectin levels. As the proportion of visceral fat increased across tertiles, percentage subcutaneous fat decreased. Notably, the risk for MS was five times greater in the adolescents with this particular fat partitioning profile compared with those with lower visceral accumulation.[103] For this reason it has been suggested that obese adolescents with a high proportion of visceral fat and relatively low subcutaneous fat have a phenotype reminiscent of partial lipodystrophy. Those who fit this profile are not necessarily the most severe obese, yet they suffer from severe metabolic complications of obesity and are at high risk of having MS.[102,103]

In conclusion, it is unclear whether hepatic steatosis is a consequence or a cause of the metabolic derangements in insulin sensitivity (MS). However, it is clear that liver steatosis represents a major metabolic concern in obese children, which is why it

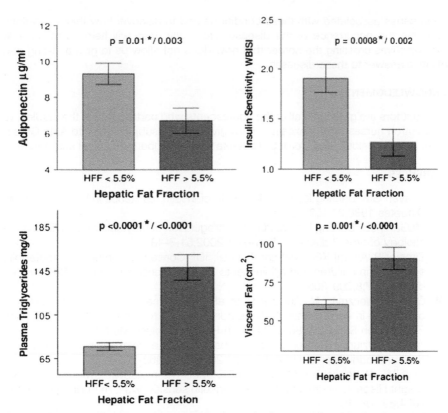

Fig. 2. Adiponectin levels, insulin sensitivity (WBISI), plasma triglycerides levels, and visceral fat in subjects with low- versus high-hepatic fat fraction (HFF). HFF was considered low when it was lower than 5.5% and high when it was higher than 5.5%. (*From* Burgert TS, Taksali SE, Dziura J, et al. Alanine aminotransferase levels fatty liver in childhood obesity: Associations with insulin resistance, adiponectin, and visceral fat. J Clin Endocrinol Metab 2006;91:2487–94; with permission. Copyright © 2006, The Endocrine Society.)

would need to be deeply and precociously investigated and identified to prevent further metabolic complications.

CONCLUSIONS AND FUTURE PERSPECTIVES

Given the relatively recent occurrence of MS in childhood, long-term follow-up studies are not available yet. However, it is reasonable to think that the metabolic derangement observed in obese children will have dramatic repercussions on their health earlier than that observed in adults, with a consequent worsening of the prognosis in terms of morbidity and mortality when they are still youth. To date, we know that the physician has few arrows in his or her quiver to fight this disease. The majority of medicines needed to treat insulin resistance, hypercholesterolemia, hypertension, or even T2D are now off-label, although more and more studies dealing with pharmacologic treatment of obesity and its complications in pediatrics are ocurring. The weight loss achieved by diet and physical exercise is still the most powerful and useful weapon against obesity and its metabolic complications.

Several genetic studies and programs dealing with childhood obesity, insulin resistance, and T2D are now ongoing all over the world. These studies have been designed to find genes associated with these conditions and to discover how their alterations determine the occurrence of the disease. Hopefully, they will help us to achieve new objectives crossing the border that now does not allow us to give a strong and definitive answer to these diseases.

ACKNOWLEDGMENTS

The authors are grateful to all of the adolescents who participated in the studies, to the research nurses for the excellent care given to our subjects, and to Aida Groszmann, Andrea Belous, and Corduta Todeasa for their superb technical assistance.

REFERENCES

1. Reaven GM. Banting lecture 1988. Role of insulin resistance in human disease. Diabetes 1988;37:1595–607.
2. McGarry JD. Banting lecture 2001: Dysregulation of fatty acid metabolism in the etiology of type 2 diabetes. Diabetes 2002;51:7–18.
3. Zimmet P, Alberti KG, Kaufman F, et al. IDF Consensus Group. The metabolic syndrome in children and adolescents—an IDF consensus report. Pediatr Diabetes 2007;8:299–306.
4. Cook S, Weitzman M, Auinger P, et al. Prevalence of a metabolic syndrome phenotype in adolescents: findings from the third National Health and Nutrition Examination Survey, 1988–1994. Arch Pediatr Adolesc Med 2003;157:821–7.
5. Weiss R, Dziura J, Burgert TS, et al. Obesity and the metabolic syndrome in children and adolescents. N Engl J Med 2004;350:2362–74.
6. Cruz ML, Weigensberg MJ, Huang TT, et al. The metabolic syndrome in overweight Hispanic youth and the role of insulin sensitivity. J Clin Endocrinol Metab 2004;89:108–13.
7. Ford ES, Ajani UA, Mokdad AH, National Health and Nutrition Examination. The metabolic syndrome and concentrations of C-reactive protein among U.S. youth. Diabetes Care 2005;28:878–81.
8. de Ferranti SD, Gauvreau K, Ludwig DS, et al. Prevalence of the metabolic syndrome in American adolescents: findings from the third national health and nutrition examination survey. Circulation 2004;110:2494–7.
9. Goodman E, Daniels SR, Morrison JA, et al. Contrasting prevalence of and demographic disparities in the World Health Organization and National Cholesterol Education Program Adult Treatment Panel III definitions of metabolic syndrome among adolescents. J Pediatr 2004;145:445–51.
10. Batey LS, Goff DC Jr, Tortolero SR, et al. Summary measures of the insulin resistance syndrome are adverse among Mexican-American versus non-Hispanic white children: the Corpus Christi Child Heart Study. Circulation 1997;96:4319–25.
11. Arslanian S, Suprasongsin C, Janosky JE. Insulin secretion and sensitivity in black versus white prepubertal healthy children. J Clin Endocrinol Metab 1997;82:1923–7.
12. Svec F, Nastasi K, Hilton C, et al. Black-white contrasts in insulin levels during pubertal development. The Bogalusa Heart Study. Diabetes 1992;41:313–7.
13. Arslanian S, Suprasongsin C. Differences in the in vivo insulin secretion and sensitivity of healthy black versus white adolescents. J Pediatr 1996;129:440–3.
14. Nguyen QM, Srinivasan SR, Xu JH, et al. Changes in risk variables of metabolic syndrome since childhood in pre-diabetic and type 2 diabetic subjects: the Bogalusa Heart Study. Diabetes Care 2008;31:2044–9.

15. World Health Organization. Obesity. Preventing and managing the global epidemic. Publication WHO/NUT/NCD/98.1.1998. Geneva, Switzerland: World Health Organization; 1998.
16. National Heart, Lung and Blood Institute. Clinical guidelines on the identification, evaluation, and treatment of overweight and obesity in adults: the evidence report. Obes Res 1998;6:S51–210.
17. Cole TJ, Bellizzi MC, Flegal KM, et al. Establishing a standard definition for child overweight and obesity worldwide: international survey. BMJ 2000;320:1240–3.
18. Himes JH, Dietz WH. Guidelines for overweight in adolescent preventive services: recommendations from an expert committee. The Expert Committee on Clinical Guidelines for Overweight in Adolescent Preventive Services. Am J Clin Nutr 1994;59:307–16.
19. Kuczmarski RJ, Ogden CL, Guo SS, et al. + 2000 CDC Growth Charts for the United States: methods and development. Vital Health Stat 11 2002;246:1–190.
20. Fernández JR, Redden DT, Pietrobelli A, et al. Waist circumference percentiles in nationally representative samples of African-American, European-American, and Mexican-American children and adolescents. J Pediatr 2004; 145:439–44.
21. Janssen I, Katzmarzyk PT, Srinivasan SR, et al. Combined influence of body mass index and waist circumference on coronary artery disease risk factors among children and adolescents. Pediatrics 2005;115:1623–30.
22. Pouliot MC, Després JP, Lemieux S, et al. Waist circumference and abdominal sagittal diameter: best simple anthropometric indexes of abdominal visceral adipose tissue accumulation and related cardiovascular risk in men and women. Am J Cardiol 1994;73:460–8.
23. Katzmarzyk PT. Waist circumference percentiles for Canadian youth 11–18 y of age. Eur J Clin Nutr 2004;58:1011–5.
24. Zannolli R, Morgese G. Waist percentiles: a simple test for atherogenic disease? Acta Paediatr 1996;85:1368–9.
25. McCarthy HD, Jarrett KV, Crawley HF. The development of waist circumference percentiles in British children aged 5.0–16.9 y. Eur J Clin Nutr 2001;55:902–7.
26. Dobbelsteyn CJ, Joffres MR, MacLean DR, et al. A comparative evaluation of waist circumference, waist-to-hip ratio and body mass index as indicators of cardiovascular risk factors. The Canadian Heart Health Surveys. Int J Obes Relat Metab Disord 2001;25:652–61.
27. Janssen I, Katzmarzyk PT, Ross R. Body mass index, waist circumference, and health risk: evidence in support of current National Institutes of Health guidelines. Arch Intern Med 2002;162:2074–9.
28. Janssen I, Heymsfield SB, Allison DB, et al. Body mass index and waist circumference independently contribute to the prediction of nonabdominal, abdominal subcutaneous, and visceral fat. Am J Clin Nutr 2002;75:683–8.
29. Thompson CJ, Ryu JE, Craven TE, et al. Central adipose distribution is related to coronary atherosclerosis. Arterioscler Thromb 1991;11:327–33.
30. Van Pelt RE, Evans EM, Schechtman KB, et al. Waist circumference vs body mass index for prediction of disease risk in postmenopausal women. Int J Obes Relat Metab Disord 2001;25:1183–8.
31. Maffeis C, Pietrobelli A, Grezzani A, et al. Waist circumference and cardiovascular risk factors in prepubertal children. Obes Res 2001;9:179–87.
32. Freedman DS, Serdula MK, Srinivasan SR, et al. Relation of circumferences and skinfold thicknesses to lipid and insulin concentrations in children and adolescents: the Bogalusa Heart Study. Am J Clin Nutr 1999;69:308–17.

33. Savva SC, Tornaritis M, Savva ME, et al. Waist circumference and waist-to-height ratio are better predictors of cardiovascular disease risk factors in children than body mass index. Int J Obes Relat Metab Disord 2000;24:1453–8.

34. Ferrannini E, Natali A, Capaldo B, et al. Insulin resistance, hyperinsulinemia, and blood pressure: role of age and obesity. European Group for the Study of Insulin Resistance (EGIR). Hypertension 1997;30:1144–9.

35. Fujimoto WY, Bergstrom RW, Boyko EJ, et al. Visceral adiposity and incident coronary heart disease in Japanese-American men. The 10-year follow-up results of the Seattle Japanese-American Community Diabetes Study. Diabetes Care 1999;22:1808–12.

36. O'Shaughnessy IM, Myers TJ, Stepniakowski K, et al. Glucose metabolism in abdominally obese hypertensive and normotensive subjects. Hypertension 1995;26:186–92.

37. Björntorp P. Portal adipose tissue as a generator of risk factors for cardiovascular disease and diabetes. Arteriosclerosis 1990;10:493–6.

38. Williamson JR, Kreisberg RA, Felts PW. Mechanism for the stimulation of gluconeogenesis by fatty acids in perfused rat liver. Proc Natl Acad Sci U S A 1966; 56:247–54.

39. Steppan CM, Bailey ST, Bhat S, et al. The hormone resistin links obesity to diabetes. Nature 2001;409:307–12.

40. Hotamisligil GS, Peraldi P, Budavari A, et al. IRS-1-mediated inhibition of insulin receptor tyrosine kinase activity in TNF-alpha- and obesity-induced insulin resistance. Science 1996;271:665–8.

41. Barzilai N, She L, Liu BQ, et al. Surgical removal of visceral fat reverses hepatic insulin resistance. Diabetes 1999;48:94–8.

42. Kim YW, Kim JY, Lee SK. Surgical removal of visceral fat decreases plasma free fatty acid and increases insulin sensitivity on liver and peripheral tissue in monosodium glutamate (MSG)-obese rats. J Korean Med Sci 1999;14:539–45.

43. Gabriely I, Ma XH, Yang XM, et al. Removal of visceral fat prevents insulin resistance and glucose intolerance of aging: an adipokine-mediated process? Diabetes 2002;51:2951–8.

44. Executive Summary of The Third Report of The National Cholesterol Education Program (NCEP) Expert Panel on Detection, Evaluation, And Treatment of High Blood Cholesterol in Adults (Adult Treatment Panel III). JAMA 2001;285:2486–97.

45. Terán-García M, Bouchard C. Genetics of metabolic syndrome. Appl Physiol Nutr Metab 2007;32:89–114.

46. Kraja AT, Hunt SC, Pankow JS, et al. An evaluation of the metabolic syndrome in the HyperGEN study. Nutr Metab 2005;18:2.

47. Weiss R, Shaw M, Savoy M, et al. Obesity dynamics and cardio-vascular risk factor stability in obese adolescents. Pediatr Diabetes, in press.

48. Steinberger J, Daniels SR, Eckel RH, et al. American Heart Association Atherosclerosis, Hypertension, and Obesity in the young committee of the council on cardiovascular disease in the young; council on cardiovascular nursing; and council on nutrition, physical activity, and metabolism. Progress and challenges in metabolic syndrome in children and adolescents: a scientific statement from the American Heart Association Atherosclerosis, Hypertension, and Obesity in the young committee of the council on cardiovascular disease in the young; council on cardiovascular nursing; and council on nutrition, physical activity, and metabolism. Circulation 2009;119:628–47.

49. Taittonen L, Uhari M, Nuutinen M, et al. Insulin and blood pressure among healthy children. Cardiovascular risk in young Finns. Am J Hypertens 1996;9:194–9.

50. Bao W, Scrinivansan SR, Berenson GS. Persistent elevation of plasma insulin levels is associated with increased cardiovascular risk in children and young adults: the Bogalusa Heart Study. Circulation 1996;93:54–9.
51. Landsberg L. Hyperinsulinemia: possible role in obesity-induced hypertension. Hypertension 1992;19:I61–6.
52. DeFronzo RA, Cooke CR, Andres R, et al. The effect of insulin on renal handling of sodium, potassium, calcium, and phosphate in man. J Clin Invest 1975;55: 845–55.
53. Stout RW, Bierman FI, Ross R. Effect of insulin on the proliferation of cultured primate arterial smooth muscle cells. Circ Res 1975;36:319–27.
54. Assimacopoulos-Jeannet F, Brichard S, Rencurel F, et al. In vivo effects of hyper-insulinemia on lipogenic enzymes and glucose transporter expression in rat liver and adipose tissues. Metabolism 1995;44:228–33.
55. Kamagate A, Dong HH. FoxO1 integrates insulin signaling to VLDL production. Cell Cycle 2008;7:3162–70.
56. Caprio S, Plewe G, Diamond MP, et al. Increased insulin secretion in puberty: a compensatory response to reductions in insulin sensitivity. J Pediatr 1989; 114:963–7.
57. Moran A, Steffen LM, Jacobs DR Jr, et al. Relation of C-reactive protein to insulin resistance and cardiovascular risk factors in youth. Diabetes Care 2005;28: 1763–8.
58. Lambert M, Delvin EE, Paradis G, et al. C-reactive protein and features of the metabolic syndrome in a population-based sample of children and adolescents. Clin Chem 2004;50:1762–8.
59. Hiura M, Kikuchi T, Nagasaki K, et al. Elevation of serum C-reactive protein levels is associated with obesity in boys. Hypertens Res 2003;26:541–6.
60. Körner A, Kratzsch J, Gausche R, et al. New predictors of the metabolic syndrome in children–role of adipocytokines. Pediatr Res 2007;61:640–5.
61. Nemet D, Wang P, Funahashi T, et al. Adipocytokines, body composition, and fitness in children. Pediatr Res 2003;53:148–52.
62. Dixon D, Goldberg R, Schneiderman N, et al. Gender differences in TNF-alpha levels among obese vs nonobese Latino children. Eur J Clin Nutr 2004;58:696–9.
63. Ruan H, Lodish HF. Insulin resistance in adipose tissue: direct and indirect effects of tumor necrosis factor-alpha. Cytokine Growth Factor Rev 2003;14: 447–55.
64. Maffeis C, Silvagni D, Bonadonna R, et al. Fat cell size, insulin sensitivity, and inflammation in obese children. J Pediatr 2007;151:647–52.
65. Hara K, Yamauchi T, Kadowaki T. Adiponectin: an adipokine linking adipocytes and type 2 diabetes in humans. Curr Diab Rep 2005;5:136–40.
66. Kadowaki T, Yamauchi T. Adiponectin and adiponectin receptors. Endocr Rev 2005;26:439–51.
67. Böttner A, Kratzsch J, Müller G, et al. Gender differences of adiponectin levels develop during the progression of puberty and are related to serum androgen levels. J Clin Endocrinol Metab 2004;89:4053–61.
68. Reinehr T, Roth C, Menke T, et al. Adiponectin before and after weight loss in obese children. J Clin Endocrinol Metab 2004;89:3790–4.
69. American Diabetes Association. Diagnosis and classification of diabetes melli-tus. Diabetes Care 2008;31:S55–60.
70. Meyer C, Pimenta W, Woerle HJ, et al. Different mechanisms for impaired fasting glucose and impaired postprandial glucose tolerance in humans. Diabetes Care 2006;29:1909–14.

71. The Writing Group for the SEARCH for Diabetes in Youth Study Group. Incidence of diabetes in youth in the United States. JAMA 2007;297:2716–24.
72. Sinha R, Fisch G, Teague B, et al. Prevalence of impaired glucose tolerance among children and adolescents with marked obesity. N Engl J Med 2002; 346:802–10.
73. Invitti C, Gilardini L, Viberti G. Impaired glucose tolerance in obese children and adolescents. N Engl J Med 2002;347:290–2.
74. Gilardini L, Girola A, Morabito F, et al. Fasting glucose is not useful in identifying obese white children with impaired glucose tolerance. J Pediatr 2006;149:282.
75. Lyssenko V, Jonsson A, Almgren P, et al. Clinical risk factors, DNA variants, and the development of type 2 diabetes. N Engl J Med 2008;359:2220–32.
76. Weiss R, Caprio S. The metabolic consequences of childhood obesity. Best Pract Res Clin Endocrinol Metab 2005;19:405–19.
77. Cali AM, Dalla Man C, Cobelli C, et al. Primary defects in beta-cell function further exacerbated by worsening of insulin resistance mark the development of impaired glucose tolerance in obese adolescents. Diabetes Care 2009;32:456–61.
78. Gungor N, Arslanian S. Progressive beta cell failure in type 2 diabetes mellitus of youth. J Pediatr 2004;44:656–9.
79. West NA, Hamman RF, Mayer-Davis EJ, et al. Cardiovascular risk factors among youth with and without type 2 diabetes: differences and possible mechanisms. Diabetes Care 2009;32:175–80.
80. Burgert TS, Taksali SE, Dziura J, et al. Alanine aminotransferase levels fatty liver in childhood obesity: Associations with insulin resistance, adiponectin, and visceral fat. J Clin Endocrinol Metab 2006;91:2487–94.
81. Manco M, Marcellini M, Devito R, et al. Metabolic syndrome and liver histology in paediatric non-alcoholic steatohepatitis. Int J Obes (Lond) 2008;32:381–7.
82. Angulo P. Nonalcoholic fatty liver disease. N Engl J Med 2002;346:1221–31.
83. Caprio S, Daniels SR, Drewnowski A, et al. Influence of race, ethnicity, and culture on childhood obesity: implications for prevention and treatment: a consensus statement of Shaping America's Health and the Obesity Society. Diabetes Care 2008;31:2211–21.
84. Tominaga K, Kurata JH, Chen YK, et al. Prevalence of fatty liver in Japanese children and relationship to obesity. An epidemiological ultrasonographic survey. Dig Dis Sci 1995;40:2002–9.
85. Franzese A, Vajro P, Argenziano A, et al. Liver involvement in obese children. Ultrasonography and liver enzymes levels at diagnosis and during follow-up in an Italian population. Dig Dis Sci 1997;42:1428–32.
86. Schwimmer JB, Deutsch R, Kahen T, et al. Prevalence of fatty liver in children and adolescents. Pediatrics 2006;118:1388–93.
87. Strauss RS, Barlow SE, Dietz WH. Prevalence of abnormal serum amino transferase values in overweight and obese adolescents. J Pediatr Gastroenterol Nutr 2000;136:727–33.
88. Ekstedt M, Franzén LE, Mathiesen UL, et al. Long-term follow-up of patients with NAFLD and elevated liver enzymes. Hepatology 2006;44:865–73.
89. Molleston JP, White F, Teckman J, et al. Obese children with steatohepatitis can develop cirrhosis in childhood. Am J Gastroenterol 2002;97:2460–2.
90. Kinugasa A, Tsunamoto K, Furukawa N, et al. Fatty liver and its fibrous changes found in simple obesity of children. J Pediatr Gastroenterol Nutr 1984;3:408–14.
91. Angelico F, Del BM, Conti R, et al. Non-alcoholic fatty liver syndrome: A hepatic consequence of common metabolic diseases. J Gastroenterol Hepatol 2003;18: 588–94.

92. Angelico F, Del BM, Conti R, et al. Insulin resistance, the metabolic syndrome and non-alcoholic fatty liver disease. J Clin Endocrinol Metab 2005;90:1578–82.
93. Mandato C, Lucariello S, Licenziati MR, et al. Metabolic, hormonal, oxidative, and inflammatory factors in pediatric obesity-related liver disease. J Pediatr 2005;147:62–6.
94. Day CP, James OFW. Steatohepatitis: a tale of two "hits". Gastroenterology 1998;114:842–5.
95. Browning JD, Horton JD. Molecular mediators of hepatic steatosis and liver injury. J Clin Invest 2004;114:147–52.
96. Berson A, De BV, Letteron P, et al. Steatohepatitis-inducing drugs cause mitochondrial dysfunction and lipid peroxidation in rat hepatocytes. Gastroenterology 1998;114:764–74.
97. Lavine JE. Vitamin E treatment of nonalcoholic steatohepatitis in children: a pilot study. J Pediatr 2000;136:734–8.
98. Pietrangelo A. Metals. Oxidative stress and hepatic fibrogenesis. Semin Liver Dis 1996;16:13–30.
99. Schwimmer JB, Pardee PE, Lavine JE, et al. Cardiovascular risk factors and the metabolic syndrome in pediatric nonalcoholic fatty liver disease. Circulation 2008;118:277–83.
100. Cali AMG, De Oliveira AM, Kim H, et al. Glucose dysregulation and hepatic steatosis in obese adolescents: Is there a link? Hepatology 2009;49:1896–903.
101. Sattar N, Scherbakova O, Ford I, et al. West of Scotland Coronary Prevention Study Elevated alanine aminotransferase predicts new-onset type 2 diabetes independently of classical risk factors, metabolic syndrome, and C-reactive protein in the west of Scotland coronary prevention study. Diabetes 2004;53:2855–60.
102. Taksali SE, Caprio S, Dziura J, et al. High visceral and low abdominal subcutaneous fat stores in the obese adolescent. Diabetes 2008;57:367–71.
103. Cali AMG, Caprio S. Ectopic fat deposition and the metabolic syndrome in obese children and adolescents. Horm Res 2009;71:2–7.

Prevention of Type 1 Diabetes

Diane K. Wherrett, MD, FRCPC, Denis Daneman, MBBCh, FRCPC*

KEYWORDS

- Type 1 diabetes • Autoimmunity • Prevention • Immunology
- Genetics • Clinical trials

Type 1 diabetes (T1D) is an autoimmune disease in which the β cells of the pancreatic islets are destroyed, rendering the individual increasingly incapable of mounting a normal insulin response to ingested nutrients.[1,2] In the early 1980s, Eisenbarth[2] enunciated the main phases in the pathogenesis of T1D (**Fig. 1**), a framework which continues to be useful in considering approaches to the prevention or cure of this disorder:

1. Susceptibility to T1D is inherited through a series of genes, the most important of which relate to the HLA class II locus on chromosome 6, with lesser contribution from several others, including the insulin gene, CTLA4 and others (see later discussion). Susceptibility genes are essential, but insufficient in explaining the immune pathogenesis of T1D, that is, most individuals with these susceptibility genes never develop the disorder.
2. Exposure to 1 or more environmental triggers alters the immune system in such a way that susceptibility is converted to pathophysiology and destruction of β cells begins. Despite intensive searches for environmental triggers, the number of candidates being assessed in clinical trials remains small, for example, cow's milk proteins, relative lack of vitamin D, and supplementation with omega-3 fatty acids.[3-7]
3. Although attack on the β cells is mediated in large part by T cells, it is the presence of humoral (B-cell) markers that punctuates the next phase: normal glucose homeostasis in the presence of 1 or more T1D-specific autoantibodies; ICA512/IA-2, insulin autoantibody (IAA) and glutamic acid decarboxylase (GAD) are the main ones available for measurement. The progression to clinical T1D is highly predictable based on the number of antibodies present.[8]
4. The earliest metabolic abnormality detected is loss of first phase insulin secretion in response to an intravenous glucose load. Glucose levels remain normal in response

Portions of this article were previously published in the *Endocrinology and Metabolism Clinics of North America*, 38:4.

Division of Endocrinology, Department of Pediatrics, The Hospital for Sick Children and University of Toronto, 555 University Avenue, Toronto, Ontario M5G 1X8, Canada

* Corresponding author.

E-mail address: denis.daneman@sickkids.ca

Pediatr Clin N Am 58 (2011) 1257–1270

doi:10.1016/j.pcl.2011.07.010

0031-3955/11/$ – see front matter © 2011 Elsevier Inc. All rights reserved.

pediatric.theclinics.com

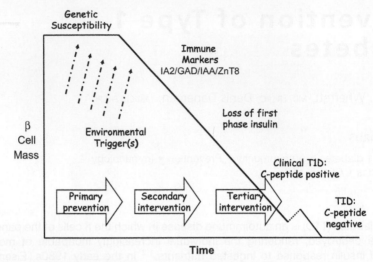

Fig. 1. The natural history of T1D.

to meal challenges at this stage. Later, impaired glucose tolerance develops. This leads inexorably to the next phases of clinical diabetes.

5. When β-cell mass is significantly decreased, insulin secretory capacity is damaged to such a degree that it is no longer sufficient to maintain normoglycemia and clinical diabetes supervenes. This phase includes the honeymoon or remission period of T1D when some β-cell function is retained, also called the C-peptide–positive phase of clinical diabetes.

6. Finally, in most, but not all, individuals with T1D, β cell function is eventually completely lost and C-peptide levels become undetectable. There is a relationship between the presence of diabetic ketoacidosis at disease onset and the rapidity of loss of β cells, and between the presence of residual β-cell function and the ability to achieve and maintain better metabolic control.

A few additional facts are important in considering targets for prevention or early intervention in the pathogenesis of T1D[9]: Firstly, the incidence of this condition is increasing by 2% to 5% per year worldwide, especially in the youngest age group (<5 years of age).[10] Secondly, there is enormous variability in incidence of T1D around the world, from less than 4 per 100,000 in a population younger than 14 years in much of Africa and Asia to more than 20, in Canada, Australia, and parts of Europe, with the highest incidence being in Finland (>50 per 100,000 in the population reported in 2008).[11] Thirdly, migrating populations take on the increased incidence of their new countries fairly rapidly, for example, Asian immigrants to the United Kingdom, immigrants from the Horn of Africa (Somalia, Eritrea, and Ethiopia) to North America.[12] Fourthly, there is evidence that genetically similar populations may have enormously dissimilar incidence rates, for example, Finland and Russian Karelia.[13] These factors strongly indicate an important role for environmental factors in the cause of T1D, because genetic drift cannot explain the rapidity of these changes. Furthermore, where incidence is increasing most rapidly, the contribution of genetic susceptibility seems to be less.[14]

GENETICS OF T1D

T1D is 15 times more common in siblings of those with T1D, with the general population prevalence of approximately 0.4% and the sibling prevalence of approximately

6%.[15] Genes located within the HLA class II region on chromosome 6p21 account for approximately 50% of genetic risk of T1D.[16,17] Haplotypes associated with T1D include DQ2 (DQB1*0201–DQA1*0501–DRB1*03) and DQ8 (DQB1*0302–DQA1*0301–DRB1*04).[18] Other HLA alleles, DQA1*0102, DQB1*0602 confer protection from T1D.[19] A region in the regulatory region of the insulin gene (INS) locus has also been shown to provide approximately 10% of the genetic susceptibility to T1D.[18] A polymorphism in the PTPN22 (protein tyrosine phosphatase non-receptor type 22) gene has been found to be associated with several autoimmune diseases, including T1D and autoimmune thyroid disease.[18] The gene product, a lymphoid tyrosine phosphatase, inhibits the T-cell receptor signaling pathway. Polymorphisms in the cytotoxic T-lymphocyte–associated gene (CTLA4) are also associated with T1D and several other autoimmune diseases.[20] Signaling through CTLA4 is critical in the down-regulation of T-cell responses. Association has also been found with the interleukin-2 receptor alpha subunit gene region. This region codes for the CD25 portion of the receptor which has a significant role in controlling T cell proliferation.[21] Over 40 genes/regions have been confirmed to be associated with T1D. Identification of these genes provides investigative targets for new understanding of disease pathogenesis.

Although there have been important discoveries in the genetics of T1D and the autoimmune processes involved, little progress has been made in identifying highly specific environmental factors pivotal in triggering this disorder. Two hypotheses remain prominent in this respect: (1) the hygiene hypothesis suggests that in modern society, the lack of exposure to pathogens early in life prevents the genetically predisposed immune system from protecting itself from autoimmune phenomena, (2) the accelerator hypothesis suggests that increasing worldwide obesity stresses the susceptible β-cell, thereby triggering its early demise.[22–28] The only environmental trigger undergoing active investigation is early exposure to cow's milk proteins, which may be important in T1D pathogenesis; conversely, breast milk may protect against triggering of the autoimmune attack. The effort to better identify environmental factors is currently being led by The Environmental Determinants of Diabetes in the Young study. This study is scheduled to enroll 7800 infants by the end of 2009 with high-risk HLA genotypes for serial assessment of islet autoimmunity and environmental exposures, such as diet, infectious diseases, and immunizations.[29]

TARGETS FOR PREVENTION OR EARLY INTERVENTION

Prevention of T1D would require interventions aimed at (1) avoiding exposure to environmental triggers early in life—primary prevention; (2) interfering with the autoimmune cascade that occurs during β-cell destruction—secondary prevention or intervention; or (3) halting or reversing β-cell loss after clinical presentation of T1D—tertiary intervention. Once full-blown clinical T1D has developed, the only approach to disease reversal would be physiologic insulin replacement using either an artificial pancreas or β-cell replacement with islet or pancreatic transplantation. T1D is seen as one of the disorders most likely to be amenable to stem cell therapy in the future.

PRIMARY PREVENTION

An environmental role in the pathophysiology of T1D is supported by a number of factors: low concordance rate of the disorder in identical twins (20%–50%); different incidence rates in populations of similar genetic makeup but significantly different socioeconomic status (eg, Finland and Russian Karelia); and rapid shifts in incidence in different areas of the world and with population migration. The specific environmental factors involved remain largely unproven, although epidemiologic and animal-model data suggest a potential role for dietary factors, more specifically, early exposure to cow's milk and low vitamin D concentrations, with much more data pointing to a role for cow's milk proteins.[3–7,30]

There are good data to indicate that the pathogenetic processes leading to T1D may begin very early in life. This data, with animal-model and epidemiologic data, has provided the impetus to evaluate carefully the role of weaning diets on the evolution of T1D, especially the role of early exposure to cow's milk proteins. A more detailed description of the supporting data is beyond the scope of this article but can be found in references.[3–7,30]

The Trial to Reduce IDDM (insulin-dependent diabetes mellitus) in the Genetically at Risk (TRIGR) is a double-blind, randomized placebo-controlled trial that is intended for definitively testing the hypothesis that weaning to a hydrolyzed diet, thereby avoiding early cow's milk protein exposure, protects high-risk newborns from initiation of the β-cell–specific autoimmune response, and therefore prevents T1D.[31] This international multicenter study is powered to meet these objectives. The recruitment of high-risk neonates allows for concentration of subjects more likely to develop T1D, the criterion being that their mother, father, or sibling has T1D. They are screened for high-risk HLA haplotypes. If results are positive, the neonates are randomly assigned to 1 of 2 groups: feeding up to 6 to 8 months of age with a regular cow's milk-based formula, or an extensively hydrolyzed cow's milk formula. Breast feeding is encouraged and noted as a potential confounder in the study. The study design is shown in **Fig. 2** and inclusion and exclusion criteria are listed below:

Neonates with a first-degree relative (ie, mother/father/sibling) with T1D are eligible.

Inclusion criteria
1. The infant has one of the following genotypes:
    a. HLA-DQB1*0302/DQA1*05-DQB1*02
    b. HLA-DQB1*0302/x (ie, excluding DQB1*02, DQB1*0301, DQB1*0602)
    c. HLA-DQA1*05–DQB1*02/y (ie, excluding DQA1*0201-DQB1*02, DQB1*001, DQB1*0602/3)
    d. HLA-DQA1*03–DQB1*02/y (ie, excluding the same ones as in [c]. above)
2. Family able to provide written informed consent.

Exclusion criteria
1. An older sibling in TRIGR intervention
2. Multiple gestation

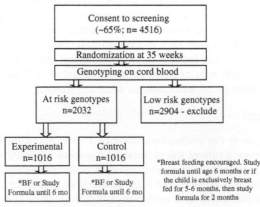

Fig. 2. TRIGR design.

3. Parents unwilling or unable to give study formula
4. Newborn has recognizable severe illness
5. Inability of family to participate in the study
6. Infant received any formula other than Nutramigen before randomization
7. Infant older than 7 days at randomization
8. No HLA sample before 8 days of age.

The major outcome for the first phase of TRIGR is the frequency of T1D-associated autoantibodies and/or development of diabetes by age 6 years. The outcome of the second phase is the manifestation of diabetes by age 10 years according to standard criteria, obviously the more definitive outcome, although the intervention may delay rather than prevent the manifestation of T1D. This latter outcome would be masked by the final outcome being measured at age 10 years.[31] Screening for TRIGR began in May 2002, with final enrollment completed by September 2006. The antibody data will be available in 2012 and the T1D outcomes in 2016.

Knip and colleagues reported results of the Finnish pilot study of TRIGR, documenting the rates of development of beta-cell autoimmunity (measured by autoantibodies to insulin, glutamic acid decarboxylase (GAD), the insulinoma-associated 2 molecule (IA-2), and zinc transporter 8) in this randomized, double-blind trial of 230 infants with HLA-conferred susceptibility to T1DM. Their data show that over a median observation period of 10 years, infants receiving the study (casein hydrolysate) formula were about half as likely to develop positivity for one or more autoantibodies compared to the infants receiving conventional, cow's-milk-based formula. Further observation is required to see whether this translates to differences in the incidence of clinical T1DM.[32]

A double-blind placebo-controlled pilot study of omega-3 fatty acid supplementation with docosahexaenoic acid (DHA) to prevent islet autoimmunity is being performed by the Type 1 Diabetes TrialNet study group.[33] Diets higher in omega-3 fatty acids have been associated with lower risk of islet autoimmunity and diabetes.[34] DHA is known to have an anti-inflammatory effect. Entry to the study was during the third trimester for pregnant mothers or during the first 5 months of life for infants with a first-degree relative with T1D. At birth, HLA typing was done on cord blood and those with high risk alleles were eligible. Enrollment of 97 infants is complete with results of compliance, levels of whole blood DHA, and inflammatory markers expected in late 2009.

A feasibility study, BABYDIET, of delay of introduction of gluten to prevent islet autoimmunity in infants with a first-degree relative with T1D and high-risk HLA genotypes did not show a reduced risk of islet autoimmunity.[35,36] The timing of introduction of cereals to infants has been associated with diabetes.[37] Infants were randomized to introduction of gluten at age 6 or 12 months with follow-up every 3 months up to 36 months of age.

Vitamin D is increasingly recognized as an immunomodulator. Its effects on the immune system are multifold:

1. In acquired immunity, Vitamin D induces an inhibitory response through reduction of T-cell proliferation, interleukin-2 and interferon-γ production, and CD8-mediated cytotoxicity. This results in a reduction of T-helper 1 responses and a promotion of T-helper 2 responses. In this way, it improves T-regulatory forces and provides for a more balanced and tolerogenic milieu[38];
2. In the innate immune system, Vitamin D inhibits dendritic cell function at multiple levels and mediates antibacterial actions through cathelicidin and the toll-like receptor 4 pathway.[38]

Animal models show that treatment with $1,25(OH)_2$Vitamin D_3 or its analogs can prevent T1D and other immune-modulated disorders.[38] Furthermore, there are data on humans that suggest that Vitamin D may also play a role. For example, the incidence of T1D increases with increasing distance from the equator suggesting a role for sun exposure. A published meta-analysis examined the association between vitamin D supplementation and the development of T1D. It found a significantly reduced risk of developing T1D in those supplemented with vitamin D (OR 0.71).[39] A definitive prospective study on the effect of vitamin D supplementation on the development of diabetes remains to be performed.

SECONDARY PREVENTION

The goal of secondary prevention studies is to prevent the progression of islet destruction that will lead to overt T1D. To carry out these studies, reliable prediction models are required. Current prediction models use combinations of autoantibodies and measures of glucose tolerance to stratify risk. It is known that autoantibodies typically develop years before onset of diabetes. These antibodies include ICA, IAA, and antibodies to GAD, tyrosine phosphatase (IA-2/ICA512), and zinc transporter 8 (ZnT8).[40] The presence of 2 or more antibodies indicates a significantly increased risk of developing diabetes, with some studies reporting increasing risk with increasing number of antibodies. One study showed that relatives with 1 or more antibodies had a 25% risk of disease development over a 5-year period, 2 or more antibodies had a 39% risk of developing T1D within 3 years, and those with 3 or more antibodies had a 75% risk of disease development over a 5-year period.[41] As β-cell destruction progresses, subclinical glucose abnormalities develop. Evidence from the Diabetes Prevention Trial - Type 1 (DPT-1), showed that fasting and 2-hour glucose levels rise gradually, as stimulated C-peptide levels slowly decline in the 30 months before diagnosis.[42] Type 1 Diabetes TrialNet, an international study group performing research in the prevention and early treatment of T1D, is running a large longitudinal observational study of relatives of those with T1D to further improve prediction.[43]

Three large multi-center trials of diabetes prevention in autoantibody-positive subjects have been completed. The European Nicotinamide Diabetes Intervention Trial used nicotinamide as a secondary preventative agent. Despite promising animal data and evidence from a previous study, nicotinamide administration in ICA-positive relatives did not delay the onset of T1D when compared with placebo.[44] In DPT-1, insulin was given orally or parenterally to alter the immune response toward insulin.[45,46] Subjects at high risk (>50% over 5 years with ICA positive and low first-phase insulin response) of developing T1D received parenteral insulin. Those at moderate risk (25%–50% over 5 years with ICA and IAA but normal first-phase insulin secretion) received insulin orally. The primary analysis of both arms of DPT-1 did not show an effect on the development of T1D.[45] Post hoc analysis of DPT-1 oral insulin arm, however, suggested a beneficial effect in the subgroup with high titers of insulin autoantibodies.[46] The results of the T1D Prediction and Prevention Study were recently published.[47] In this study, newborns from the general population and siblings of those with diabetes had HLA genotyping done at birth. Those with 2 or more islet antibodies and high-risk HLA alleles were treated with nasal insulin or placebo. The study was stopped early as the treatment had no effect. The results of these studies, though disappointing, demonstrate that large scale prevention studies are feasible and provide significant insight into planning for future studies.

There are currently 3 diabetes prevention trials underway. The first is the Type 1 Diabetes TrialNet study, "Oral Insulin For Prevention of Diabetes In Relatives at Risk for

Type 1 Diabetes Mellitus." This study is further investigating the suggestion of oral insulin benefit as seen in the DPT-1 subjects with high IAA titers. Subjects have insulin autoantibodies and one of ICA, GAD antibodies, or ICA512 antibodies. The study intervention is oral insulin 7.5 mg/d or placebo for the study's duration with the endpoint, the development of diabetes. Recruitment began in 2007. The Pre-POINT trial is an international multicenter study that is examining intervention with nasal and oral insulin in children aged 18 months to 7 years who have a sibling or 2 or more relatives with T1D.[48] These children also have high-risk HLA alleles but no islet autoantibodies. The effects of 4 doses of oral and nasal insulin are being studied to determine whether autoimmunity will be affected. If the study is successful, a larger trial is planned.

The Intranasal Insulin Trial is based in Australia and New Zealand and is assessing the effect of intranasal insulin in first- and second-degree relatives aged 4 to 30 years who are at increased risk of diabetes based on data from an earlier pilot study.[49] Treatment continues for one year with follow-up for the development of diabetes for 4 years.

TERTIARY PREVENTION

It has long been recognized that most individuals presenting with T1D have little residual insulin secretion (as measured by C-peptide secretion) at the time of diagnosis.[50,51] However, in the weeks to months after diagnosis and initiation of insulin treatment, there can be substantial recovery of β-cell function with falling insulin requirements, increasing C-peptide concentrations, and easily controlled blood glucose levels.[50,51] This "honeymoon" or remission period of diabetes may last from weeks to months and occasionally years.[52] The honeymoon period is believed to be the result of the recovery of residual β cells unable to cope with the metabolic demands of the body. With institution of insulin treatment and reestablishment of glycemic control, these cells recover their capacity for insulin secretion only to be finally destroyed by the underlying autoimmune process. In addition, changes in insulin sensitivity probably also play a role in the expression of the honeymoon period, with decreased sensitivity at the time of diagnosis due to the hyperglycemia, with improvement after establishment of metabolic control.[53]

The ability to measure C-peptide concentrations in those receiving insulin therapy allows an accurate assessment of residual β-cell function, and it can be used as a marker of the efficacy of therapeutic intervention.[54] Prolongation of the honeymoon period has the potential to have significant beneficial effects in those with T1D. Metabolic control is much easier to establish in the presence of some residual insulin secretion. As a result, long-term diabetes-related complications are significantly less prevalent in those with residual insulin secretion. This was well demonstrated in the Diabetes Control and Complications Trial in which those subjects with sustained C-peptide production were found to have rates of nephropathy, retinopathy, and hypoglycemia that were half that of those without any residual insulin.[55] The population of newly diagnosed T1D patients therefore represents an important group for future study of promising new interventions. Therapies that can safely maintain endogenous insulin secretion in the longer term would represent an important clinical advance.

Several agents, including, cyclosporine, azathioprine, and prednisone, were studied in the 1980s for their efficacy in maintaining insulin production after the diagnosis of diabetes.[56–59] Some beneficial effects were observed, but toxicity concerns made further use of these agents unfavorable. Several immunomodulatory monoclonal antibodies have been studied. The monoclonal antibody hOKT3γ1 (Ala-Ala), interferes with T-cell activation by binding the T-cell receptor, CD3.[60] Herold and colleagues[61,62] showed that this modified anti-CD3 monoclonal antibody maintained C-peptide production over 2 years after 1 course administered in newly diagnosed patients within 6 weeks of diagnosis. A reduction in HbA1c and lower insulin doses were found in the treated group when compared with the untreated group. A European multicenter trial showed that a single course of a very similar modified anti-CD3 antibody, ChA-glyCD3, in newly diagnosed patients resulted in higher C-peptide production and reduced insulin doses for 18 months following treatment when compared with placebo.[63] These results were most pronounced among patients with C-peptide production at, or higher than, the 50th percentile. Another study of this modified CD3 molecule has recently completed enrollment through the Immune Tolerance Network. In this study, new onset subjects between 3 and 30 years of age within 8 weeks of diagnosis will receive 2 doses of hOKT3γ1 (Ala-Ala), one at the initiation of the study and a second dose one year later. The study will follow C-peptide production over 2 years from the initiation of treatment. In addition, the manufacturers of these modified CD3 molecules are sponsoring trials of these agents, the DEFEND-1 and Protégé studies, in recent-onset patients. The Protégé study reported that it did not meet this primary endpoint of insulin dose <0.5 units/kg and HbA1c <6.5% at one year.[64]

The TrialNet study group is performing several trials in individuals newly diagnosed with T1D. The first such TrialNet study assessed the role of mycophenolate mofetil (MMF) and dacluzimab (DZB) in maintaining C-peptide production. MMF and DZB have been shown to be effective in transplantation regimens and are well character-ized and tolerated. This study was stopped early when analysis of C-peptide produc-tion one year after initiation of treatment revealed no difference between the groups receiving both drugs or placebo.

TrialNet is also investigated the use of the anti-B lymphocyte monoclonal antibody, rituximab, in preserving C-peptide production in 8- to 40-year-olds with new onset diabetes. Rituximab depletes mature B cells thereby reducing antigen presentation to T cells. It has been shown to be effective in other autoimmune diseases including lupus and rheumatoid arthritis.[65] This study showed a reduced loss of C-peptide with improved HbA1c and lower insulin dose at one year.[66]

CTLA4, a costimulatory molecule expressed on T cells is an important negative regulator of T-cell activation. CTLA4-Ig is a monoclonal antibody that binds to the cos-timulatory molecules CD80 and CD86, blocking the costimulation that is required for full T-cell activation. This antibody is approved for use in rheumatoid arthritis. In the ongoing TrialNet study, CTLA4-Ig (abatacept) is being used in a placebo-controlled study in new-onset subjects. Treatment was being given to 112 subjects with two-thirds receiving active therapy and one-third receiving placebo infusions over 2 years, with results showing a slower loss of insulin secretion in the treated group with lower HbA1c and smaller insulin doses.[67]

GAD is an important antigen in T1D. Animal studies have shown that administration of GAD to induce immune tolerance can prevent diabetes.[68] A recent study showed that 2 doses of GAD formulated in alum given within 6 months of diagnosis slowed the decrease of C-peptide production over the first 30 months after initiation of therapy.[69] This study involved 70 subjects aged between 10 and 18 years with fasting C-peptide greater than 0.1 mmol/L. TrialNet is completing a trial of 2 or 3 injections of GAD in alum versus placebo in 126 new-onset subjects that will include children as young as 3 years. The loss of C-peptide was not altered in either treatment group.[70]

A small randomized placebo-controlled pilot study of the antitumor necrosis factor drug, etanercept, was recently reported.[71] The drug was given by subcutaneous injec-tion twice weekly for 24 weeks in 18 children within 4 weeks of diagnosis. C-peptide production was significantly greater in the treatment group with lower HbA1c and

Table 1
Active studies with results to be reported

Natural History Study of the Development of Type 1 Diabetes Sponsor: TrialNet Study Group	• Does not have diabetes • 1–45 years of age and first-degree relative of a person with T1D • 1–20 years of age and second- or third-degree relative of a person with T1D
Oral Insulin For Prevention of Diabetes In Relatives at Risk for Type 1 Diabetes Mellitus Sponsor: TrialNet Study Group	• 3–45 years of age with a relative with T1D • Insulin autoantibodies and one other diabetes autoantibody • Normal glucose tolerance
Effects of Recombinant Human Glutamic Acid Decarboxylase Formulated in Alum on the Progression of T1D in New Onset Subjects Sponsor: TrialNet Study Group	• 3–45 years of age • Within 3 months of diagnosis of diabetes • GAD antibodies • Stimulated C-peptide levels $\geq$0.2 pmol/mL
Study of Thymoglobulin to Arrest Newly Diagnosed Type 1 Diabetes (START) Sponsor: Immune Tolerance Network	• 12–35 years of age • Diagnosis of diabetes within the 12 weeks before study entry • Positive for 1 or more autoantibodies (anti-GAD, anti-insulin, or IA-2 autoantibodies) • Stimulated C-peptide level >0.4 pmol/mL
Trial of Intranasal Insulin in Children and Young Adults at Risk of Type 1 Diabetes (INIT II) Sponsor: Melbourne Health/Diabetes Vaccine Development Center	• Age 4–30 years if first-degree relative of a person with T1D • Age 4–20 years if second-degree relative of a person with T1D • Two or more diabetes autoantibodies • Normal glucose tolerance • First phase insulin relase more than threshold
Primary Intervention with Oral/Nasal Insulin for Prevention of Type 1 Diabetes in Infants at High Genetic Risk to Develop Type 1 Diabetes (Pre-POINT) Sponsor: Juvenile Diabetes Research Foundation	• Ages between 18 months and 7 years • High-risk HLA genotype • Sibling or both parents with diabetes • Does not have diabetes or diabetes autoantibodies
Phase 3 Trial of Otelixizumab for Adults With Newly Diagnosed Type 1 Diabetes Mellitus (Autoimmune): DEFEND-1 Sponsor: Tolerx/Juvenile Diabetes Research Foundation	• Ages 18–35 years • Diagnosis of diabetes mellitus, no more than 90 days between diagnosis and administration of study drug • Stimulated C-peptide level greater than 0.20 nmol/L and less than or equal to 3.50 nmol/L • Positive for one or both of the following antibodies: ICA (anti-IA2) and/or GAD autoantibodies
The Protégé Study - Clinical Trial of Teplizumab in Children and Adults With Recent-Onset Type 1 Diabetes Mellitus Sponsor: MacroGenics Effects of Canakinumab On the Progression of Type1 Diabetes in New Onset Subjects Sponsor: TrialNet Study Group	• Ages 8–35 years • Diagnosis of T1D mellitus within 12 weeks • Detectable fasting or stimulated C-peptide level • Positive for ICA512/IA-2, GAD autoantibodies, or IAA (if present during the first 2 weeks, but not beyond 2 weeks, of insulin treatment)

smaller insulin doses. Other interventions currently under investigation or planned for study in this patient population, are anakinra, thymoglobulin, antithymocyte globulin, GAD/lansoprazole/sitagliptin, efalizumab, intensive metabolic control, and atorvastatin. **Table 1** lists active studies and their eligibility criteria.

"Curing" Established T1D

Once full-blown T1D has developed, immune interventions are unlikely to be effective because the vast majority of β cells have been destroyed. At this stage, effective interventions would include β-cell implantation as part of pancreatic or islet cell transplantation, or of gene therapy using implanted cells capable of producing insulin in response to glycemia, or of stem-cell–derived β cells. Pancreatic transplantation has been successfully applied, particularly in combination with kidney transplantation necessitated by diabetes-related end-stage renal failure. The paucity of donors and the need for lifelong immune suppression to prevent organ rejection have limited the application of these transplants. Islet cell transplantation enjoyed a period of success when investigators in Edmonton were able to show prolonged graft survival and an insulin-free period. However, limited supply of islets, side effects of the immunosuppression, and eventual return to insulin dependence all challenge the ability of this approach to have a broad impact.

Genetic engineering and stem cell biology hold out the most hope in the long run for a cure for T1D and elimination of the need to inject insulin. With respect to gene therapy, cells have been created in which insulin secretion is possible. However, insulin is produced in small amounts and unregulated by blood sugar concentrations. Stem cells are currently under intensive evaluation; however, successful therapy for diabetes and other immune disorders remains elusive.

REFERENCES

1. Devendra D, Liu E, Eisenbarth GS, et al. Type 1 diabetes: recent developments. BMJ 2004;328(7442):750–4.
2. Eisenbarth GS. Type I diabetes mellitus. A chronic autoimmune disease. N Engl J Med 1986;314(21):1360–8.
3. Akerblom HK, Vaarala O, Hyoty H, et al. Environmental factors in the etiology of type 1 diabetes. Am J Med Genet 2002;115(1):18–29.
4. Helgason T, Jonasson MR. Evidence for a food additive as a cause of ketosis-prone diabetes. Lancet 1981;2(8249):716–20.
5. Thorsdottir I, Ramel A. Dietary intake of 10- to 16-year-old children and adolescents in central and northern Europe and association with the incidence of type 1 diabetes. Ann Nutr Metab 2003;47(6):267–75.
6. Vaarala O, Knip M, Paronen J, et al. Cow's milk formula feeding induces primary immunization to insulin in infants at genetic risk for type 1 diabetes. Diabetes 1999;48(7):1389–94.
7. Virtanen SM, Laara E, Hypponen E, et al. Cow's milk consumption, HLA-DQB1 genotype, and type 1 diabetes: a nested case-control study of siblings of children with diabetes. Childhood diabetes in Finland study group [erratum appears in Diabetes 2000;49(9):1617]. Diabetes 2000;49(6):912–7.
8. Barker JM, Yu J, Yu L, et al. Autoantibody "subspecificity" in type 1 diabetes: risk for organ-specific autoimmunity clusters in distinct groups. Diabetes Care 2005; 28(4):850–5.
9. Daneman D. State of the world's children with diabetes. Pediatr Diabetes 2009; 10(2):120–6.

10. International Diabetes Federation. Diabetes atlas. 3rd edition. Brussels. (Belgium): International Diabetes Federation; 2006. Available at:. http://www.eatlas.idf.org.

11. Tuomilehto J, Karvonen M, Pitkaniemi J, et al. Record-high incidence of type I (insulin-dependent) diabetes mellitus in Finnish children. The Finnish Childhood Type I Diabetes Registry Group. Diabetologia 1999;42(6):655–60.

12. Raymond NT, Jones JR, Swift PG, et al. Comparative incidence of type I diabetes in children aged under 15 years from South Asian and White or other ethnic backgrounds in Leicestershire, UK, 1989 to 1998. Diabetologia 2001;44(Suppl 3): B32–6.

13. Kondrashova A, Reunanen A, Romanov A, et al. A six-fold gradient in the incidence of type 1 diabetes at the eastern border of Finland. Ann Med 2005;37(1):67–72.

14. Gillespie KM, Bain SC, Barnett AH, et al. The rising incidence of childhood type 1 diabetes and reduced contribution of high-risk HLA haplotypes. Lancet 2004; 364(9446):1699–700.

15. Redondo MJ, Eisenbarth GS. Genetic control of autoimmunity in type I diabetes and associated disorders. Diabetologia 2002;45(5):605–22.

16. Atkinson MA, Eisenbarth GS. Type 1 diabetes: new perspectives on disease pathogenesis and treatment. Lancet 2001;358(9277):221–9.

17. Achenbach P, Bonifacio E, Koczwara K, et al. Natural history of type 1 diabetes. Diabetes 2005;54(Suppl 2):S25–31.

18. Huber A, Menconi F, Corathers S, et al. Joint genetic susceptibility to type 1 diabetes and autoimmune thyroiditis: from epidemiology to mechanisms. Endocr Rev 2008;29(6):697–725.

19. Barker JM. Clinical review: type 1 diabetes-associated autoimmunity: natural history, genetic associations, and screening. J Clin Endocrinol Metab 2006; 91(4):1210–7.

20. Cooper JD, Smyth DJ, Smiles AM, et al. Meta-analysis of genome-wide association study data identifies additional type 1 diabetes risk loci. Nat Genet 2008; 40(12):1399–401.

21. Barrett JC, Clayton DG, Concannon P, et al. Genome-wide association study and meta-analysis find that over 40 loci affect risk of type 1 diabetes. Nat Genet 2009; 41:703–7.

22. Ball TM, Castro-Rodriguez JA, Griffith KA, et al. Siblings, day-care attendance, and the risk of asthma and wheezing during childhood. N Engl J Med 2000; 343(8):538–43.

23. Betts P, Mulligan J, Ward P, et al. Increasing body weight predicts the earlier onset of insulin-dependant diabetes in childhood: testing the 'accelerator hypothesis' (2). Diabet Med 2005;22(2):144–51.

24. Daneman D. Is the 'Accelerator Hypothesis' worthy of our attention? Diabet Med 2005;22(2):115–7.

25. Gale EA. A missing link in the hygiene hypothesis? Diabetologia 2002;45(4):588–94.

26. Kaila B, Taback SP. The effect of day care exposure on the risk of developing type 1 diabetes: a meta-analysis of case-control studies. Diabetes Care 2001;24(8): 1353–8.

27. von Mutius E, Martinez FD, Fritzsch C, et al. Skin test reactivity and number of siblings. BMJ 1994;308(6930):692–5.

28. Wilkin TJ. The accelerator hypothesis: weight gain as the missing link between type I and type II diabetes. Diabetologia 2001;44(7):914–22.

29. Group TS. The environmental determinants of diabetes in the young (TEDDY) study. Ann N Y Acad Sci 2008;1150:1–13.

30. Merriman TR, Merriman TR. Type 1 diabetes, the A1 milk hypothesis and vitamin D deficiency. Diabetes Res Clin Pract 2009;83(2):149–56.
31. Group TS. Study design of the trial to reduce IDDM in the genetically at risk (TRIGR). Pediatr Diabetes 2007;8(3):117–37.
32. Knip M, Virtanen SM, Seppä K, et al. Dietary Intervention in Infancy and Later Signs of Beta-Cell Autoimmunity. N Engl J Med 2010;363:1900–8.
33. Chase HP, Lescheck E, Rafkin-Mervis L, et al. Nutritional Intervention to Prevent (NIP) type 1 diabetes a Pilot Trial. ICAN: Infant, Child, Adolescent Nutrition 2009;1(2):98–107.
34. Norris JM, Yin X, Lamb MM, et al. Omega-3 polyunsaturated fatty acid intake and islet autoimmunity in children at increased risk for type 1 diabetes. JAMA 2007; 298(12):1420–8.
35. Schmid S, Buuck D, Knopff A, et al. BABYDIET, a feasibility study to prevent the appearance of islet autoantibodies in relatives of patients with Type 1 diabetes by delaying exposure to gluten. Diabetologia 2004;47(6):1130–1.
36. Bonifacio E, Hummel M, Hummel S, et al. Primary dietary intervention study to reduce the risk of islet autoimmunity in children at increased risk for type 1 diabetes: The BABYDIET study. Diabetes Care 2011;34(6):1301–5.
37. Norris JM, Barriga K, Klingensmith G, et al. Timing of initial cereal exposure in infancy and risk of islet autoimmunity. JAMA 2003;290(13):1713–20.
38. Moro JR, Iwata M, von Andriano UH, et al. Vitamin effects on the immune system: vitamins A and D take centre stage. Nat Rev Immunol 2008;8(9):685–98.
39. Zipitis CS, Akobeng AK. Vitamin D supplementation in early childhood and risk of type 1 diabetes: a systematic review and meta-analysis. Arch Dis Child 2008; 93(6):512–7.
40. Wenzlau JM, Juhl K, Yu L, et al. The cation efflux transporter ZnT8 (Slc30A8) is a major autoantigen in human type 1 diabetes. Proc Natl Acad Sci U S A 2007; 104(43):17040–5.
41. Verge CF, Gianani R, Kawasaki E, et al. Number of autoantibodies (against insulin, GAD or ICA512/IA2) rather than particular autoantibody specificities determines risk of type I diabetes. J Autoimmun 1996;9(3):379–83.
42. Sosenko JM, Palmer JP, Greenbaum CJ, et al. Patterns of metabolic progression to type 1 diabetes in the Diabetes Prevention trial-type 1. Diabetes Care 2006; 29(3):643–9.
43. Mahon JL, Sosenko JM, Rafkin-Mervis L, et al. The TrialNet Natural History Study of the Development of Type 1 Diabetes: objectives, design, and initial results. Pediatr Diabetes 2009;10(2):97–104.
44. Gale EA, Bingley PJ, Emmett CL, et al. European Nicotinamide Diabetes Intervention Trial (ENDIT): a randomised controlled trial of intervention before the onset of type 1 diabetes. Lancet 2004;363(9413):925–31.
45. Diabetes Prevention Trial–Type 1 Diabetes Study Group. Effects of insulin in relatives of patients with type 1 diabetes mellitus. N Engl J Med 2002;346(22): 1685–91.
46. Skyler JS, Krischer JP, Wolfsdorf J, et al. Effects of oral insulin in relatives of patients with type 1 diabetes: the diabetes prevention trial–type 1. Diabetes Care 2005;28(5):1068–76.
47. Nanto-Salonen K, Kupila A, Simell S, et al. Nasal insulin to prevent type 1 diabetes in children with HLA genotypes and autoantibodies conferring increased risk of disease: a double-blind, randomised controlled trial. Lancet 2008; 372(9651):1746–55.

48. Achenbach P, Barker J, Bonifacio E, et al. Modulating the natural history of type 1 diabetes in children at high genetic risk by mucosal insulin immunization. Curr Diab Rep 2008;8(2):87–93.
49. Harrison LC, Honeyman MC, Steele CE, et al. Pancreatic beta-cell function and immune responses to insulin after administration of intranasal insulin to humans at risk for type 1 diabetes. Diabetes Care 2004;27(10):2348–55.
50. Bonfanti R, Bazzigaluppi E, Calori G, et al. Parameters associated with residual insulin secretion during the first year of disease in children and adolescents with Type 1 diabetes mellitus. Diabet Med 1998;15(10):844–50.
51. Sochett EB, Daneman D, Clarson C, et al. Factors affecting and patterns of residual insulin secretion during the first year of type 1 (insulin-dependent) diabetes mellitus in children. Diabetologia 1987;30(7):453–9.
52. Pozzilli P, Manfrini S, Buzzetti R, et al. Glucose evaluation trial for remission (GE-TREM) in type 1 diabetes: a European multicentre study. Diabetes Res Clin Pract 2005;68(3):258–64.
53. Yki-Jarvinen H, Koivisto VA. Natural course of insulin resistance in type I diabetes. N Engl J Med 1986;315(4):224–30.
54. Palmer JP, Fleming GA, Greenbaum CJ, et al. C-peptide is the appropriate outcome measure for type 1 diabetes clinical trials to preserve beta-cell function: report of an ADA workshop, 21–22 October 2001. Diabetes 2004;53(1):250–64. [Erratum appears in Diabetes 2004;53(7):1934].
55. Steffes MW, Sibley S, Jackson M, et al. Beta-cell function and the development of diabetes-related complications in the diabetes control and complications trial. Diabetes Care 2003;26(3):832–6.
56. Cyclosporin-induced remission of IDDM after early intervention. Association of 1 yr of cyclosporin treatment with enhanced insulin secretion. The Canadian-European Randomized Control Trial Group. Diabetes 1988;37(11):1574–82.
57. Feutren G, Papoz L, Assan R, et al. Cyclosporin increases the rate and length of remissions in insulin-dependent diabetes of recent onset. Results of a multicentre double-blind trial. Lancet 1986;2(8499):119–24.
58. Harrison LC, Colman PG, Dean B, et al. Increase in remission rate in newly diagnosed type I diabetic subjects treated with azathioprine. Diabetes 1985;34(12):1306–8.
59. Silverstein J, Maclaren N, Riley W, et al. Immunosuppression with azathioprine and prednisone in recent-onset insulin-dependent diabetes mellitus. N Engl J Med 1988;319(10):599–604.
60. Chatenoud L, Bluestone JA, Chatenoud L, et al. CD3-specific antibodies: a portal to the treatment of autoimmunity. Nat Rev Immunol 2007;7(8):622–32.
61. Herold KC, Gitelman SE, Masharani U, et al. A single course of anti-CD3 monoclonal antibody hOKT3gamma1(Ala-Ala) results in improvement in C-peptide responses and clinical parameters for at least 2 years after onset of type1 diabetes. Diabetes 2005;54(6):1763–9.
62. Herold KC, Hagopian W, Auger JA, et al. Anti-CD3 monoclonal antibody in new-onset type 1 diabetes mellitus. N Engl J Med 2002;346(22):1692–8.
63. Keymeulen B, Vandemeulebroucke E, Ziegler AG, et al. Insulin needs after CD3-antibody therapy in new-onset type 1 diabetes. N Engl J Med 2005;352(25):2598–608.
64. Sherry N, Hagopian W, Ludvigsson J, et al. Teplizumab for treatment of type 1 diabetes (Protégé study): 1-year results from a randomised, placebo-controlled trial. The Lancet 2011;378(9790):487–97.

65. Levesque MC, St Clair EW, Levesque MC, et al. B cell-directed therapies for auto-immune disease and correlates of disease response and relapse. J Allergy Clin Immunol 2008;121(1):13–21 [quiz 22–3].
66. Pescovitz MD, Greenbaum CJ, Krause-Steinrauf H, et al. Rituximab, B-lympho-cyte depletion, and preservation of beta-cell function. N Engl J Med 2009; 361(22):2143–52.
67. Orban T, Bundy B, Becker DJ, et al. Co-stimulation modulation with abatacept in patients with recent-onset type 1 diabetes: a randomised, double-blind, placebo-controlled trial. The Lancet 2011;378(9789):412–9.
68. Tisch R, Wang B, Serreze DV. Induction of glutamic acid decarboxylase 65-specific Th2 cells and suppression of autoimmune diabetes at late stages of disease is epitope dependent. J Immunol 1999;163(3):1178–87.
69. Ludvigsson J, Faresjo M, Hjorth M, et al. GAD treatment and insulin secretion in recent-onset type 1 diabetes. N Engl J Med 2008;359(18):1909–20.
70. Wherrett DK, Bundy B, Becker DJ, et al. Antigen-based therapy with glutamic acid decarboxylase (GAD) vaccine in patients with recent-onset type 1 diabetes: a randomised double-blind trial. The Lancet 2011;378(9788):319–27.
71. Mastrandrea L, Yu J, Behrens T, et al. Etanercept treatment in children with new onset type 1 diabetes: pilot randomized, placebo-controlled, double blind study. Diabetes Care 2009;32(7):1244–9.

Pediatric Disorders of Water Balance

Sayali A. Ranadive, MD[a], Stephen M. Rosenthal, MD[b],*

KEYWORDS

• Hyponatremia • Hypernatremia • Diabetes insipidus • SIADH

PEDIATRIC DISORDERS OF WATER BALANCE

Under normal circumstances, plasma osmolality is maintained within a relatively narrow range (280–295 mOsm/kg). This homeostasis requires adequate water intake, regulated by an intact thirst mechanism and appropriate free water excretion by the kidneys, mediated by appropriate secretion of arginine vasopressin (AVP, also known as antidiuretic hormone). AVP is produced by a subset of magnocellular neurons in the paraventricular nuclei (PVN) and supraoptic nuclei (SON) of the hypothalamus. Axons from these neurons project via the pituitary stalk to the posterior pituitary gland.[1] The terminals of these axons contain neurosecretory granules that store AVP for release.[2] A gene on chromosome 20p13 encodes AVP and its carrier protein, neurophysin II (NPII). AVP and NPII are synthesized as a single polypeptide, cleaved within the neurosecretory granules and then reassembled into AVP-NPII complexes before secretion.[3] Stores of preformed AVP in the posterior pituitary can last for 30 to 50 days under basal circumstances or for 5 to 10 days during maximal stimulation.[4] This significant storage capacity explains why a defect in AVP synthesis may not become clinically apparent until weeks after a causal insult, and a partial defect may only be revealed after prolonged water deprivation.

AVP synthesis, transport, and secretion are regulated primarily by changes in plasma osmolality and, to a lesser degree, by changes in circulating volume.[1,5] Osmoreceptors in the hypothalamus (organum vasculosum of the lamina terminalis and anterior hypothalamus) stimulate secretion of AVP when plasma osmolality increases by as little as 1% in healthy individuals. Basal AVP levels are normally low, 0.5 to 2 pg/mL, and do not increase until plasma osmolality exceeds 280 mOsm/kg.[2] Maximum urine concentration (urine osmolality 900–1200 mOsm/kg) is

Portions of this article were previously published in the *Endocrinology and Metabolism Clinics of North America*, 38:4.

[a] Department of Endocrinology, Children's Hospital and Research Center Oakland, 747 52nd Street, Oakland, CA 94609, USA
[b] Department of Pediatrics, Division of Endocrinology, University of California San Francisco, 513 Parnassus Avenue, Room S672, San Francisco, CA 94143, USA
* Corresponding author.
E-mail address: rosenthals@peds.ucsf.edu

Pediatr Clin N Am 58 (2011) 1271–1280
doi:10.1016/j.pcl.2011.07.013
0031-3955/11/$ – see front matter © 2011 Elsevier Inc. All rights reserved.

attained at plasma AVP levels of 5 to 6 pg/mL. Although plasma AVP can continue to rise above 6 pg/mL with ongoing plasma hyperosmolality, further increases in urine osmolality cannot be achieved because of limits of the renal medullary gradient.[2] Changes in blood volume inversely affect AVP secretion such that 8% to 10% of decrease in circulating blood volume stimulates AVP secretion and increases in intravascular volume inhibit AVP release.[6] Baroreceptors in the carotid sinus and aortic arch (high-pressure baroreceptors) and in the atria and pulmonary venous circulation (low-pressure baroreceptors) relay pressure and volume information via the glossopharyngeal and vagus nerves, respectively, to the brain stem. These baroreceptors become activated when stretched by increases in intravascular volume, leading to inhibition of AVP secretion through fibers projecting from the brain stem to the PVN and SON of the hypothalamus.[6] In addition, many other factors affect AVP secretion; it is stimulated by pain, nausea, stress, and various drugs and is inhibited by multiple factors.[2,6]

Adequate water intake, governed by an intact thirst mechanism, is also regulated predominantly by changes in plasma osmolality, intravascular volume, and blood pressure. Thirst is consistently stimulated when plasma osmolality increases by 2% to 3% or when circulating blood volume decreases by 4% to 10%.[2,7] Because the thresholds that trigger thirst are higher than those that trigger AVP secretion, adequate thirst becomes essential during pathologic states of AVP deficiency or insensitivity.[2] Challenges in the management of adipsic diabetes insipidus, resulting from damage to thirst centers and to AVP-secreting neurons, highlight the critical role of thirst in the maintenance of plasma osmolality when AVP secretion or responsiveness is inadequate.

AVP exerts its antidiuretic action by binding to the X chromosome-encoded V2 vasopressin receptor (V2R), a G protein-coupled receptor on the basolateral membrane of renal collecting duct epithelial cells. After V2R activation, increased intracellular cyclic adenosine monophosphate (cAMP) mediates shuttling of the water channel aquaporin 2 (AQP-2) to the apical membrane of collecting duct epithelial cells, resulting in increased water permeability and antidiuresis (**Fig. 1**).[8]

Clinical disorders of water balance are common, and abnormalities in many steps involving AVP secretion and responsiveness have been described. This article focuses on the principal disorders of water balance, diabetes insipidus (DI), and the syndrome of inappropriate antidiuretic hormone secretion (SIADH).

DIABETES INSIPIDUS

DI results from the inability to reabsorb free water. Polyuria, polydipsia, and hypoosmolar urine are the hallmarks of this disorder, although hypernatremia may be present, particularly in infants, at the time of diagnosis. DI can be central, due to deficiency of AVP, or nephrogenic, due to a defect in AVP action in the kidneys (**Box 1**).[9,10]

Nephrogenic DI (NDI) may be genetic or acquired. The genetic causes are inactivating mutations of the *AVPR2* gene, located on the X chromosome (Xq28), or autosomal recessive or dominant mutations in the *AQP-2* gene, located on chromosome 12 (12q13). Acquired NDI can be caused by various conditions, including some forms of primary renal disease, obstructive uropathy, hypokalemia, hypercalcemia, sickle cell disease, and drugs such as lithium and demeclocycline.[2,9–11] Prolonged polyuria of any cause can also lead to some degree of NDI because of a reduction of tonicity in the renal medullary interstitium and a subsequent decrease in the gradient necessary to concentrate urine.

X-linked NDI (XNDI) is rare, affecting approximately 4 in 1,000,000 males worldwide, and it accounts for about 90% of the genetic causes of NDI. Of the 211 reported *AVPR2* mutations causing XNDI, approximately half are missense, and 31 of these

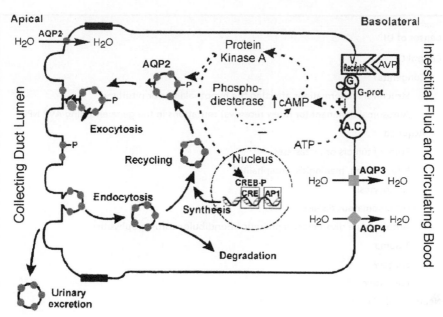

Fig. 1. Antidiuretic action of AVP on the renal collecting duct epithelial cell. AVP binding to the V2R, located on the basolateral membrane, results in an increase in cAMP and activation of protein kinase A (PKA). Ser256 on the C terminal of AQP-2 is phosphorylated by PKA, resulting in the shuttling of AQP-2 to the apical membrane, allowing the normally impermeable apical membrane to become permeable to water. In addition, acting through a cAMP-response element in the AQP-2 promoter, chronic exposure of these cells to AVP results in increased synthesis of AQP-2. AQP-3 and AQP-4, constitutively located on the basolateral border of the collecting duct membrane, provide channels for the transport of water out of the collecting duct cells and into the interstitium and circulation. ATP, adenosine triphosphate; CRE, cAMP response element; CREB, cAMP response element binding protein. (*From* Nielsen S, Kwon TH, Christensen B, et al. Physiology and pathophysiology of renal aquaporins. J Am Soc Nephrol 1990;10:647–63; with permission.)

have been characterized functionally.[12] Most *AVPR2* missense mutations result in a translated but misfolded V2R protein that remains trapped in the endoplasmic reticulum.[13–15] Pharmacologic chaperones can partially rescue the cell-surface expression and functional activity of misfolded mutant V2Rs that would otherwise be targeted for degradation.[16–18]

Infants with congenital (X-linked or autosomal) NDI typically present within the first several weeks of life with nonspecific symptoms, such as fever, vomiting, dehydration, and growth failure, associated with polyuria and hypo-osmolar urine (50–100 mOsm/kg). Mental retardation of variable severity and intracerebral calcifications of the frontal lobes and basal ganglia can result from repeated episodes of dehydration if the condition remains untreated.[19] Longstanding polyuria and polydipsia can lead to nonobstructive hydronephrosis, hydroureter, and megabladder.[20,21] Thiazide diuretics, along with low sodium intake, were historically used to treat NDI,[22] as this combination decreases glomerular filtration rate and results in decreased urine output. During the last 20 years, thiazide diuretics in combination with either amiloride or indomethacin have become the mainstay of congenital NDI treatment.[19,23,24] In vitro studies have demonstrated that pharmacologic chaperones, which are cell permeable, nonpeptide

---

Box 1
Causes of DI

Central DI

  Congenital

    Structural malformations affecting the hypothalamus or pituitary

    Autosomal dominant (or rarely recessive) mutations in the gene encoding AVP-NPII

  Acquired

    Primary tumors or metastases

    Infection (eg, meningitis, encephalitis)

    Histiocytosis

    Granulomatous diseases

    Autoimmune disorders (lymphocytic infundibuloneurohypophysitis)

    Trauma

    Surgery

    Idiopathic

Nephrogenic DI

  Congenital

    X-linked: inactivating mutations in *AVPR2*

    Autosomal: recessive or dominant mutations in *AQP-2*

  Acquired

    Primary renal disease

    Obstructive uropathy

    Metabolic causes (eg, hypokalemia, hypercalcemia)

    Sickle cell disease

    Drugs (eg, lithium, demeclocycline)

    Prolonged polyuria of any cause

---

small molecules, can restore the cell-surface expression and function of misfolded mutant V2Rs.[16–18,25] One such compound is orally active, well tolerated, and effective in decreasing urine volume in adults with severe XNDI.[18,26] Thus, pharmacologic chaperones represent a new, safe, and targeted therapy for XNDI caused by protein misfolding due to missense mutations of *AVPR2*.

Central DI is rarely congenital and more frequently, acquired. Congenital central DI may be caused by structural malformations affecting the hypothalamus or by autosomal dominant or recessive mutations in the gene encoding AVP-NPII. The autosomal dominant causes are more common and result from heterozygous *AVP-NPII* gene mutations.[3] The proposed mechanism for the dominant negative effect is that the heterozygous mutation disrupts the processing of the mutant precursor.[27,28] The accumulation of this misfolded protein in the vasopressinergic neurons causes a gradual destruction of these neurons.[3,27] In such patients, clinical DI usually develops several months to years after birth. A rare autosomal recessive form of central DI has been reported in association with a mutation in the *AVP-NPII* gene, resulting in a biologically inactive AVP.[29]

Acquired forms of central DI occur in association with a variety of disorders in which there is destruction or degeneration of vasopressinergic neurons. Causes include primary tumors (eg, craniopharyngioma, germinoma) or metastases, infection (meningitis, encephalitis), histiocytosis, granuloma, vascular disorders, autoimmune disorders (lymphocytic infundibuloneurohypophysitis), and trauma or surgery.[9,10,30] Idiopathic DI is a diagnosis of exclusion, and one that is made with decreasing frequency as a result of improved sensitivity of magnetic resonance imaging (MRI) of the brain and of tests for cerebral spinal fluid (CSF) and serum tumor markers.[30,31]

The principal presenting sign of DI is polyuria, which, in addition to deficiency or impaired responsiveness to AVP, may result from an osmotic agent (eg, hyperglycemia in diabetes mellitus) or from excessive water intake (primary polydipsia). Hypernatremia usually does not occur if patients have an intact thirst mechanism, adequate access to fluids, and no additional ongoing fluid loss (eg, diarrhea). Infants with DI, in addition to polyuria and polydipsia, may be irritable and may have fever of unknown origin, growth failure secondary to inadequate caloric intake, and hydronephrosis. Older children may also have nocturia and enuresis. DI may not be apparent in patients with coexisting untreated anterior pituitary-mediated adrenal glucocorticoid insufficiency, as cortisol is required to generate normal free water excretion.[2]

A diagnosis of DI can be made if simultaneous screening laboratory studies reveal hyperosmolality concurrent with urine that is inappropriately dilute. If DI is present, it is more likely to be uncovered by these screening tests if they are obtained as soon as possible after awakening and before any fluid intake (assuming that the patient has not consumed fluids overnight). However, because most patients with DI have intact thirst and can drink to prevent hyperosmolality and hypernatremia, a standardized water deprivation test is often necessary to make the diagnosis. The patient is monitored with serial measurements of weight, serum sodium level, serum osmolality, urine volume, and urine osmolality while being fasted and deprived of water for 8 to 10 hours. If urine osmolality greater than 750 mOsm/kg is achieved with any degree of water deprivation, DI can be excluded.[6,9] The diagnosis of DI is established if serum osmolality rises above 300 mOsm/kg and urine osmolality remains below 300 mOsm/kg. Urine osmolality in the 300 to 750 mOsm/kg range during water deprivation may indicate partial DI.[9] If DI is suspected, a plasma sample should be obtained for AVP radioimmunoassay. AVP or a synthetic analog (desmopressin) should then be administered to distinguish AVP deficiency from AVP unresponsiveness.

MRI of the brain, with particular attention to the hypothalamic-pituitary region, is indicated in patients with central DI. The posterior pituitary hyperintensity ("bright spot") on T1-weighted magnetic resonance images is often absent in central DI.[30,32–35] However, the bright spot can be absent in normal individuals,[36] and conversely, children with central DI can have a normal bright spot at the time of diagnosis.[37–39] Therefore, the presence of the bright spot does not establish neurohypophyseal integrity, and its absence does not always indicate central nervous system (CNS) pathology. In central DI patients with or without the posterior pituitary bright spot, an otherwise normal MRI warrants close follow-up with CSF tumor markers and cytology, serum tumor markers, and serial contrast-enhanced brain MRIs for early detection of an evolving occult hypothalamic-stalk lesion.[31]

The management of central DI includes treating the primary disease, correction of a fluid deficit, if present, and normalization of urine output with desmopressin. This AVP analog has markedly reduced pressor activity in comparison with native AVP, has a prolonged half-life, and can be administered orally, intranasally, or by subcutaneous injection. In infancy, if polyuria is not excessive, DI may be best managed with fluid intake alone to avoid a potential risk of hyponatremia with desmopressin treatment.

Box 2
Causes of SIADH

1. Neurologic and psychiatric disorders

   a. Infections: meningitis, encephalitis, brain abscess

   b. Vascular: thrombosis, subarachnoid or subdural hemorrhage, temporal arteritis, cavernous sinus thrombosis, stroke

   c. Neoplasm: primary or metastatic

   d. Skull fracture, traumatic brain injury

   e. Psychosis, delirium tremens

   f. Other: Guillain-Barré syndrome, acute intermittent porphyria, autonomic neuropathy, postpituitary surgery, multiple sclerosis, epilepsy, hydrocephalus, lupus erythematosus.

2. Drugs

   a. Intravenous cyclophosphamide

   b. Carbamazepine

   c. Vincristine or vinblastine

   d. Thiothixene

   e. Thioridazine, other phenothiazines

   f. Haloperidol

   g. Amitriptyline, other tricyclic antidepressants or serotonin-reuptake inhibitors

   h. Monoamine oxidase inhibitors

   i. Bromocriptine

   j. Lorcainide

   k. Clofibrate

   l. General anesthesia

   m. Narcotics, opiate derivatives

   n. Nicotine

   o. Desmopressin overtreatment of DI or eneuresis

3. Lung diseases and interventions

   a. Pneumonia

   b. Tuberculosis

   c. Lung abscess, empyema

   d. Acute respiratory failure

   e. Positive pressure ventilation

4. Non-CNS tumors with ectopic production of AVP

   a. Carcinoma of lung (small cell, bronchogenic), duodenum, pancreas, thymus, olfactory neuroblastoma, bladder, prostate, uterus

   b. Lymphoma

   c. Sarcoma

   d. Leukemia

5. Miscellaneous

  a. AIDS

  b. Postoperative state

  c. Glucocorticoid deficiency

  d. Hypothyroidism

  e. Idiopathic

SYNDROME OF INAPPROPRIATE ANTIDIURETIC HORMONE SECRETION

SIADH, caused by the inability to excrete free water, is characterized by hyponatremia and hypo-osmolality with inappropriately concentrated urine and natriuresis.[40–42] Following the original criteria established by Bartter and Schwartz,[40] a diagnosis of SIADH is made when the following occur: (1) plasma hypo-osmolality (<275 mOsm/kg), (2) less than maximally dilute urine (urine osmolality>100 mOsm/kg), (3) euvolemia (secondary to regulatory adaptations), (4) natriuresis, (5) normal renal function, and (6) no evidence of thyroxine or cortisol deficiency. Although most patients with SIADH have inappropriately measurable or elevated levels of plasma AVP relative to plasma osmolality, 10% to 20% of patients with SIADH do not have measurable AVP levels. This may reflect issues of assay sensitivity or may indicate a syndrome resembling SIADH, such as the recently described nephrogenic syndrome of inappropriate anti-diuresis (NSIAD) associated with an activating mutation in the X-linked G protein-coupled V2R and unmeasurable circulating levels of AVP.[43]

Euvolemia in chronic SIADH is an important distinguishing factor in the evaluation of a patient with serum hypo-osmolality and has a bearing on treatment issues, as discussed subsequently. Euvolemia in chronic SIADH is thought to represent an adaptation to water overload. This adaptation is mediated, in part, at the cellular level through depletion of intracellular electrolytes (potassium) and organic osmolytes.[41] The loss of brain solutes is thought to allow effective regulation of brain volume during chronic hyponatremia and SIADH. Natriuresis, thought to be mediated in part through secretion of atrial natriuretic peptide, also contributes to volume regulation in chronic SIADH.[44] Cerebral salt wasting (CSW), associated with some intracranial diseases (eg, subarachnoid hemorrhage), is often considered in the differential diagnosis of SIADH. However, the hypo-osmolality, hyponatremia, and natriuresis in CSW are associated with volume contraction, which distinguishes this disorder from the euvolemic condition of SIADH.[41]

Several disorders and conditions are associated with SIADH and can be grouped into 5 categories (**Box 2**): (1) neurologic and psychiatric disorders, (2) a large variety of drugs (eg, phenothaiozines, tricyclic antidepressants), (3) various pulmonary disorders and interventions (eg, pneumonia, asthma, positive pressure ventilation), (4) non-CNS tumors with ectopic production of AVP, and (5) miscellaneous causes (eg, AIDS, postoperative state, glucocorticoid deficiency, severe hypothyroidism).[41,42]

Therapy for SIADH includes treatment of the underlying disorder (or discontinuation of an offending drug) and fluid restriction. Replacement of sodium loss may also be necessary, but it can usually be achieved through normal dietary salt intake. Severe hyponatremia (serum sodium<120 mEq/L) may be associated with CNS abnormalities, including seizures, and may require treatment with hypertonic (3%) intravenous sodium chloride solution. Concurrent use of a diuretic, such as furosemide, may be indicated when volume expansion is severe. Other therapeutic approaches include the use of agents that induce NDI, such as demeclocycline and lithium, although both are contraindicated particularly in younger pediatric patients because of untoward side effects. Urea has been used as an osmotic diuretic in pediatric SIADH and NSIAD.[45] A variety of nonpeptide V2R antagonists are in various stages of clinical trials or have been approved by the Food and Drug Administration for use in adults.[41]

If SIADH and hyponatremia are acute (<48 hours), it is thought that hyponatremia can be corrected quickly. However, if SIADH and hyponatremia are chronic (>48 hours), overzealous treatment can result in CNS damage, including central pontine myelinolysis (CPM).[41] Brain solute loss, although an important regulatory mechanism in chronic SIADH, may predispose to the development of CPM with rapid correction of serum osmolality. It is generally recommended that plasma sodium be corrected to a safe level of approximately 120 to 125 mEq/L at a rate of no greater than 0.5 mEq/L/h, with an overall correction that does not exceed 12 mEq/L in the initial 24 hours and 18 mEq/L in the initial 48 hours of treatment.[41]

REFERENCES

1. Robertson GL. Antidiuretic hormone. Normal and disordered function. Endocrinol Metab Clin North Am 2001;30(3):671–94, vii.
2. Robinson AG, Verbalis JG. Posterior pituitary gland. In: Larsen PR, Kronenberg HM, Melmed S, et al, editors. Williams textbook of endocrinology. 10th edition. Philadelphia: Saunders; 2003. p. 281–329.
3. Rutishauser J, Kopp P, Gaskill MB, et al. Clinical and molecular analysis of three families with autosomal dominant neurohypophyseal diabetes insipidus associated with a novel and recurrent mutations in the vasopressin-neurophysin II gene. Eur J Endocrinol 2002;146(5):649–56.
4. Lederis K, Jayasena K. Storage of neurohypophysial hormones and the mechanism for their release. In: Heller H, Pickering BT, editors. Pharmacology of the endocrine system and related drugs. London: Pergamon; 1970. p. 111–54.
5. Roberts MM, Robinson AG, Hoffman GE, et al. Vasopressin transport regulation is coupled to the synthesis rate. Neuroendocrinology 1991;53(4):416–22.
6. Muglia LJ, Majzoub JA. Disorders of the posterior pituitary. In: Sperling MA, editor. Pediatric endocrinology. Philadelphia: Saunders; 2002. p. 289–322.
7. Baylis PH, Thompson CJ. Osmoregulation of vasopressin secretion and thirst in health and disease. Clin Endocrinol (Oxf) 1988;29(5):549–76.
8. Schrier RW, Cadnapaphornchai MA. Renal aquaporin water channels: from molecules to human disease. Prog Biophys Mol Biol 2003;81(2):117–31.
9. Baylis PH, Cheetham T. Diabetes insipidus. Arch Dis Child 1998;79(1):84–9.
10. Verbalis JG. Diabetes insipidus. Rev Endocr Metab Disord 2003;4(2):177–85.
11. Morello JP, Bichet DG. Nephrogenic diabetes insipidus. Annu Rev Physiol 2001; 63:607–30.
12. Spanakis E, Milord E, Gragnoli C. AVPR2 variants and mutations in nephrogenic diabetes insipidus: review and missense mutation significance. J Cell Physiol 2008;217(3):605–17.
13. Bichet DG, Birnbaumer M, Lonergan M, et al. Nature and recurrence of AVPR2 mutations in X-linked nephrogenic diabetes insipidus. Am J Hum Genet 1994; 55(2):278–86.
14. Wenkert D, Schoneberg T, Merendino JJ Jr, et al. Functional characterization of five V2 vasopressin receptor gene mutations. Mol Cell Endocrinol 1996; 124(1–2):43–50.

15. Pasel K, Schulz A, Timmermann K, et al. Functional characterization of the molecular defects causing nephrogenic diabetes insipidus in eight families. J Clin Endocrinol Metab 2000;85(4):1703–10.
16. Bernier V, Bichet DG, Bouvier M. Pharmacological chaperone action on G-protein-coupled receptors. Curr Opin Pharmacol 2004;4(5):528–33.
17. Morello JP, Salahpour A, Laperriere A, et al. Pharmacological chaperones rescue cell-surface expression and function of misfolded V2 vasopressin receptor mutants. J Clin Invest 2000;105(7):887–95.
18. Bernier V, Morello JP, Zarruk A, et al. Pharmacologic chaperones as a potential treatment for X-linked nephrogenic diabetes insipidus. J Am Soc Nephrol 2006; 17(1):232–43.
19. Kirchlechner V, Koller DY, Seidl R, et al. Treatment of nephrogenic diabetes insipidus with hydrochlorothiazide and amiloride. Arch Dis Child 1999;80(6):548–52.
20. van Lieburg AF, Knoers NV, Monnens LA. Clinical presentation and follow-up of 30 patients with congenital nephrogenic diabetes insipidus. J Am Soc Nephrol 1999;10(9):1958–64.
21. Knoers NV, Deen PM. Molecular and cellular defects in nephrogenic diabetes insipidus. Pediatr Nephrol 2001;16(12):1146–52.
22. Kennedy GC, Crawford JD. Treatment of diabetes insipidus with hydrochlorothiazide. Lancet 1959;1(7078):866–7.
23. Alon U, Chan JC. Hydrochlorothiazide-amiloride in the treatment of congenital nephrogenic diabetes insipidus. Am J Nephrol 1985;5(1):9–13.
24. Knoers N, Monnens LA. Amiloride-hydrochlorothiazide versus indomethacin-hydrochlorothiazide in the treatment of nephrogenic diabetes insipidus. J Pediatr 1990;117(3):499–502.
25. Ranadive SA, Ersoy B, Favre H, et al. Identification, characterization and rescue of a novel vasopressin-2 receptor mutation causing nephrogenic diabetes insipidus. Clin Endocrinol (Oxf) 2009;71:388–93.
26. Serradeil-Le Gal C, Wagnon J, Valette G, et al. Nonpeptide vasopressin receptor antagonists: development of selective and orally active V1a, V2 and V1b receptor ligands. Prog Brain Res 2002;139:197–210.
27. Miller WL. Molecular genetics of familial central diabetes insipidus. J Clin Endocrinol Metab 1993;77(3):592–5.
28. Gagliardi PC, Bernasconi S, Repaske DR. Autosomal dominant neurohypophyseal diabetes insipidus associated with a missense mutation encoding Gly23→Val in neurophysin II. J Clin Endocrinol Metab 1997;82(11):3643–6.
29. Willcutts MD, Felner E, White PC. Autosomal recessive familial neurohypophyseal diabetes insipidus with continued secretion of mutant weakly active vasopressin. Hum Mol Genet 1999;8(7):1303–7.
30. Maghnie M, Cosi G, Genovese E, et al. Central diabetes insipidus in children and young adults. N Engl J Med 2000;343(14):998–1007.
31. Mootha SL, Barkovich AJ, Grumbach MM, et al. Idiopathic hypothalamic diabetes insipidus, pituitary stalk thickening, and the occult intracranial germinoma in children and adolescents. J Clin Endocrinol Metab 1997;82(5):1362–7.
32. Alter CA, Bilaniuk LT. Utility of magnetic resonance imaging in the evaluation of the child with central diabetes insipidus. J Pediatr Endocrinol Metab 2002; 15(Suppl 2):681–7.
33. Ghirardello S, Garre ML, Rossi A, et al. The diagnosis of children with central diabetes insipidus. J Pediatr Endocrinol Metab 2007;20(3):359–75.
34. Fujisawa I, Nishimura K, Asato R, et al. Posterior lobe of the pituitary in diabetes insipidus: MR findings. J Comput Assist Tomogr 1987;11(2):221–5.

35. Gudinchet F, Brunelle F, Barth MO, et al. MR imaging of the posterior hypophysis in children. AJR Am J Roentgenol 1989;153(2):351–4.

36. Brooks BS, el Gammal T, Allison JD, et al. Frequency and variation of the posterior pituitary bright signal on MR images. AJNR Am J Neuroradiol 1989;10(5):943–8.

37. Alonso G, Bergada I, Heinrich JJ. Magnetic resonance imaging in central diabetes insipidus in children and adolescents. findings at diagnosis and during follow-up. An Esp Pediatr 2000;53(2):100–5 [in Spanish].

38. Kubota T, Yamamoto T, Ozono K, et al. Hyperintensity of posterior pituitary on MR T1WI in a boy with central diabetes insipidus caused by missense mutation of neurophysin II gene. Endocr J 2001;48(4):459–63.

39. Maghnie M, Genovese E, Bernasconi S, et al. Persistent high MR signal of the posterior pituitary gland in central diabetes insipidus. AJNR Am J Neuroradiol 1997;18(9):1749–52.

40. Bartter FC, Schwartz WB. The syndrome of inappropriate secretion of antidiuretic hormone. Am J Med 1967;42(5):790–806.

41. Verbalis JG, Goldsmith SR, Greenberg A, et al. Hyponatremia treatment guidelines 2007: expert panel recommendations. Am J Med 2007;120(11 Suppl 1): S1–21.

42. Baylis PH. The syndrome of inappropriate antidiuretic hormone secretion. Int J Biochem Cell Biol 2003;35(11):1495–9.

43. Feldman BJ, Rosenthal SM, Vargas GA, et al. Nephrogenic syndrome of inappropriate antidiuresis. N Engl J Med 2005;352(18):1884–90.

44. Cogan E, Debieve MF, Pepersack T, et al. Natriuresis and atrial natriuretic factor secretion during inappropriate antidiuresis. Am J Med 1988;84(3 Pt 1):409–18.

45. Huang EA, Feldman BJ, Schwartz ID, et al. Oral urea for the treatment of chronic syndrome of inappropriate antidiuresis in children. J Pediatr 2006;148(1):128–31.

Steroid 21 Hydroxylase Deficiency Congenital Adrenal Hyperplasia

Saroj Nimkarn, MD, Karen Lin-Su, MD, Maria I. New, MD*

KEYWORDS

• Congenital adrenal hyperplasia • Adrenal steroid
• 21 hydroxylase • 21 OHD

Congenital adrenal hyperplasia (CAH) refers to a group of genetic enzyme deficiencies that impair normal steroid synthesis by the adrenal cortex. The most common form is 21 hydroxylase deficiency (21 OHD), accounting for more than 90% of the cases. Less frequent causes of CAH include deficiencies of 11β-hydroxylase, 3β-hydroxysteroid dehydrogenase, 17α-hydroxylase/17,20-lyase, steroidogenic acute regulatory (StAR) protein (lipoid hyperplasia) and the newly described form of CAH owing to P450 oxido-reductase defect. In almost all cases, each of these deficiencies results from recessive mutations in the respective genes that encode the enzymes and has distinctive clinical phenotypes. This article focuses on CAH owing to 21 OHD.

STEROID 21 HYDROXYLASE DEFICIENCY

CAH owing to 21 OHD is divided into classical and nonclassical (NC) CAH. Patients affected with the classical form have more severe symptoms of hyperandrogenism. Beginning in utero, prenatal exposure to potent androgens such as testosterone and Δ^4-androstenedione at critical stages of sexual differentiation virilizes the external genitalia of genetic females, often resulting in genital ambiguity at birth in female patients. The classical form is subdivided into the simple virilizing form (SV) and the salt-wasting form (SW), based on the patient's ability to produce adequate salt-retaining hormone, aldosterone. Salt-wasters account for most of classical 21 OHD CAH patients ($\geq$75%) whereas approximately 25% of individuals are simple virilizers. Newborns who are salt wasters are at risk for life-threatening salt-wasting crises.

Individuals with the NC form of 21 OHD CAH have only mild enzyme deficiency and present postnatally with signs of hyperandrogenism; therefore, females with the NC

Portions of this article were previously published in the *Endocrinology and Metabolism Clinics of North America*, 38:4.
Adrenal Steroid Disorders Program, Division of Pediatric Endocrinology, Mount Sinai School of Medicine, 1 Gustave L. Levy Place, Box 1198, New York, NY 10029, USA
* Corresponding author.
E-mail address: maria.new@mssm.edu

form are not virilized at birth and do not present with genital ambiguity. Clinical features distinguishing classical and nonclassical forms are shown in **Table 1**. In males, the clinical distinction between SV and NC-CAH may not be readily apparent, but genetic analysis and adrenocorticotropic hormone (ACTH) stimulation results may clarify the diagnosis.

Screening studies indicate that the worldwide incidence of classical 21 OHD is 1:15,000 to 1:16,000 live births,[1–3] of which approximately 75% are salt wasters. The worldwide incidence of NC-CAH is much higher at 1:1000, with a frequency as high as 1:27 among Ashkenazi Jews.[4,5]

PATHOPHYSIOLOGY

Adrenal steroid production occurs in three major pathways: glucocorticoids, mineralocorticoids, and sex steroids, as shown in **Fig. 1**. ACTH regulates adrenal steroid production via a rate-limiting step that results in pregnanolone, the principal substrate for the steroidogenic pathway (see **Fig. 1**). It promotes StAR protein function in transporting free cholesterol to the inner mitochondrial membrane, the site where a side chain cleavage occurs and the first step in steroidogenesis takes place. The central nervous system controls the secretion of ACTH, its diurnal variation, and its increase during periods of physiologic stress via the hypothalamus-produced corticotropin-releasing factor (CRF).[6,7] The hypothalamic-pituitary-adrenal feedback system is mediated through the circulating level of plasma cortisol by its negative feedback on CRF and ACTH secretion. Hence, impeded cortisol secretion in 21 OHD CAH leads to increased ACTH production, which in turn, stimulates (1) excessive synthesis of adrenal products in those pathways unimpaired by the enzyme deficiency and (2) a build-up of precursor molecules, mainly 17 hydroxyprogesterone, in pathways blocked by the enzyme deficiency. The excess 17-OHP is shunted into the intact androgen pathway, where the 17,20-lyase enzyme converts the 17-OHP to Δ^4-androstenedione, which is converted into androgens. Because the mineralocorticoid pathway requires minimal 21 hydroxylase activity, mineralocorticoid deficiency (salt wasting) is a feature of the most severe form of the disease.

CLINICAL PRESENTATION AND FEATURES
External Genitalia

Adrenocortical function begins around the seventh week of gestation[8]; thus, a female fetus with classical CAH is exposed to adrenal androgens at the critical time of sexual differentiation (approximately 9 to 15 weeks gestational age). In classical CAH patients, the degree of genital virilization may range from mild clitoral enlargement alone to, in rare cases, a penile urethra. Degrees of genital virilization are classified into five Prader stages (**Fig. 2**).[9]

Table 1		
Clinical features in individuals with classical and nonclassical 21 OHD CAH		
Feature	Classical 21 OHD CAH	Nonclassical 21 OHD CAH
Prenatal virilization	Present in females	Absent
Postnatal virilization	Males and females	Variable
Salt wasting	~75% of all individuals	Absent
Cortisol deficiency	~100%	Rare

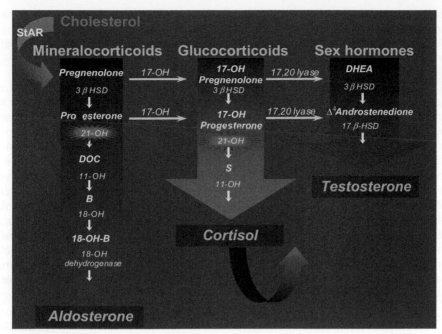

Fig. 1. Adrenal steroidogenetic pathways.

Stage I: clitoromegaly without labial fusion

Stage II: clitoromegaly and posterior labial fusion

Stage III: greater degree of clitoromegaly, single perineal urogenital orifice, and almost complete labial fusion

Stage IV: increasingly phallic clitoris, urethra-like urogenital sinus at base of clitoris, and complete labial fusion

Stage V: penile clitoris, urethral meatus at tip of phallus, and scrotum-like labia (appear like males without palpable gonads).

Internal Genitalia

As the androgens interact with the receptors on genital skin, they induce changes in the developing external female genitalia such as clitoral enlargement, fusion of the labial folds, and rostral migration of the urethral/vaginal perineal orifice. However,

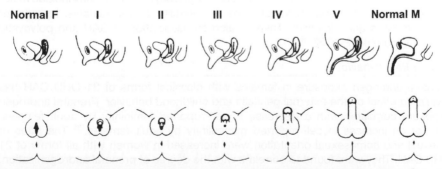

Fig. 2. Different degrees of virilization according to the scale developed by Prader.[9]

internal female genitalia (uterus, fallopian tubes, and ovaries) are normal, as females cannot produce Müllerian-inhibiting hormone because they do not have testicular Sertoli cells. Therefore the Müllerian ducts do not regress, and the internal female internal genitalia develop normally.

Postnatal Effects and Growth

Lack of appropriate postnatal treatment in boys and girls results in continued exposure to excessive androgens, causing progressive penile or clitoral enlargement, the development of premature pubic (pubarche) and axillary hair and acne. Hyperandrogenism during childhood often leads to rapid linear growth accompanied by premature epiphyseal maturation and closure, resulting in a final adult height that is typically below that expected from parental heights (on average −1.1 to −1.5 SD below the midparental target height).[10–13] On the other hand, poor growth can occur in patients with 21 OHD as a result of glucocorticoid treatment when replacement therapy exceeds physiologic requirements.

Final height in classical 21 OHD (as well as NC 21 OHD) is one of the features least amenable to glucocorticoid therapy even among patients with excellent adrenal control. A study of growth hormone therapy alone or in combination with a GnRH analog in CAH patients with compromised height prediction showed improvement in short- and long-term growth to reduce the height deficit.[13,14]

Puberty and Secondary Sexual Characteristics

In most patients treated adequately from early life, the onset of puberty in both girls and boys with classical 21 OHD occurs at the expected chronologic age.[15,16] However, a recent careful study showed that the mean ages at onset of puberty in both males and females were somewhat younger than the general population, but did not differ significantly among the three forms of 21 OHD.[17] Following the onset of puberty, in most successfully treated patients, the milestones of further development of secondary sex characteristics in general appear to be normal.[15–17]

Inadequate treatment leads to an advanced epiphyseal development. This can result in precocious puberty. Also in cases where a significant body maturation at the initial presentation, such as simple virilizing males who were not detected by newborn screening, the exposure to elevated androgens followed by the sudden decreased androgen levels after initiation of glucocorticoid treatment may cause an early activation of the hypothalamic-pituitary-gonadal axis. Studies suggest that excess adrenal androgens (aromatized to estrogens) inhibit the pubertal pattern of gonadotropin secretion by the hypothalamic-pituitary axis.[18] This inhibition, which probably takes place via a negative feedback effect can be reversed by glucocorticoid treatment.

In adolescents and adults, signs of hyperandrogenism in females may include male-pattern alopecia (temporal balding), acne, or infertility, and in females, irregular or absent menses and hirsutism. There is also an association of CAH and polycystic ovarian syndrome (PCOS).[19]

Gender Role Behavior

Prenatal androgen exposure in females with classical forms of 21 OHD CAH has a virilizing effect on the external genitalia and childhood behavior. Prenatal androgen exposure correlates with a decrease in self-reported femininity by adult females, but not an increase in self-reported masculinity by adult females.[20] The rates of bisexual and homosexual orientation were increased in women with all forms of 21 OHD CAH. They were found to correlate with the degree of prenatal androgenization. Of interest, bisexual/homosexual orientation was correlated with global measures of masculinization of nonsexual behavior and predicted independently by the degree of both prenatal androgenization and masculinization of childhood behavior.[21]

Changes in childhood play behavior correlated with reduced female gender satisfaction and reduced heterosexual interest in adulthood. Affected adult females are more likely to have gender dysphoria, and experience less heterosexual interest and reduced satisfaction with the assignment to the female sex. In contrast, males with 21 OHD CAH do not show a general alteration in childhood play behavior, core gender identity, or sexual orientation.[22]

Fertility

Difficulty with fertility in females with CAH may arise for various reasons, including anovulation, secondary polycystic ovarian syndrome, irregular menses, nonsuppressible serum progesterone levels, or an inadequate introitus. Fertility is reduced in SW 21 OHD with rare reports of pregnancy. In a retrospective survey of fertility rates in a large group of females with classical CAH, simple virilizers were shown to be more likely to become pregnant and carry the pregnancy to term.[23] However, more recent data suggest that fertility rates have significantly improved from 60% in SW and 80% in SV patients.[24] Adequate glucocorticoid therapy is probably an important variable with respect to fertility outcome. The development of PCOS in CAH patients is not uncommon and may be related to both prenatal and postnatal excess androgen exposure, which can affect the hypothalamic-pituitary-gonadal axis.

In male patients with classical CAH, several long-term studies indicate that those who have been adequately treated undergo normal pubertal development, have normal testicular function, and normal spermatogenesis and fertility.[17,25–27] However, small testes and reduced sperm count can occur in patients as a result of inadequately controlled disease.[28–32] A complication in postpubertal boys with inadequate control of CAH is hyperplastic nodular testes. Almost all these patients were found to have adenomatous adrenal rests within the testicular tissue, so-called testicular adrenal rest tumor (TART), as indicated by the presence of specific 11β-hydroxylated steroids in the blood from gonadal veins.[33] TART can lead to end-stage damage of testicular perenchyma, most probably as a result of long-standing obstruction of the seminiferous tubules.[34] These tumors have been reported to be ACTH dependent and to regress following adequate steroid therapy.[35–39]

Ironically, some investigators have reported normal testicular maturation as well as normal spermatogenesis and fertility in patients who had never received glucocorticoid treatment.[20,25,27,40]

Salt Wasting in 21 OHD

When the loss of 21 hydroxylase function is severe, adrenal aldosterone secretion is not sufficient for sodium reabsorption by the distal renal tubules, and individuals suffer from salt wasting, in addition to cortisol deficiency and androgen excess. Classical CAH patients who make adequate aldosterone are considered to have SV-CAH. Infants with renal salt wasting have poor feeding, weight loss, failure to thrive, vomiting, dehydration, hypotension, hyponatremia, and hyperkalemic metabolic acidosis progressing to adrenal crisis (azotemia, vascular collapse, shock, and death). Adrenal crisis can occur as early as age 1 to 4 weeks. The salt wasting is presumed to result from inadequate secretion of salt-retaining steroids, primarily aldosterone. In addition, hormonal precursors of the 21 OH enzyme may act as antagonists to mineralocorticoid action in the sodium-conserving mechanism of the immature newborn renal tubule.[41–43] The adrenal medulla may also be incompletely formed in some CAH patients. Merke and colleagues[44] noted that the epinephrine and metanephrine concentrations in CAH patients who manifested salt-wasting crisis was approximately 50% of that of controls, in line with adrenal gland histopathologic studies that showed depleted secretory vesicles.

Affected males who are not detected in a newborn screening program are at high risk for a salt-wasting adrenal crisis because their normal male genitalia do not alert medical professionals to their condition; they are often discharged from the hospital after birth without diagnosis and experience a salt-wasting crisis at home. On the other hand, salt-wasting females are born with ambiguous genitalia that trigger the diagnostic process and appropriate treatment. It is important to recognize that the extent of virilism may not differ among the two classical CAH SV and SW forms. Thus, even a mildly virilized newborn with 21 OHD should be observed carefully for signs of a potentially life-threatening crisis within the first few weeks of life.

It has been observed that an aldosterone biosynthetic defect apparent in infancy may be ameliorated with age.[45,46] Speiser and colleagues[47] reported the spontaneous partial recovery in adulthood of a patient with documented severe salt wasting in infancy. Therefore, it is desirable to follow the sodium and mineralocorticoid requirements carefully by measuring plasma renin activity (PRA) in patients who have been diagnosed in the neonatal period as salt wasters.

Although insufficient aldosterone biosynthesis is clinically apparent only in the SW form of the disease, impaired adrenal capacity to produce aldosterone in response to renin stimulation appeared to be a spectrum in all forms of 21 OHD CAH.[48]

Nonclassical Congenital Adrenal Hyperplasia

Individuals with the NC form of 21 OHD, also known as late-onset 21 OHD, have only mild to moderate enzyme deficiency and present postnatally with signs of hyperandrogenism. NC-CAH may present at any age after birth with a variety of hyperandrogenic symptoms, excluding ambiguous genitalia. This form of CAH results from a mild deficiency of the 21 hydroxylase enzyme. Similar to classical CAH, NC-CAH may cause premature development of pubic hair, advanced bone age, and accelerated linear growth velocity in both males and females. Severe cystic acne has also been attributed to NC-CAH.

Women may present with symptoms of androgen excess, including hirsutism, temporal baldness, and infertility.[49] Menarche in females may be normal or delayed, and secondary amenorrhea is a frequent occurrence. Further virilization may include hirsutism, male habitus, deepening of the voice, or male-pattern alopecia (temporal recession). Clinical course of NC form varies among individuals[50] and it is difficult to predict the appearance of any virilization symptoms.[51]

Polycystic ovarian syndrome may also be seen as a secondary complication in these patients. Possible reasons for the development of PCOS include reprogramming of the hypothalamic-pituitary-gonadal axis from prenatal exposure to androgens, or chronic levels of excess adrenal androgens that disrupt gonadotropin release and have direct effects on the ovary, ultimately leading to the formation of cysts. Because of the overlap of hyperandrogenic symptoms, it is important to consider NC 21 OHD in a patient diagnosed with PCOS. Of note, NC 21 OHD CAH was identified in 2.2% to 10.0% among women who presented with hyperandrogenic symptoms.[50,52,53]

Symptoms in adult males with NC-CAH may include short stature, acne, or oligozoospermia and diminished fertility.[54] Infertility is often caused by TART,[55] although some untreated men have been fertile,[28] as discussed before.

A subset of individuals with NC 21 OHD are completely asymptomatic[56] when detected (usually as part of a family study). Based on longitudinal follow-up of such patients, we observed that symptoms of hyperandrogenism wax and wane with time. The presence of 21 OHD can also be discovered during the evaluation of an incidental adrenal mass.[57] An increased incidence of adrenal incidentalomas has been found, reported as high as 82% in patients with 21 OHD and up to 45% in subjects heterozygous for 21 OHD mutations. This probably arises from hyperplastic tissue areas and does not require surgical intervention.[58]

DIAGNOSIS OF CONGENITAL ADRENAL HYPERPLASIA
Hormonal Diagnosis

Biochemical diagnosis of 21 OHD can be confirmed by hormonal evaluation. In a randomly timed blood sample, a very high concentration of 17-hydroxyprogesterone (17-OHP), the precursor of the defective enzyme, is diagnostic of classical 21 OHD. The gold standard to establish hormonal diagnosis for NC 21 OHD and for certain enigmatic cases is the corticotropin stimulation test (250 μg cosyntropin intravenously), measuring levels of 17-OHP and Δ^4-androstenedione at baseline and 60 minutes. The 17-OHP values can then be plotted in the published nomogram to ascertain disease severity (**Fig. 3**).[59] The corticotropin stimulation test is crucial in establishing hormonal diagnosis of the NC form of the disease, as even early-morning values of 17-OHP may not be sufficiently elevated to allow accurate diagnosis. For example, an NC patient may have a normal baseline 17-OHP of 100 ng/dL, yet stimulate to greater than 2000 ng/dL, and that would be diagnostic for NC-CAH. Patients with classical CAH typically have stimulated 17-OHP levels of 20,000 to 100,000 ng/dL. The corticotropin stimulation test may also be helpful in males for distinguishing between the NC and SV forms, as males with 21 OHD have normal genitalia.

Molecular Genetics

Hormonally and clinically defined forms of 21 OHD CAH are associated with distinct genotypes characterized by varying enzyme activity demonstrated though in vitro expression studies. The gene encoding 21 hydroxylase is a microsomal cytochrome P450-termed cytochrome P450, family 21, subfamily A, polypeptide 21 (*CYP21A2*) (Online Mendelian Inheritance in Man [OMIM] database number 201,910) located on the short arm of chromosome 6, within the human leukocyte antigen (HLA) complex.[60,61]*CYP21A2* and its homolog, the pseudogene *CYP21A1P* alternate with two genes, *C4B* and *C4A*, that encode the two isoforms of the fourth component of the serum complement system.[62]

More than 100 mutations have been described including point mutations, small deletions, small insertions, and complex rearrangements of the gene.[63] **Table 2** demonstrates the common mutations in *CYP21A2* and their related phenotypes. In recessive disorders, the less severe mutation of the two alleles typically dictates phenotype. Classical 21 OHD is most often caused by two alleles with severe mutations. In contrast to the classical form, patients with NC 21 OHD are predicted to have mild mutations on both alleles or one severe and one mild mutation (compound heterozygosity) of *CYP21A2*. It is not always possible, however, to accurately predict the phenotype on the basis of the genotype—such predictions have been shown to be 79% to 88% accurate[59,76,77] with some nonconcordance. Studies have demonstrated that there is often a divergence in phenotypes within mutation-identical groups, the reason for which requires further investigation.[78,79]

TREATMENT AND MANAGEMENT OF CONGENITAL ADRENAL HYPERPLASIA
Hormone Replacement

The goal of therapy in CAH is to both correct the deficiency in cortisol secretion and suppresses ACTH overproduction. Proper treatment with glucocorticoid reduces

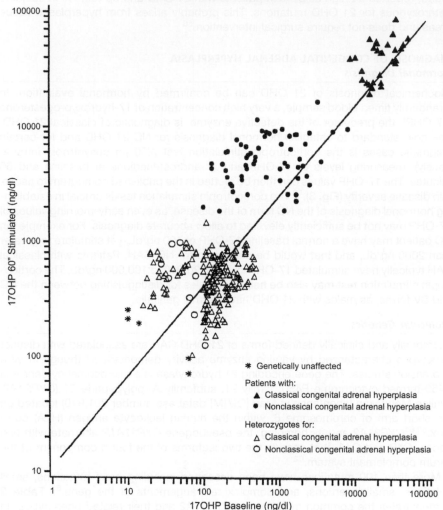

Fig. 3. Nomogram of 17 OHP.

stimulation of the androgen pathway, thus preventing further virilization and allowing normal growth and development. The usual requirement of hydrocortisone (or its equivalent) for the treatment of classical CAH is about 10 to 15 mg/m^2/day divided into 2 or 3 doses per day. Dosage requirements for patients with NC-CAH may be less. Adults may be treated with the longer-acting dexamethasone or prednisone, alone or in combination with hydrocortisone. A small dose of dexamethasone at bedtime (0.25 to 0.5 mg) is usually adequate for androgen suppression in NC patients. The goal of corticosteroid therapy is to give the lowest dose required for optimal control. Antiandrogen treatment may be useful as adjunctive therapy in adult women who continue to have hyperandrogenic signs despite good adrenal suppression.

Table 2
Common mutations in CYP21A2 gene and their related phenotypes

Study	Exon/Intron	Mutation Type	Mutation	Phenotype	Severity of Enzyme Defect (% Enzyme Activity)	References
Nonclassical mutations						
Tusie-Luna, 1991	Exon 1	Missense mutation	P30L	NC	Mild (30–60)	64
Speiser, 1988	Exon 7	Missense mutation	V281L	NC	Mild (20–50)	65
Helmberg, 1992	Exon 8	Missense mutation	R339H	NC	Mild (20–50)	66
Helmberg, 1992; Owerbach, 1992	Exon 10	Missense mutation	P453S	NC	Mild (20–50)	66,67
Classical mutations						
White, 1984	Deletion	30kb Deletion	—	SW	Severe (0)	68
Higashi, 1988	Intron 2	Aberrant splicing of Intron 2	656 A/C-G	SW, SV	Severe (ND)	69
White, 1994	Exon 3	Eight-base deletion	G110 Δ8nt	SW	Severe (0)	70
Tusie-Luna, 1990; Amor, 1988	Exon 4	Missense mutation	I172N	SV	Severe (1)	71,72
Tusie-Luna, 1990; Amor, 1988	Exon 6	Cluster	I236N, V237E, M239K	SW	Severe (0)	71,72
Globerman, 1988	Exon 8	Nonsense mutation	Q318X	SW	Severe (0)	73
Chiou, 1990	Exon 8	Missense mutation	R356W	SW, SV	Severe (0)	74
Wedell, 1993	Exon 10	Missense mutation	R483P[a]	SW	Severe (1–2)	75

Abbreviations: NC, nonclassical; ND, not defined; SV, simple virilizing; SW, salt wasting.

Females with concomitant PCOS may benefit from an oral contraceptive, although this treatment would not be appropriate for patients trying to get pregnant. Most adult males with NC-CAH are asymptomatic and often remain undiagnosed; therefore, treatment is generally not necessary.[56] For certain cases, however, our group has found that treatment may be helpful in preventing TARTs and preserving fertility. Glucocorticoid treatment may also prevent the development of adrenal adenomas.[80]

Titration of the dose should be aimed at maintaining androgen levels at age and sex-appropriate levels and 17-OHP levels of less than 1000 ng/dL to normalize growth in growing children. Concurrently, overtreatment should be avoided because it can lead to Cushing syndrome and in linear growth suppression in children. Patients with SW-CAH have elevated PRA in response to the sodium-deficient state, and they require treatment with the salt retaining steroid 9α-fludrocortisone acetate. It has not been customary to supplement conventional glucocorticoid replacement therapy with the administration of salt-retaining steroids in the SV and NC forms of CAH, although there has been some suggestion that adding fludrocortisone to patients with elevated PRA may improve hormonal control of the disease.[81] The requirement for fludrocortisone appears to diminish with age, and oversuppression of the PRA should be avoided, to prevent complications from hypertension and excessive mineralocorticoid activity.

Monitoring of glucocorticoid/mineralocorticoid replacement therapy is recommended every 3 to 4 months while children are actively growing, and less often thereafter; and monitoring for TART in males every 3 to 5 years after onset of puberty. In adulthood, long-term follow-up in the following areas is recommended: overweight/obesity, bone mineral density, fertility, and cardiovascular risks.

Stress Dosing

In non–life-threatening periods of illness or physiologic stress, the corticosteroid dose should be increased to two or three times the maintenance dose for the duration of that period. We recommend that each family should be given injection kits of hydrocortisone for emergency use (25 mg for infants, 50 mg for children, and 100 mg for adults). In the event of a surgical procedure, our protocol indicated that a total of 5 to 10 times the daily maintenance dose is required during the first 24 to 48 hours. The doses can then be tapered over the following days to the normal preoperative schedule. Stress doses of dexamethasone should not be given because of the delayed onset of action. It is not necessary for increased mineralocorticoid doses during these periods of stress.

It is imperative for all patients who are receiving corticosteroid replacement therapy such as these patients with CAH to wear a Medic-Alert or other identifying bracelets that will enable correct and appropriate therapy in case of emergencies. Additionally, all responsible family members should be trained in the intramuscular administration of hydrocortisone.

Surgery

In the past, it was routine to recommend early corrective surgery for neonates born with ambiguous genitalia. In recent years, the implementation of early corrective surgery has become increasingly controversial because of lack of data on long-term functional outcome.[82] Thus, the role of the parents in sex assignment becomes crucial in all aspects of the decision-making process, and should include full discussion of the controversy and all possible therapeutic options for the intersex child, particularly early versus delayed surgery. Furthermore, a multidisciplinary case-by-case approach, involving pediatric endocrinology, urology, genetics, and psychoendrocrinology, is imperative when considering sex assignment and possible surgical repair.[83,84]

The aim of surgical repair in females with ambiguous genitalia caused by CAH, when the decision is made by parents or patients themselves, is generally to remove the redundant erectile tissue, preserve the sexually sensitive glans clitoris, and provide a normal vaginal orifice that functions adequately for menstruation, intromission, and delivery. A medical indication for early surgery other than for sex assignment is recurrent urinary tract infections as a result of pooling of urine in the vagina or urogenital sinus. The extent of surgery depends on the degree of genital virilization. For female patients with greater degrees of virilization (an enlarged phallus, fused labia, and a single perineal opening), surgical procedures may include reduction of the enlarged clitoris, separation of the labia, and opening of the lower vagina. Further procedures may be required in adolescence and adulthood to provide an adequate introitus for menstruation, tampon use, and coitus. A cross-sectional study of 24 adult women with classical CAH who had undergone genital surgery showed that there was significant impairment to sensitivity in the clitoris compared with unaffected controls and CAH women who had not undergone genital surgery. Sexual function difficulties were also reported, including vaginal penetration, anorgasmia, and intercourse frequency.[85]

A review of sexual and reproductive outcomes in 35 adult women with CAH found that none of the subjects expressed doubts about their gender assignment. Twenty percent had homosexual inclinations; 23% were married; and 37% reported never having had heterosexual intercourse with vaginal penetration. Eighty-one percent of the subjects who had experienced vaginal intercourse reported pain during penetration. Past pregnancy was reported in 8 of the 35 women; 6 of them had children.[86]

Another study of 62 women with CAH demonstrated that they were often less satisfied with their genital function and appearance than controls, regardless of whether or not they had surgery. Half of the CAH women reported that CAH affected their sex life. Clitoral surgery was frequently associated with dissatisfaction with clitoral size and/or sensation. Of the women who had vaginoplasty, 37.5% underwent reoperation because of vaginal stenosis. Painful intercourse was reported in 30% of the subjects. Embarrassment regarding the cosmetic appearance of the external genitalia was also quite common.[87]

Bone Mineral Density

Bone mineral density (BMD) is affected by the competing actions of androgen excess (from undertreatment) and glucocorticiod excess (from overtreatment), which can both occur simulataneously in a patient. To adequately suppress androgen production in patients with CAH, the usual requirement of hydrocortisone is generally higher than the endogenous secretory rate of cortisol. Chronic therapy with glucocorticoids at supraphysiologic levels can result in diminished bone accrual and lead to osteopenia and osteoporosis. Glucocorticoid-induced bone loss is a well-known phenomenon and is the most prevalent form of secondary osteoporosis.[88]

Unlike other diseases treated with chronic glucocorticoid therapy, however, the effect of glucocorticoid replacement in CAH on BMD is unclear. Several studies of patients with 21 OHD have reported decreased BMD,[89,90] whereas other studies have reported increased or normal BMD.[91,92] The discrepancies may be attributable to differences in age and gender, as well as varying treatment regimens. Generally, studies that have included males and older females, particularly postmenopausal women with CAH, have shown a higher incidence of osteopenia and osteoporosis, whereas studies limited to younger patients have not shown such a decrease. It has been postulated that the elevated androgens typically found in young adult women with CAH may have a protective effect on bone integrity, but the precise mechanism is unknown. The increased adrenal androgens, which are converted to estrogens, may counteract the detrimental effects of glucocorticoids on bone mass. This may explain why older CAH women, particularly those who are postmenopausal, are at higher risk for osteoporosis than younger CAH patients. A study is currently under way to examine a potential mechanism by which certain CAH patients are protected against glucocorticoid-induced bone loss.

Metabolic Aspects

Long-term glucocorticoid treatment coupled with increased androgens may lead to undesirable metabolic effects in patients with CAH. Increased body mass index and body fat mass have been described in CAH.[91,93–95] Higher fasting plasma insulin with reduced insulin sensitivity and elevated serum leptin have also been reported in CAH patients,[96–98] as has a higher frequency of gestational diabetes.[99] Other cardiovascular risk factors, such as increased carotid intima-media thickness[98] and hypertension,[95,100] have been described as well.

A decrease in epinephrine reserve with resulting defects in leptin, insulin, and glucose control has been shown during both high- and moderate-intensity exercise in adolescents with classical CAH.[101,102]

Fertility and Management during Pregnancy

Management of congenital adrenal hyperplasia during pregnancy

As described previously, females with CAH have normal internal female structures and reproductive capability. Although barriers to fertility exist, many CAH females are able to achieve pregnancy with or without medical assistance. Despite genital reconstruction of the external genitalia, many females with classical CAH may have difficulty with a vaginal delivery and will require Caesarean section. Females with NC-CAH should be able to deliver vaginally in the absence of other complications. Because of the physical stress of labor and delivery, particularly if anesthesia is administered, all females with known CAH, who are being treated with glucocorticoid replacement, should receive stress dose hydrocortisone during labor and delivery.

Preferably, the carrier status of the partner should be ascertained before pregnancy. If the partner is found to be genetically unaffected, then the glucocorticoid of choice is hydrocortisone, which does not cross the placenta, as it is inactivated by placental 11β-hydroxysteroid dehydrogenase type 2.[103] Although harm to the fetus from prednisone has not been documented in humans, inactivation of prednisone by the placenta is unpredictable[104]; therefore, prednisone is usually not the preferred treatment for CAH during pregnancy. Our group monitors adrenal hormones, including 17-OHP and androgens, throughout the pregnancy. However, 17-OHP is a necessary hormone for the maintenance of pregnancy, and the serum level of androgens increase during pregnancy owing to increased sex hormone binding globulin (SHBG); therefore, the target levels to maintain during pregnancy should not be as rigid as in the nonpregnant state. For the most part, the prepregnancy dose of hydrocortisone (or the equivalent dose) is adequate to continue throughout pregnancy, although in some instances, dose increases may be necessary.

Prenatal treatment with dexamethasone

In pregnancies at risk of the offspring having classical forms of CAH, prenatal diagnosis and treatment can be offered. Conventionally, this occurs in the family where there is a previously affected sibling or first-degree relative with known mutations causing classical CAH, proven by DNA analysis. If the CAH patient's partner is a carrier of a severe mutation, placing the fetus at risk for classical 21 OHD, the patient should be offered prenatal diagnosis and treatment with dexamethasone until chorionic villus sampling or amniocentesis is performed. Prenatal dexamethasone (at a dose of 0.02 mg/kg/day, based on prepregnancy weight, divided into two or three doses), administered at or before 9 weeks of gestation to the mother, has been shown to be effective in reducing virilization in females affected with classical CAH.[105,106] In these studies, no significant or enduring side effects were noted in either the mothers (other than greater weight gain and a higher incidence of striae and edema than untreated mothers) or the fetuses. There was no statistically significant difference between treated and untreated mothers in hypertension or gestational diabetes. All mothers who took partial or full treatment stated they would take dexamethasone again in the event of a future pregnancy. In our report and in others, no cases have been reported of cleft palate, placental degeneration, or fetal death, which have been observed in a rodent model of in utero exposure to high-dose glucocorticoids.[107,108] Another study, in contrast, noted some significant maternal side effects, including excessive weight gain, cushingoid facial features, severe striae resulting in permanent scarring, and hyperglycemic response to oral glucose administration.[109]

A long-term follow-up study of 44 children treated prenatally in Scandinavia demonstrated normal pre- and postnatal growth compared with matched controls.[110] In our study, prenatally treated newborns also did not differ in weight, length, or head circumference from untreated, unaffected newborns.[105,106] Moreover, a survey of 174 prenatally dexamethasone (DEX)-exposed children, ages 1 month to 12 years (including 48 with CAH), compared with 313 unexposed children (including 195 with CAH) found no differences in cognitive or motor development between the two groups.[111] Another report from Sweden suggested that there may be long-term cognitive effects of prenatal treatment with dexamethasone.[112] In their study, DEX-treated CAH children performed less well than unaffected controls on tests measuring verbal processing speed; however, no comparison was made with CAH children who were not DEX-exposed. Full-scale IQ was not different from healthy controls. Another long-term follow-up study of DEX- exposed children did not show any statistically significant differences in measures of psychopathology, behavioral problems, and adaptive functioning. In addition, DEX-exposed children were described by their parents as being more sociable than controls.[113] These studies have prompted imperative further investigation into the psychological, cognitive, and medical outcome of patients treated prenatally with dexamethasone; more long-term studies are currently under way.

Transitioning the Pediatric Patient to Adulthood

Transitioning the pediatric patient to adulthood is a very important aspect of caring for CAH patients. There are several issues to consider for a smooth transition. During the pediatric period, children with CAH are typically brought to doctor visits by their parents and are monitored very frequently. Once patients reach adulthood, however, they must assume responsibility for understanding their medical condition and for compliance. Medical visits tend to decrease in frequency, and patients are at risk for poor follow-up. Another issue to take into account is that the goals of treatment are different in children compared with adults. Although prevention of Addisonian and salt-wasting crises are critical at any age, the goals in childhood focus on reducing virilization and optimizing growth. Once growth and development are completed, however, the goals of treatment shift toward preventing symptoms of hyperandrogenism in women, preserving fertility, and satisfactory sexual function. The dose and type of glucocorticoid may require adjustment once growth is completed, as growth suppression is no longer a concern. Mineralocorticoid requirements tend to decrease with age.

Although some endocrinologists are trained in both pediatric and adult endocrinology, allowing them to continue caring for their pediatric patients into adulthood, most patients will require some form of transitioning into an adult endocrinology practice. A program of transitioning the pediatric patient into adulthood was developed at the University of Kiel in Germany (the "Kieler Model") as a means for providing a smooth transition.[114] In this program, there is an outpatient clinic staffed by both a pediatric and an adult endocrinologist. The transition usually takes place around 17 to 18 years of age, at which time the CAH patient sees both endocrinologists, and the pediatric endocrinologist provides the adult endocrinologist with an extensive summary of treatment up to that time. Depending on the complexity, the patient is seen several times by both the pediatric and adult endocrinologist in joint appointments until the transition is complete. Similar programs of transitioning may help to optimize the care of CAH patients into adulthood.

SUMMARY

The pathophysiology of the various types of CAH (the most common being 21 OHD) can be traced to discrete, inherited defects in the genes encoding enzymes for adrenal steroidogenesis. Treatment of CAH is targeted to replace the insufficient adrenal hormones. With proper hormone replacement therapy, normal and healthy development may often be expected. Glucocorticoid and, if necessary, mineralocorticoid replacement, has been the mainstay of treatment for CAH, but new treatment strategies continue to be developed and studied to improve care.

REFERENCES

1. Pang S, Clark A. Congenital adrenal hyperplasia due to 21-hydroxylase deficiency: newborn screening and its relationship to the diagnosis and treatment of the disorder. Screening 1993;2:105–39.
2. Therrell BJ, Berenbaum S, Manter-Kapanke V, et al. Results of screening 1.9 million Texas newborns for 21-hydroxylase-deficient congenital adrenal hyperplasia. Pediatrics 1998;101:583–90.
3. Balsamo A, Cacciari E, Piazzi S, et al. Congenital adrenal hyperplasia: neonatal mass screening compared with clinical diagnosis only in the Emilia-Romagna region of Italy, 1980–1995. Pediatrics 1996;98:362–7.
4. Speiser PW, Dupont B, Rubinstein P, et al. High frequency of nonclassical steroid 21-hydroxylase deficiency. Am J Hum Genet 1985;37:650–67.
5. Sherman SL, Aston CE, Morton NE, et al. A segregation and linkage study of classical and nonclassical 21-hydroxylase deficiency. Am J Hum Genet 1988; 42:830–8.
6. Ganong W. The central nervous system and the synthesis and release of adrenocorticotrophic hormone. In: Nalbandov A, editor. Advances in neuroendocrinology. Urbana: University of Illinois Press; 1963. p. 92.
7. Guillemin R, Schally A. Recent advances in the chemistry of neuroendocrine mediators originating in the central nervous system. In: Nalbandov A, editor. Advances in neuroendocrinology. Urbana: University of Illinois Press; 1963. p. 314.
8. Goto M, Piper Hanley K, Marcos J, et al. In humans, early cortisol biosynthesis provides a mechanism to safeguard female sexual development. J Clin Invest 2006;116:953–60.

9. Prader A, Gurtner HP. [The syndrome of male pseudohermaphrodism in congenital adrenocortical hyperplasia without overproduction of androgens (adrenal male pseudohermaphrodism)]. Helv Paediatr Acta 1955;10:397–412.

10. Eugster EA, Dimeglio LA, Wright JC, et al. Height outcome in congenital adrenal hyperplasia caused by 21-hydroxylase deficiency: a meta-analysis. J Pediatr 2001;138:26–32.

11. Muirhead S, Sellers EA, Guyda H. Indicators of adult height outcome in classical 21-hydroxylase deficiency congenital adrenal hyperplasia. J Pediatr 2002;141: 247–52.

12. Brunelli V, Russo G, Bertelloni S, et al. Final height in congenital adrenal hyperplasia due to 21-hydroxylase deficiency: the Italian experience. J Pediatr Endocrinol Metab 2003;16(Suppl 2):277–83.

13. Lin-Su K, Vogiatzi MG, Marshall I, et al. Treatment with growth hormone and luteinizing hormone releasing hormone analog improves final adult height in children with congenital adrenal hyperplasia. J Clin Endocrinol Metab 2005;90:3318–25.

14. Quintos JB, Vogiatzi MG, Harbison MD, et al. Growth hormone therapy alone or in combination with gonadotropin-releasing hormone analog therapy to improve the height deficit in children with congenital adrenal hyperplasia. J Clin Endocrinol Metab 2001;86:1511–7.

15. Jones H, Verkauf B. Congenital adrenal hyperplasia: age at menarche and related events at puberty. Am J Obstet Gynecol 1971;109:292.

16. Ghali I, David M, David L. Linear growth and pubertal development in treated congenital adrenal hyperplasia due to 21-hydroxylase deficiency. Clin Endocrinol (Oxf) 1977;6:425–36.

17. Trinh L, Nimkarn S, Obeid J, et al. Growth and pubertal characteristics in patients with congenital adrenal hyperplasia due to 21-hydroxylase deficiency. ENDO 2006 The Endocrine Society's 88th Annual Meeting. Boston, Massachusetts, June 24–27, 2006. p. 368.

18. Klingensmith G, Garcia S, Jones H, et al. Glucocorticoid treatment of girls with congenital adrenal hyperplasia: effects on height, sexual maturation, and fertility. J Pediatr 1977;90:996–1004.

19. Barnes RB, Rosenfield RL, Ehrmann DA, et al. Ovarian hyperandrogynism as a result of congenital adrenal virilizing disorders: evidence for perinatal masculinization of neuroendocrine function in women. J Clin Endocrinol Metab 1994; 79:1328–33.

20. Long DN, Wisniewski AB, Migeon CJ. Gender role across development in adult women with congenital adrenal hyperplasia due to 21-hydroxylase deficiency. J Pediatr Endocrinol Metab 2004;17:1367–73.

21. Meyer-Bahlburg HF, Dolezal C, Baker SW, et al. Sexual orientation in women with classical or non-classical congenital adrenal hyperplasia as a function of degree of prenatal androgen excess. Arch Sex Behav 2008;37:85–99.

22. Hines M, Brook C, Conway GS. Androgen and psychosexual development: core gender identity, sexual orientation and recalled childhood gender role behavior in women and men with congenital adrenal hyperplasia (CAH). J Sex Res 2004; 41:75–81.

23. Mulaikal RM, Migeon CJ, Rock JA. Fertility rates in female patients with congenital adrenal hyperplasia due to 21-hydroxylase deficiency. N Engl J Med 1987; 316:178–82.

24. Premawardhana L, Hughes I, Read G, et al. Longer term outcome in females with congenital adrenal hyperplasia (CAH): the Cardiff experience. Clin Endocrinol (Oxf) 1997;46:327–32.

25. Prader A, Zachmann M, Illig R. Normal spermatogenesis in adult males with congenital adrenal hyperplasia after discontinuation of therapy. In: Lee P, Platnick L, Kowarski A, et al, editors. Congenital adrenal hyperplasia. Baltimore (MD): University Park Press; 1977. p. 397.

26. Stewart J. A fertile male with untreated congenital adrenal hyperplasia. Acta Endocrinol Suppl 1960;51:661.

27. Urban M, Lee P, Migeon C. Adult height and fertility in men with congenital virilizing adrenal hyperplasia. N Engl J Med 1978;299:1392.

28. Cabrera M, Vogiatzi M, New M. Long term outcome in adult males with classic congenital adrenal hyperplasia. J Clin Endocrinol Metab 2001;86:3070–80.

29. Sugino Y, Usui T, Okubo K, et al. Genotyping of congenital adrenal hyperplasia due to 21-hydroxylase deficiency presenting as male infertility: case report and literature review. J Assist Reprod Genet 2006;23:377–80.

30. Bonaccorsi A, Adler I, Figueiredo J. Male infertility due to congenital adrenal hyperplasia: testicular biopsy findings, hormonal evaluation, and therapeutic results in three patients. Fertil Steril 1987;47:664–70.

31. Claahsen-van der Grinten HL, Sweep FC, Blickman JG, et al. Prevalence of testicular adrenal rest tumours in male children with congenital adrenal hyperplasia due to 21-hydroxylase deficiency. Eur J Endocrinol 2007;157:339–44.

32. Molitor J, Chertow B, Fariss B. Long-term follow-up of a patient with congenital adrenal hyperplasia and failure of testicular development. Fertil Steril 1973;24: 319.

33. Blumberg-Tick J, Boudou P, Nahoul K, et al. Testicular tumors in congenital adrenal hyperplasia: steroid measurements from adrenal and spermatic veins. J Clin Endocrinol Metab 1991;73:1129–33.

34. Claahsen-van der Grinten HL, Otten BJ, Hermus AR, et al. Testicular adrenal rest tumors in patients with congenital adrenal hyperplasia can cause severe testicular damage. Fertil Steril 2008;89:597–601.

35. Schoen E, DiRaimondo V, Dominguez O. Bilateral testicular tumors complicating congenital adrenocortical hyperplasia. J Clin Endocrinol Metab 1961;21:518.

36. Miller E, Murray H. Congenital adrenocortical hyperplasia: case previously reported as "bilateral interstitial cell tumor of the testicle". J Clin Endocrinol Metab 1962;22:655.

37. Glenn J, Boyce W. Adrenogenitalism with testicular adrenal rests simulating interstitial cell tumor. J Urol 1963;89:456.

38. Srikanth M, West B, Ishitani M, et al. Benign testicular tumors in children with congenital adrenal hyperplasia. J Pediatr Surg 1992;27:639–41.

39. Rutgers J, Young R, Scully R. The testicular "tumor" of the adrenogenital syndrome. A report of six cases and review of the literature on testicular masses in patients with adrenocortical disorders. Am J Surg Pathol 1988;12:503–13.

40. Wilkins L, Crigler J, Silverman S, et al. Further studies on the treatment of congenital adrenal hyperplasia with cortisone. II. The effects of cortisone on sexual and somatic development, with a hypothesis concerning the mechanism of feminization. J Clin Endocrinol Metab 1952;12:277.

41. Klein R. Evidence for and evidence against the existence of a salt-losing hormone. J Pediatr 1960;57:452.

42. Kowarski A, Finkelstein JW, Spaulding JS, et al. Aldosterone secretion rate in congenital adrenal hyperplasia. A discussion of the theories on the pathogenesis of the salt-losing form of the syndrome. J Clin Invest 1965;44:1505–13.

43. Kuhnle U, Land M, Ulick S. Evidence for the secretion of an antimineralocorticoid in congenital adrenal hyperplasia. J Clin Endocrinol Metab 1986;62:934–40.

44. Merke D, Chrousos G, Eisenhofer G, et al. Adrenomedullary dysplasia and hypofunction in patients with classic 21-hydroxylase deficiency. N Engl J Med 2000;343:1362–8.
45. Stoner E, Dimartino-Nardi J, Kuhnle U, et al. Is salt-wasting in congenital adrenal hyperplasia due to the same gene as the fasciculata defect? Clin Endocrinol (Oxf) 1986;24:9–20.
46. Luetscher JA. Studies of aldosterone in relation to water and electrolyte balance in man. Recent Prog Horm Res 1956;12:175.
47. Speiser PW, Agdere L, Ueshiba H, et al. Aldosterone synthesis in salt-wasting congenital adrenal hyperplasia with complete absence of adrenal 21-hydroxylase. N Engl J Med 1991;324:145–9.
48. Nimkarn S, New MI. Prenatal diagnosis and treatment of congenital adrenal hyperplasia owing to 21-hydroxylase deficiency. Nat Clin Pract Endocrinol Metab 2007;3:405–13.
49. New MI. Nonclassical 21-hydroxylase deficiency. J Clin Endocrinol Metab 2006; 91:4205–14.
50. New MI. Extensive clinical experience: nonclassical 21-hydroxylase deficiency. J Clin Endocrinol Metab 2006;91:4205–14.
51. Kashimada K, Ono M, Onishi T, et al. Clinical course of patients with nonclassical 21-hydroxylase deficiency (21-OHD) diagnosed in infancy and childhood. Endocr J 2008;55:397–404.
52. Fanta M, Cibula D, Vrbikova J. Prevalence of nonclassic adrenal hyperplasia (NCAH) in hyperandrogenic women. Gynecol Endocrinol 2008;24:154–7.
53. Escobar-Morreale HF, Sanchon R, San Millan JL. A prospective study of the prevalence of nonclassical congenital adrenal hyperplasia among women presenting with hyperandrogenic symptoms and signs. J Clin Endocrinol Metab 2008;93:527–33.
54. Claahsen-van der Grinten HL, Otten BJ, Sweep FC, et al. Repeated successful induction of fertility after replacing hydrocortisone with dexamethasone in a patient with congenital adrenal hyperplasia and testicular adrenal rest tumors. Fertil Steril 2007;88:705, e5–8.
55. Jaaskelainen J, Tiitinen A, Voutilainen R. Sexual function and fertility in adult females and males with congenital adrenal hyperplasia. Horm Res 2001;56: 73–80.
56. Clayton PE, Miller WL, Oberfield SE, et al. Consensus statement on 21-hydroxylase deficiency from the European Society for Paediatric Endocrinology and the Lawson Wilkins Pediatric Endocrine Society. Horm Res 2002;58:188–95.
57. Mokshagundam S, Surks M. Congenital adrenal hyperplasia diagnosed in a man during workup for bilateral adrenal masses. Arch Intern Med 1993;153: 1389–91.
58. Jaresch S, Kornely E, Kley H, et al. Adrenal incidentaloma and patients with homozygous or heterozygous congenital adrenal hyperplasia. J Clin Endocrinol Metab 1992;74:685–9.
59. Wilson RC, Mercado AB, Cheng KC, et al. Steroid 21-hydroxylase deficiency: genotype may not predict phenotype. J Clin Endocrinol Metab 1995;80:2322–9.
60. Dupont B, Oberfield SE, Smithwick EM, et al. Close genetic linkage between HLA and congenital adrenal hyperplasia (21-hydroxylase deficiency). Lancet 1977;2:1309–12.
61. Nebert DW, Nelson DR, Coon MJ. The P450 superfamily: update on new sequences, gene mapping, and recommended nomenclature. DNA Cell Biol 1991;10:1–14.

62. White PC, New MI, Dupont B. Structure of the human steroid 21-hydroxylase genes. Proc Natl Acad Sci U S A 1986;83:5111–5.

63. Stenson PD, Ball EV, Mort M, et al. Human Gene Mutation Database (HGMD): 2003 update. Hum Mutat 2003;21:577–81.

64. Tusie-Luna MT, Speiser PW, Dumic M, et al. A mutation (Pro-30 to Leu) in CYP21 represents a potential nonclassic steroid 21-hydroxylase deficiency allele. Mol Endocrinol 1991;5:685–92.

65. Speiser PW, New MI, White PC. Molecular genetic analysis of nonclassic steroid 21-hydroxylase deficiency associated with HLA-B14, DR1. N Engl J Med 1988; 319:19–23.

66. Helmberg A, Tusie-Luna M, Tabarelli M, et al. R339H and P453S: CYP21 mutations associated with nonclassic steroid 21-hydroxylase deficiency that are not apparent gene conversions. Mol Endocrinol 1992;6:1318–22.

67. Owerbach D, Sherman L, Ballard AL, et al. Pro-453 to Ser mutation in CYP21 is associated with nonclassic steroid 21-hydroxylase deficiency. Mol Endocrinol 1992;6:1211–5.

68. White PC, New MI, Dupont B. HLA-linked congenital adrenal hyperplasia results from a defective gene encoding a cytochrome P-450 specific for steroid 21-hydroxylation. Proc Natl Acad Sci U S A 1984;81:7505–9.

69. Higashi Y, Tanae A, Inoue H, et al. Aberrant splicing and missense mutations cause steroid 21-hydroxylase [P-450(C21)] deficiency in humans: possible gene conversion products. Proc Natl Acad Sci U S A 1988;85:7486–90.

70. White PC, Tusie-Luna MT, New MI, et al. Mutations in steroid 21-hydroxylase (CYP21). Hum Mutat 1994;3:373–8.

71. Tusie-Luna M, Traktman P, White PC. Determination of functional effects of mutations in the steroid 21-hydroxylase gene (CYP21) using recombinant vaccinia virus. J Biol Chem 1990;265:20916–22.

72. Amor M, Parker KL, Globerman H, et al. Mutation in the CYP21B gene (Ile-172-Asn) causes steroid 21-hydroxylase deficiency. Proc Natl Acad Sci U S A 1988; 85:1600–7.

73. Globerman H, Amor M, Parker KL, et al. Nonsense mutation causing steroid 21-hydroxylase deficiency. J Clin Invest 1988;82:139–44.

74. Chiou SH, Hu MC, Chung BC. A missense mutation at Ile172–Asn or Arg356–Trp causes steroid 21-hydroxylase deficiency. J Biol Chem 1990;265:3549–52.

75. Wedell A, Luthman H. Steroid 21-hydroxylase (P450c21): a new allele and spread of mutations through the pseudogene. Hum Genet 1993;91:236–40.

76. Speiser PW, Dupont J, Zhu D, et al. Disease expression and molecular genotype in congenital adrenal hyperplasia due to 21-hydroxylase deficiency. J Clin Invest 1992;90:584–95.

77. Wedell A, Ritzen EM, Haglund-Stengler B, et al. Steroid 21-hydroxylase deficiency: three additional mutated alleles and establishment of phenotype-genotype relationships of common mutations. Proc Natl Acad Sci U S A 1992;89:7232–6.

78. Krone N, Braun A, Roscher A, et al. Predicting phenotype in steroid 21-hydroxylase deficiency? Comprehensive genotyping in 155 unrelated, well defined patients from southern Germany. J Clin Endocrinol Metab 2000;85:p1059–65.

79. Chemaitilly W, Betensky B, Marshal I, et al. Case report: the natural history and genotype-phenotype nonconcordance of HLA identical siblings with the same mutations of the 21-hydroxylase gene. J Pediatr Endocrinol Metab 2005;18: 143–54.

80. Rohana AG, Ming W, Norlela S, et al. Functioning adrenal adenoma in association with congenital adrenal hyperplasia. Med J Malaysia 2007;62:158–9.

81. Jansen M, Wit JM, van den Brande JL. Reinstitution of mineralocorticoid therapy in congenital adrenal hyperplasia. Effects on control and growth. Acta Paediatr Scand 1981;70:229–33.

82. Forest MG, Dorr HG. Prenatal therapy in congenital adrenal hyperplasia due to 21-hydroxylase deficiency: retrospective follow-up study of 253 treated pregnancies in 215 families. Endocrinologist 2003;13:252–9.

83. Schachter SC. Handedness in women with intrauterine exposure to diethystilbestrol. Neuropsychologia 1994;32:619–23.

84. Schnitzer J, Donahoe P. Surgical treatment of congenital adrenal hyperplasia. Endocrinol Metab Clin North Am 2001;30:137–54.

85. Crouch NS, Liao LM, Woodhouse CR, et al. Sexual function and genital sensitivity following feminizing genitoplasty for congenital adrenal hyperplasia. J Urol 2008;179:634–8. [Epub 2007 Dec 21].

86. Gastaud F, Bouvattier C, Duranteau L, et al. Impaired sexual and reproductive outcomes in women with classical forms of congenital adrenal hyperplasia. Clin Endocrinol Metab 2007;92:1391–6.

87. Nordenskjold A, Holmdahl G, Frisen L, et al. Type of mutation and surgical procedure affect long-term quality of life for women with congenital adrenal hyperplasia. J Clin Endocrinol Metab 2008;93:380–6.

88. Mazziotti G, Giustina A, Canalis E, et al. Glucocorticoid-induced osteoporosis: clinical and therapeutic aspects. Arq Bras Endocrinol Metabol 2007;51:1404–12.

89. Falhammar H, Filipsson H, Holmdahl G, et al. Fractures and bone mineral density in adult women with 21-hydroxylase deficiency. J Clin Endocrinol Metab 2007;92:4643–9.

90. King JA, Wisniewski AB, Bankowski BJ, et al. Long-term corticosteroid replacement and bone mineral density in adult women with classical congenital adrenal hyperplasia. J Clin Endocrinol Metab 2006;91:865–9.

91. Stikkelbroeck N, Oyen W, van der Wilt GJ, et al. Normal bone mineral density and lean body mass, but increased fat mass, in young adult patients with congenital adrenal hyperplasia. J Clin Endocrinol Metab 2003;88:1036–42.

92. Christiansen P, Molgaard C, Muller J. Normal bone mineral content in young adults with congenital adrenal hyperplasia due to 21-hydroxylase deficiency. Horm Res 2004;61:133–6.

93. Cornean RE, Hindmarsh PC, Brook CG. Obesity in 21-hydroxylase deficient patients. Arch Dis Child 1998;78:261–3.

94. Charmandari E, Chrousos GP. Metabolic syndrome manifestations in classic congenital adrenal hyperplasia: do they predispose to atherosclerotic cardiovascular disease and secondary polycystic ovary syndrome? Ann N Y Acad Sci 2006;1083:37–53.

95. Volkl TM, Simm D, Beier C, et al. Obesity among children and adolescents with classic congenital adrenal hyperplasia due to 21-hydroxylase deficiency. Pediatrics 2006;117:e98–105.

96. Speiser PW, Serrat J, New MI, et al. Insulin insensitivity in adrenal hyperplasia due to nonclassical steroid 21-hydroxylase deficiency. J Clin Endocrinol Metab 1992;75:1421–4.

97. Charmandari E, Weise M, Bornstein S, et al. Children with classic congenital adrenal hyperplasia have elevated serum leptin concentrations and insulin resistance: potential clinical implications. J Clin Endocrinol Metab 2002;87:2114–20.

98. Sartorato P, Zulian E, Benedini S, et al. Cardiovascular risk factors and ultrasound evaluation of intima-media thickness at common carotids, carotid bulbs,

and femoral and abdominal aorta arteries in patients with classic congenital adrenal hyperplasia due to 21-hydroxylase deficiency. J Clin Endocrinol Metab 2007;92:1015–8.

99. Falhammar H, Filipsson H, Holmdahl G, et al. Metabolic profile and body composition in adult women with congenital adrenal hyperplasia due to 21-hydroxylase deficiency. J Clin Endocrinol Metab 2007;92:110–6.

100. Roche EF, Charmandari E, Dattani MT, et al. Blood pressure in children and adolescents with congenital adrenal hyperplasia (21-hydroxylase deficiency): a preliminary report. Clin Endocrinol (Oxf) 2003;58:589–96.

101. Weise M, Drinkard B, Mehlinger SL, et al. Stress dose of hydrocortisone is not beneficial in patients with classic congenital adrenal hyperplasia undergoing short-term, high-intensity exercise. J Clin Endocrinol Metab 2004;89:3679–84.

102. Green-Golan L, Yates C, Drinkard B, et al. Patients with classic congenital adrenal hyperplasia have decreased epinephrine reserve and defective glycemic control during prolonged moderate-intensity exercise. J Clin Endocrinol Metab 2007;92:3019–24.

103. Burton PJ, Waddell BJ. Dual function of 11beta-hydroxysteroid dehydrogenase in placenta: modulating placental glucocorticoid passage and local steroid action. Biol Reprod 1999;60:234–40.

104. Rennick GJ. Use of systemic glucocorticosteroids in pregnancy: be alert but not alarmed. Australas J Dermatol 2006;47:34–6.

105. Carlson AD, Obeid JS, Kanellopoulou N, et al. Prenatal treatment and diagnosis of congenital adrenal hyperplasia owing to steroid 21-hydroxylase deficiency. In: New MI, editor. Diagnosis and treatment of the unborn child. Reddick (FL): Idelson-Gnocchi Ltd. Publisher; 1999. p. 75–84.

106. New M, Carlson A, Obeid J, et al. Update: Prenatal diagnosis for congenital adrenal hyperplasia in 595 pregnancies. Endocrinologist 2003;13:233–9.

107. Goldman A, Sharpior B, Katsumata M. Human foetal palatal corticoid receptors and teratogens for cleft palate. Nature 1978;272:464–6.

108. Nimkarn S, New MI. Prenatal diagnosis and treatment of congenital adrenal hyperplasia owing to 21-hydroxylase deficiency. Nat Clin Pract Endocrinol Metab 2007;3:405–13.

109. Pang S, Clark AT, Freeman LO, et al. Maternal side-effects of prenatal dexamethasone therapy for fetal congenital adrenal hyperplasia. J Clin Endocrinol Metab 1992;76:249–53.

110. Lajic S, Wedell A, Bui T, et al. Long-term somatic follow-up of prenatally treated children with congenital adrenal hyperplasia. J Clin Endocrinol Metab 1998;83:3872–80.

111. Meyer-Bahlburg HF, Dolezal C, Baker SW, et al. Cognitive and motor development of children with and without congenital adrenal hyperplasia after early-prenatal dexamethasone. J Clin Endocrinol Metab 2004;89:610–4.

112. Hirvikoski T, Nordenstrom A, Lindholm T, et al. Cognitive functions in children at risk for congenital adrenal hyperplasia treated prenatally with dexamethasone. J Clin Endocrinol Metab 2007;92:542–8.

113. Hirvikoski T, Nordenstrom A, Lindholm T, et al. Long-term follow-up of prenatally treated children at risk for congenital adrenal hyperplasia: does dexamethasone cause behavioural problems? Eur J Endocrinol 2008;159:309–16.

114. Kruse B, Riepe FG, Krone N, et al. Congenital adrenal hyperplasia—how to improve the transition from adolescence to adult life. Exp Clin Endocrinol Diabetes 2004;112:343–55.

Recent Consensus Statements in Pediatric Endocrinology: A Selective Review

Michelle Klein, MD*, Anpalakan Sathasivam, MD,
Yeray Novoa, MD, Robert Rapaport, MD*

KEYWORDS

- Consensus statements • Diabetic ketoacidosis
- Small for gestational age • Idiopathic short stature
- Intersex disorders

Jo Rycroft-Malone,[1] PhD, a leading expert in the field of evidence-based medicine, said, "to achieve clinically effective care we must access three strands of evidence: knowledge from research findings, knowledge from clinical experience, and patient-specific information (including preferences and acceptability of an intervention to individuals."

Clinical guidelines and consensus statements serve to summarize and organize current knowledge on diverse subjects, and provide practical guidelines for proper clinical management. Recommendations should be based on research and evidence derived from appropriate sources. Randomized controlled trials and systematic reviews of randomized controlled trials are usually the preferred sources.[2] When a certain aspect of treatment or care has not been covered adequately in the literature, expert opinion is considered in developing guidelines.

In 2008, more than 20 consensus statements were published in the pediatric literature alone. To acquaint the reader in pediatric endocrinology with some of the major findings, the authors summarize the salient points of the latest consensus statements jointly developed by multiple endocrine societies including the Lawson Wilkins Society for Pediatric Endocrinology (LWPES) and the European Society for Pediatric Endocrinology (ESPS). Common to all of the reviewed consensus statements is the bringing

Portions of this article were previously published in the *Endocrinology and Metabolism Clinics of North America*, 38:4.
Division of Pediatric Endocrinology and Diabetes, Mount Sinai Hospital, One Gustave Levly Place, Box 1616, New York, NY 10029, USA
* Corresponding authors.
E-mail addresses: michelle.klein@mssm.edu (M. Klein); robert.rapaport@mssm.edu (R. Rapaport).

Pediatr Clin N Am 58 (2011) 1301–1315
doi:10.1016/j.pcl.2011.07.014
0031-3955/11/$ – see front matter © 2011 Elsevier Inc. All rights reserved.

together of experts in the field to review the literature, evaluate the evidence, and formulate statements representing the views of many. As much as possible, the original intent and language of the statements was respected and paraphrased. For more information and for review of sources used for the consensus statements, the reader is referred to the original published articles.

CONSENSUS STATEMENT ON THE MANAGEMENT OF DIABETIC KETOACIDOSIS IN CHILDREN AND ADOLESCENTS

The purpose was to explore management and complications of diabetic ketoacidosis (DKA) in children and adolescents to formulate a consensus on prevention and reduction of DKA.[3]

The statement was endorsed by LWPES, ESPS, International Society for Pediatric and Adolescent Diabetics (ISPAD), Juvenile Diabetes Research Foundation International (JDRF), World Federation of Pediatric Intensive and Critical Care Societies (WFPICCS), European Society for Pediatric Critical Care (ESPCC), European Society for Pediatric and Neonatal Intensive Care (ESPNIC), and Australian Pediatric Endocrine Group (APEG).

Later guidelines published by the American Diabetes Association (ADA)[4] and by the ISPAD[5] included recommendations of this consensus statement.

Definition of DKA

DKA occurs when there is a disruption in the homeostatic balance between insulin and counter-regulatory hormones secondary to a deficiency in circulating insulin and an increase in levels of catecholamines, glucagon, growth hormone, and cortisol. The result is a state of hyperglycemia, hyperosmolarity, increased lipolysis, ketonemia, and metabolic acidosis secondary to increased ketone body production. Osmotic diuresis, dehydration, and loss of electrolytes are further consequences of the hyperglycemia and acidosis.

The major biochemical diagnostic criteria for DKA include hyperglycemia (blood glucose: >11 mmol/L [approximately 200 mg/dL]) with a venous pH less than 7.3 or bicarbonate less than 15 mmol/L.[6] There are associated minor criteria including glycosuria, ketonuria, and ketonemia. DKA is classified further by the degree of the acidosis:

Mild (venous pH: <7.30; HCO3: <15 mmol/L)
Moderate (pH: <7.2; HCO3: <10 mmol/L)
Severe (pH: <7.1; HCO3: <5 mmol/L)

Clinical features of DKA include dehydration, Kussmaul breathing, severe abdominal pain, nausea, and vomiting; additionally, patients may have fever if infection is also present.[4]

Frequency of DKA

The more prevalent type I diabetes mellitus (TIDM) is in a given region, the less likely it is for DKA to be present at diagnosis. It is more common to see DKA at the onset of diabetes in children less than 4 years of age, children who do not have a first-degree relative with TIDM, and children from families of lower socioeconomic status or without ready access to medical care. Certain medications including glucocorticoids, atypical antipsychotics, and Diazoxide have been indicted as causative agents of DKA in patients not previously diagnosed with TIDM.

Factors such as poor metabolic control, a history of DKA, poor family structure, a psychiatric history, or being a peripubertal or adolescent female increase the risk of DKA in patients with TIDM. The most common reason for the occurrence of DKA (75% of cases) in these patients is either incorrect insulin dosing or absence of insulin. Other causes include insufficient amounts of insulin during stress or illness to balance counter-regulatory hormones and inappropriate cessation of insulin pump therapy.

Cerebral Edema

The first signs of cerebral edema (CE) can be subtle and nonspecific and include headache, mental status changes, bradycardia, and hypertension. Studies have shown that CE usually occurs 4 to 12 hours after management of DKA has begun, but it can occur any time before or during treatment. The incidence of CE is up to 1% in all cases of DKA.

Increased risk for CE is seen in patients who present with DKA at diagnosis, are younger, and have symptoms of DKA for a longer amount of time. Other risk factors include degree of acidosis at presentation, greater hypocapnia at presentation after adjusting for the severity of acidosis, bicarbonate treatment during DKA, elevated serum urea nitrogen at presentation, and a slower rise in measured serum sodium concentrations during treatment of DKA. Neither the severity of hyperglycemia at presentation of DKA nor the concentration of sodium in intravenous fluids has been shown to increase the risk of cerebral edema.

Management of DKA

Mild cases of DKA, in which patients have hyperglycemia and ketosis, but can tolerate oral (PO) and are not dehydrated, do not require inpatient or emergency room management. Patients who are vomiting, cannot tolerate fluids by mouth, or are dehydrated should be evaluated in an emergency room or inpatient setting. Admission to an ICU should be advised in children with severe DKA (prolonged duration of symptoms, mental status changes, or vascular compromise) or patients who are at increased risk of cerebral edema.

The initial assessment of DKA requires a detailed history and physical examination. Degree of dehydration should be assessed using weight, pulse, blood pressure and respiratory effort, capillary refill, and skin turgor. Samples for measurement of glucose, electrolytes, osmolality, venous or arterial pH and pCO2, hemoglobin and hematocrit, and HbA1c should be obtained, as well as a urinalysis for ketones.

Management of DKA in the ICU should include hourly measurement of the vital signs including strict fluid input and output, capillary blood glucose, and neurologic examinations (looking for Cushing's triad and other signs of cerebral edema). Every 2 to 4 hours, blood gases and chemistries should be done to evaluate electrolytes, serum urea nitrogen (BUN), hematocrit, and blood glucose. More frequent testing is warranted if the patient is critically ill. An electrocardiogram should be considered if potassium measurement is delayed.

Hydration Status and Fluid Replacement

Hemodynamic instability and shock are rare in pediatric DKA. Chemical measurements, as a means of assessing fluid deficit, can be unreliable at diagnosis. The extracellular fluid has higher osmolality and fluid shifts from the intracellular to extracellular compartments. Therefore, sodium measured on a blood chemistry is usually lower than the total body sodium. The effective osmolality at the time of presentation is usually in the range of 300 to 350 mOsm/L. Hemoconcentration leads to an increased BUN and hematocrit and may help to differentiate severe extracellular fluid (ECF) contraction from true hyponatremia.

Goals of therapy in DKA include replacement of diminished circulatory volume, repletion of electrolytes, recovery of the glomerular filtration rate (GFR) to further eliminate glucose and ketones from the circulation, and avoidance of complications including cerebral edema. Slower correction of overall fluid deficit with isotonic or near-isotonic fluids can lead to quicker resolution of acidosis. The risk of using large amounts of normal saline is hyperchloremic metabolic acidosis. There is no evidence supporting the use of colloids over crystalloids for DKA therapy.

Fluids given to the child before assessment should be factored into calculation of deficit. Initial intravenous fluid administration should begin immediately with an isotonic solution, which can be given if needed in a 10 to 20 cc/kg bolus over 1 to 2 hours. The remainder replacement intravenous fluid should be given evenly over at least 48 hours. Subsequent fluid management should be with a solution with a tonicity greater than or equal to 0.45% saline. In addition to clinical assessment of dehydration, calculation of effective osmolality may be valuable to guide fluid and electrolyte therapy. Because the severity of dehydration may be difficult to determine and can be overestimated, fluid infusion should not exceed a rate of 1.5 to 2 times the usual daily requirement based on age, weight, or body surface area. Urinary losses should not be added to the calculation of replacement fluids.

Insulin

After the fluid deficit and electrolyte losses are calculated, low-dose intravenous insulin administration is standard of care. The goal of insulin therapy is to inhibit lipolysis and ketogenesis and decrease the blood glucose levels. A bolus of insulin is not necessary, and its use is controversial. The dose of insulin should be maintained at 0.1 U/kg/h until resolution of ketoacidosis (pH: >7.30; HCO3: >15 mmol/L) or until the anion gap is closed. If the patient has hypoglycemia on maximum amounts of intravenous dextrose, then the insulin drip should be lowered, but not less than 0.05 U/kg/h.

To prevent hypoglycemia, glucose should be added to the intravenous fluid when the plasma glucose falls to approximately 14 to 17 mmol/L (250 to 300 mg/dL), because the resolution of acidemia usually takes longer than the normalization of blood glucose. Five percent glucose can be used initially and then slowly increased to maintain euglycemia on the insulin drip. Reassessment of the patient, review of insulin therapy, and consideration of other possible causes of impaired response to insulin should be considered (eg, infection, errors in insulin preparation, or adhesion of insulin to tubing with very dilute solutions) if biochemical parameters of ketoacidosis do not improve. In the rare event that intravenous insulin cannot be given, insulin may be administered subcutaneously or intramuscularly every hour at the same dose.

Electrolyte Replacement

In DKA, potassium is lost from the intracellular compartment as a result of insulin deficiency, hypertonicity, and the exchange of hydrogen ions within the cell. Potassium also is lost secondary to vomiting and osmotic diuresis. Therefore, serum levels of potassium are not reliable in the initial work-up of DKA. Once insulin is given, potassium will move from the extracellular to intracellular space, and serum levels will decrease. Repletion of potassium is necessary and should be started once the serum levels are no longer elevated and the patient has urinated.

In DKA, phosphate deficit also occurs as a result of osmotic diuresis and movement across the cell. Treatment with insulin results in movement of phosphate back into the intracellular space and a subsequent drop in serum phosphate. Although studies have not shown significant clinical benefit from phosphate repletion in DKA and its use remains controversial, potassium phosphate may be used safely together with potassium chloride to avoid hyperchloremia. Calcium levels should be monitored closely.

Acidosis

Fluid replacement and insulin are the first-line agents for treating acidosis. Insulin prevents ketoacid production and breaks it down into bicarbonate. Fluid replacement improves tissue perfusion and increases GFR to aid in acid excretion.

The use of bicarbonate in treating DKA remains controversial. Some studies have shown that bicarbonate may worsen electrolyte abnormalities in DKA by contributing to hypokalemia and hypernatremia via increased sodium load. Bicarbonate also can increase the synthesis of ketones in the liver and thereby slow down the time to recovery from ketoacidosis. Still, a subset of patients with severe DKA (arterial pH: <6.9) who have impaired cardiac contractility, peripheral vasodilatation, poor tissue perfusion, and life-threatening hyperkalemia may benefit from judicious use of bicarbonate.

Treatment of Cerebral Edema

The clinician should have high suspicion for CE in patients with DKA, and therapy should commence immediately once diagnosed. The head of the bed should be elevated. Intravenous fluids should be reduced, and intravenous mannitol should be given. If Mannitol is not available, 3% hypertonic saline may be used instead. Mechanical ventilation may be required if the patient's respiratory status is compromised. Studies have shown poor outcomes in patients with CE associated with DKA who were aggressively ventilated (pCO2 <22 mm Hg). The role of glucocorticoids in treatment of CE in DKA has not been supported.

Prevention of DKA

Education and early detection remain the ultimate tools in prevention. Genetic and immunologic diagnostic testing in patients at higher risk for T1DM has been shown to decrease the occurrence of DKA at onset of diabetes. In patients with TIDM, studies have shown that comprehensive health care and education including plans for sick day management and continuous subcutaneous insulin pump malfunction can help to decrease the incidence of DKA.

CONSENSUS STATEMENT ON IDIOPATHIC SHORT STATURE

The purpose was to summarize the advances in the management of children with idiopathic short stature (ISS).[7]

The statement was endorsed by: Growth Hormone Research Society (GHRS), LWPES, European Society for Pediatric Endocrinology (ESPE), Latin American Society of Pediatric Endocrinology (SLEP), Japanese Society of Pediatric Endocrinology (JSPE), Canadian Pediatric Endocrine Group (CPEG), Asia Pacific Pediatric Endocrine Society (APPES), and APEG.

Definition

ISS was defined as

> "a height more than two standard deviation scores (SDS) below the corresponding mean for a given age, sex, and population group without evidence of systemic, endocrine, nutritional, or chromosomal abnormalities"

This includes constitutional delay of growth and puberty (CDGP) and familial short stature. Children born small for gestational age, children with syndromes involving short stature, and children with chronic medical conditions that interfere with growth should be excluded from this definition.

ISS can be subdivided into two groups based on the midparental height (calculated by average of parents' heights + 6.5 cm for boys/- 6.5 cm for girls.)[8] One group is children whose adult height is about the same as the midparental height, and the other is children whose adult height is below the midparental height.

Assessment of the Short Child

Each evaluation of a short child should begin with a comprehensive history:

- Birth history (including in utero events, anthropomorphic data at birth, amniocentesis, gestational age, and complications)
- Medical history including hospitalizations, surgeries, medications, chronic diseases, dietary history, developmental history including dentition, which can parallel bone maturation
- Family history focusing on stature, onset of puberty, and chronic diseases of first- and second-degree family members; consanguinity should be documented
- Pubertal history of the patient
- Prior growth point or curves

The physical examination should include the general appearance, any dysmorphic features, and body disproportions. A length should be obtained in all children under 3 years of age with a recumbent stadiometer. A standing stadiometer can be used in cooperative children over 3 years of age. Arm span, sitting height or upper-to-lower segment ratios, body mass index (BMI), and for children younger than 4 years measurement of the head circumference should be included. Pubertal status using Tanner staging should be documented.

DIAGNOSTIC STUDIES

If the history and physical examination do not reveal a specific diagnosis, the following screening tests are indicated:

A complete blood count
Sedimentation rate
A complete metabolic panel
Screening for celiac disease
Thyroid function tests
Insulin-like growth factor (IGF)-1 level
A radiograph for bone age (BA).

In a female with unexplained short stature or in any male with genital abnormalities, a karyotype should be done. Skeletal survey should be reserved for patients with suspicion of a skeletal dysplasia.

It is strongly recommended that IGF-1 levels be obtained as part of the evaluation. Insulin-like growth factor binding protein (IGFBP-3) measurements add little to the evaluation of short stature except in children younger than 3 years. Measures of spontaneous growth hormone (GH) secretion are not indicated. GH stimulation testing should be performed in any patient with a history and physical examination suggestive of GH deficiency, a low growth velocity or low IGF-1 levels. A peak stimulated GH value less than 10 ng/dL is considered GH deficiency (and thus excludes ISS). If a diagnosis of ISS is made, a head magnetic resonance imaging (MRI) scan is not indicated.

Genetic testing including short stature homeobox (SHOX) gene analysis should be considered in appropriate clinical settings.

TREATMENT

The primary goal of treatment is to reach a normal adult height. A secondary goal is to reach a more socially acceptable height during childhood. In the United States, GH treatment has been approved for children shorter than -2.25 SDS (1.2 percentile). Children whose heights are -2 SDS and who are more than 2 SDS below their midparental target height (TH) or their predicted adult height (PAH) also should be considered for treatment. There are no laboratory criteria for starting GH therapy. Optimal age for initiating treatment is 5 years to early puberty (most studies examined children older than 3 to 4 years). The role of PAH in the decision to treat with GH is unclear. The PAH may be inaccurate, but it can be a helpful tool together with other factors (BA, family height and pubertal history, and midparental target height) in deciding to treat.

Dosing and Duration of GH Treatment

Current US Food and Drug Administration (FDA)-approved dosing for GH in children with ISS is up to 0.3 to 0.37 mg/kg/wk (42 to 52 µg/k/d).[9] There are no data on long-term safety of doses higher than 0.35 mg/k/wk (50 µg/k/d) in children with ISS. The dose of GH is adjusted based on weight gain and interval growth velocity. IGF-1 measurements are also useful in assessing efficacy, safety, and compliance. Increased short-term growth is achieved with higher IGF-1 values, but there are no long-term studies to asses the safety or ultimate effect of these elevated levels. The current recommendation is if IGF-1 levels are consistently above 2.5 SDS, the dose of GH should be reduced.

There are two groups with differing ideas about when to stop treatment with GH. One group recommends stopping GH when near-adult height is reached (height velocity <2 cm/y or BA >16 years in boys or >14 years in girls). The other group recommends stopping GH when the height is in the normal adult range (above -2 SDS) or has reached another cut-off for the reference adult population. The individual patient's desire to terminate treatment should be considered at each visit.

Response to GH

Change in height SDS of more than 0.3 to 0.5, height velocity increase of more than 3 cm/y, and height velocity SDS increase of more than 1 suggest a successful first-year response to GH. The dose of GH can be increased if the growth velocity is decreased, and compliance is assured. If the rate of growth is still suboptimal after 1 to 2 years of higher doses of GH, then GH treatment should be stopped and other treatment options considered.

Children with ISS on GH therapy (average duration 4 to 7 years) have a mean increase in adult height of 3.5 to 7.5 cm. Responses are highly variable and are dose-dependent. Children who are younger, heavier, who receive higher doses per kilogram, and who are shortest relative to target height have the best growth response. Adult height outcome is influenced negatively by older age at the start of treatment and is influenced positively by a taller midparental height, a taller height at the start of treatment, a greater BA delay, and a greater first-year response to GH therapy.

Monitoring

Adverse effects noted in children receiving GH for ISS are generally the same as those previously reported in children receiving GH for other indications, although they occur less frequently.[10] Height, weight, pubertal development, and adverse effects to GH should be monitored every 3 to 6 months in children treated with GH. Regular evaluations for scoliosis, tonsillar hypertrophy, papilledema, and slipped capital femoral epiphysis should be performed. After 1 year of treatment, the response to GH should be assessed by calculating height velocity SDS and the change in height SDS. A BA may be obtained periodically. No instances of elevated blood glucose in GH-treated patients with ISS have been reported.

Alternative to GH Treatment

Anabolic steroids, such as oxandrolone (given orally) and testosterone (patch or gel) are alternative treatment options. Both have been shown useful in boys with CDGP and short stature greater than -2.5 SDS. If the adult height prediction is close to the target height, then testosterone has been shown to be the most appropriate treatment. Oxandrolone has not been shown to significantly increase predicted or measured adult height.

IGF-1 is FDA-approved for short stature associated with severe IGF deficiency and normal GH secretion. Children first should be given a trial of GH, and if they do not respond, IGF-1 should be considered. Data are lacking regarding efficacy and safety.

GnRH analogs (GnRHa) are not recommended to be used alone in children with ISS, but in combination with GH it has potential value if it is used for at least 3 years. Its use might be considered if the PAH is below 2 SDS at the time of onset of puberty. When using GnRHa, one must consider the psychological effects of delaying puberty.

Studies using aromatase inhibitors (AIs) for at least 2 years have shown that males with ISS on GH have an increase in PAH.[11,12] The long-term efficacy and safety of AI in males have not been demonstrated. No data support the use of AI in females.

CONSENSUS STATEMENT ON THE MANAGEMENT OF THE CHILD BORN SMALL FOR GESTATIONAL AGE THROUGH TO ADULTHOOD

The purpose was to identify key health issues facing children born small for gestational age (SGA) and to propose management strategies.[13]

The statement was endorsed by: ESPE, LWPES, GHRS, SLEP, APPES, APEG, JSPE.

Definition

To diagnose a child as SGA the following information must be obtained:

Gestational age (preferably calculated from the first trimester ultrasound examination)
Birth weight, length, and head circumference
Reference cut-off defined by a comparable population of patients, below which the definition lies.

The definition of SGA is birth weight or birth length less than -2 SD below the mean specific for the population. Children born SGA must be monitored for many health issues including heart disease, perinatal morbidity, associated neurodevelopmental disorders, poor growth/short stature, and metabolic irregularities.

Early Growth and Development

Longitudinal studies of growth in children born SGA have shown weight catch-up usually occurs in the first 6 months, while height catch-up can take up to 2 years. Ninety percent of children born SGA do catch-up. Factors that decrease the chance of catch-up growth include severe prematurity, growth retardation, and very low birth weight, while having tall parents increases the likelihood of catch-up.

Children born SGA should be monitored with measurements of length, weight, and head circumference every 3 months for the first year of life and every 6 months thereafter. Pediatricians should be aware of children who do not catch-up in the first 6 months of life or remain short by 2 years of age. These children should be referred to a pediatric endocrinologist.

Children born SGA have increased central adiposity and decreased lean mass. Studies have shown rapid weight gain in infancy is associated with obesity as an adult; therefore earlier dense feedings for SGA infants may not be appropriate.

Endocrinopathies and Metabolic Disorders

Overall, there are no true endocrinopathies associated with SGA. Classic growth GH deficiency usually is not seen. IGF1 and IGFBP3 levels are decreased 1 SDS in SGA children; however, they are not predictive of growth velocity or adult height. Routine evaluation of the hypothalamic-pituitary-adrenal and the thyroid axes are not recommended.

Being born SGA is not associated with late or early puberty. The small population of children who do have early puberty also have rapid puberty, leading to faster bone maturation and ultimately decreased adult height. Bone age is unreliable in children born SGA, and height prediction based on it is not routinely recommended. Hypospadias and cryptorchidism are observed in children born SGA.

Type 2 diabetes mellitus, adolescent hypertension, impaired glucose tolerance, and dyslipidemia have not been shown to occur more frequently in children born SGA. Insulin resistance, however, has been shown to occur as early as 1 year of age. Although the overall prevalence of risk factors is low, young adults born SGA have a higher incidence of metabolic risk factors (2.3%), especially if they are obese, of a certain ethnicity, and have strong family history.

Management of Growth and Puberty

Early evaluation of short children born SGA is recommended. There are over 40 years of research on the use of GH in children with SGA, and its use has been approved by the FDA and the European Agency for the Evaluation of Medicinal Products. The general consensus is that children between the ages of 2 to 4 years born SGA who have not caught up with a height less than 2.5 SD should be treated with GH. If the child is over the age of 4 years and does not show catch-up growth, then a height of 2 SD should be used as the cut-off. The starting dose of GH is 0.24 to 0.49 mg/kg/wk (35 to 70 μg/kg/d), with the higher doses used in those with the most marked growth retardation.[14]

Age and height SDS at the start of treatment, midparental height, and dose of GH all influence the response during the first 2 to 3 years. Children with recognized syndromes respond less well to GH than those with nonsyndromic SGA. A growth velocity of more than + 0.5 SDS in the first year of treatment is considered a positive response to GH treatment. If there is a poor response, re-evaluation is indicated, including consideration of compliance, dose of GH, diagnosis, and the decision to discontinue treatment. In those with a positive response, withdrawal of GH therapy after 2 to 3 years leads to catch-down growth and is not recommended. GH should be stopped in adolescence when the growth velocity falls to less than 2 cm/y.

There is no evidence that the addition of a GnRH analog is associated with additional height gain in children born SGA. Pre-treatment IGF-1 levels may have a role in predicting responsiveness to GH, and in those receiving treatment, IGF-1 monitoring may be a useful tool for dose optimization. Some syndromes, such as Bloom's syndrome or Fanconi syndrome may carry risks that may contraindicate the use of GH therapy. Adverse effects from GH treatment are not seen more commonly in children born SGA compared with other conditions.

Consequences in Adulthood

Studies have shown that children born SGA are at increased risk for metabolic consequences later on in life. Most of the evidence, however, comes from observational studies not limited to children born SGA. A rapid weight gain in infancy has been associated with an increased risk of obesity. Both small and large sizes at birth have been reported to be associated with increased risk of type 2 diabetes and glucose intolerance. Women born SGA are at an increased risk of having an SGA infant, preeclampsia, and gestational diabetes.

CONSENSUS STATEMENT ON MANAGEMENT OF INTERSEX DISORDERS

The purpose was to review the management of intersex disorders and devise a consensus statement on definitions, diagnosis, and management, and formulated proposals for future studies.[15]

The consensus statement was endorsed by LWPES, ESPE.

Introduction and Definitions

The definitions and nomenclature for intersex disorders are being reviewed and reworked continually as a result of dissatisfaction amongs health care professionals, families, and patients with the current terminology. The term disorders of sex development (DSD), as defined by congenital conditions in which development of chromosomal, gonadal, or anatomic sex is atypical was proposed by the consensus committee. This phrase would replace terminology such as intersex, pseudohermaphroditism, hermaphroditism, and sex reversal, as these terms are potentially imprecise and derogatory (**Table 1**).

Psychosexual development is shaped by both biologic and environmental influences including exposure to androgens, genetics, neuro-anatomy, and family and social history. To understand psychosexual development, one must define its three components:

1. Gender identity—a person's self-representation as male or female (some individuals may not identify exclusively with either)

Table 1 Proposed revised nomenclature	
Previous	**Proposed**
Intersex	Disorders of sex development (DSD)
Male pseudohermaphrodite, undervirilization of an XY male	46, XY DSD
Female pseudohermaphrodite, overvirilization of an XX female, and masculinization of an XX female	46, XX DSD
True hermaphrodite	Ovotesticular DSD
XX male or XX sex reversal	46, XX testicular DSD
XY sex reversal	46, XY complete gonadal dysgenesis

2. Gender role—the psychological characteristics that are sexually dimorphic within the general population, such as toy preferences and physical aggression
3. Sexual orientation—the direction(s) of erotic interest (heterosexual, bisexual, homosexual).

Gender dissatisfaction occurs more often in people with DSD than in the general population and signifies discontent with sex assignment. Psychosocial care, like medical and surgical care, is an integral part of DSD management.

Clinical Management of DSD

DSD usually is diagnosed in newborns with atypical genitalia, with congenital adrenal hyperplasia (CAH) remaining the most common cause.[16] DSD, however, may be diagnosed in the older child or adult who presents with) gynecomastia or hematuria in a male, inguinal hernia, virilization, or primary amenorrhea in a female, or delayed/partial puberty or previously unrecognized genital ambiguity.

Specifically, criteria suggestive of DSD include:

Obvious genital ambiguity
Female genitalia with an enlarged clitoris, posterior labial fusion, or an inguinal/labial mass
Male genitalia with bilateral undescended testes, micropenis, isolated perineal hypospadias, or mild hypospadias with undescended testis
Family history of DSD
Discordance between genital appearance and a prenatal karyotype.

In newborns with DSD, gender assignment should not occur until an evaluation is performed by an experienced multidisciplinary team including a pediatric endocrinologist, surgeon/urologist, psychologist/psychiatrist, geneticist, gynecologist, and neonatologist. All individuals should receive a gender assignment. The families should be involved in the decision-making process, and in the case of older children, the patient should be involved also.

A comprehensive history including prenatal and family history should be obtained followed by a complete physical examination. The examination of the genitalia must be thorough and documented well. Anatomy should be compared with published norms.

Initial testing should be tailored to clinical findings depends on availability of testing at the individual center. First-line testing should include:

Fluorescence in situ hybridization (FISH) with X- and Y-specific probe detection (even when prenatal karyotype is available)
A full karyotype
Imaging of the abdomen and pelvis via sonography
Measurement of 17-hydroxyprogesterone
Testosterone
Gonadotropins
Anti-Müllerian Hormone
Serum electrolytes
Urinalysis.

The results obtained from these tests should be sufficient for making a diagnosis within the category of DSD. Should the diagnosis remain elusive, additional testing can include

Human chorionic gonadotropin- and adrenocorticotropin-stimulation tests (to assess testicular and adrenal steroid biosynthesis)

Urinary steroid analysis by gas chromatography mass spectroscopy

Imaging studies

Gonadal biopsies

DNA analysis of the main genes in the pathway of testis differentiation and functionality.

Despite all of the available testing, only 20% of cases of DSD have an identified molecular diagnosis. Only 50% of 46,XY children with DSD will receive a definitive diagnosis.

Assigning Gender in Newborns

After a comprehensive evaluation, deciding on gender assignment is a daunting and stressful task for both the health care team and family. The following evidence from patients with DSD should be used along with individual factors including opinions of the family and their cultural practices, genital appearance and surgical options, a need for lifelong replacement therapy, and potential for fertility . Evidence to assist in sex assignment includes

Markedly virilized 46, XX infants with CAH should be raised as female, because more than 90% of patients with 46XX CAH identify as female.

60% of patients with 5-alpha-reductase-deficiency assigned female as a newborn and who then virilized at puberty lived as males. This along with the potential for fertility as a male should be discussed when deciding on gender assignment. Although fertility is less well documented in 17-beta-hydroxysteroid dehydrogenase deficiency, the same considers should be made.

25% of patients with partial androgen insensitivity syndrome (PAIS), androgen biosynthetic defects, and incomplete gonadal dysgenesis were dissatisfied with their assigned sex whether male of female.

Available data support male rearing in all patients with micropenis, again taking into consideration fertility.

Potential for fertility on the basis of gonadal differentiation and genital development should be considered in patients with ovotesticular DSD

Prenatal androgen exposure, testicular function at and after puberty, phallic development, and gonadal location should be considered in patients with mixed gonadal dysgenesis (MGD).

65% of individuals with cloacal exostrophy lived as female, but there was still variability in gender identity outcome.

Surgical Management

Surgeons should have both pediatric training and expertise in DSD surgery. Early genitoplasty is acceptable if the cause of DSD has been identified, and severe virilization (Prader 3 to 4) exists. Genitoplasty should be performed in concordance with repair of the common urogenital sinus. The surgical procedure should focus on preservation of erectile function and the innervation of the clitoris. Vaginal dilatation should not be used in childhood. It is expected that revision of surgeries done in infancy will be necessary at the time of puberty or shortly after.

If there is less severe clitoromegaly and no involvement of the urogenital sinus, then surgery should be postponed until adolescence. Once a patient with an absent or inadequate vagina is psychologically motivated and a full partner is involved, then vaginoplasty should be performed. Unfortunately, self-dilatation, skin substitution, and bowel vaginoplasty all have pros and cons, and none has been universally successful.

If hypospadias is associated with a DSD, then surgical repair and testosterone supplementation are recommended. There is no evidence that removal of asymptomatic discordant structures prophylactically is necessary. Symptoms in the future may suggest the need for surgical removal.

The testes in patients with DSD raised female should be removed to prevent malignancy in adulthood. Because the earliest reported malignancy was at 14 years of age, a parents' right to refuse removal of the testes until adolescence is supported. The availability of estrogen-replacement therapy allows for the option of early removal at the time of diagnosis. The streak gonad in a patient with MGD raised male should be removed in early childhood. Females with gonadal dysgenesis (bilateral streak gonads) and Y-chromosome material should have bilateral gonadectomy performed in early childhood. Gonadectomy should be performed before puberty in patients with androgen biosynthetic defects raised female.

Testicular biopsy should be performed at puberty in patients with gonadal dysgenesis to monitor for premalignant lesion termed carcinoma in situ or undifferentiated intratubular germ cell neoplasia. If the biopsy is positive, the patient should be given the option of sperm banking. Treatment with local low-dose radiation is curative.

Replacement of Sex Steroids

The goal of replacement of sex steroids in patients with DSD is to mimic normal pubertal maturation so that the patient experiences a normal pubertal growth spurt, secondary sexual characteristics, and appropriate bone mineral accumulation. Testosterone is available as an intramuscular depot injection, an oral preparation, and transdermal preparations. The depot injection is the most commonly used. Patients with PAIS may require supraphysiologic doses of testosterone for optimal effect.

Females with hypogonadism require estrogen supplementation to induce a pubertal growth spurt, secondary sexual characteristics such as breasts, and menarche. A progestin usually is added after breakthrough bleeding develops or within 1 to 2 years of continuous estrogen. In women without a uterus, there is no evidence that the addition of cyclic progesterone is beneficial.

Psychosocial Management and Long-Term Outcomes

Psychosocial care provided by mental health staff with expertise in DSD is an integral part of management of DSD. The earliest age at which gender identity can be assessed accurately remains unclear, but it is thought to begin before the age of 3 years. Atypical gender role behavior is more common in children with DSD. In affected children and adolescents who report significant gender dysphoria, a specialist in psychosexual development is crucial to help the patient identify feelings about gender. If the patient expresses a desire to change gender, the patient's wish should be supported. Patients with DSD often complain of sexual aversion and lack of arousability, which often are misinterpreted as decreased libido. A support network including medical and psychological professionals is crucial to identifying and treating these important issues.

There is much needed follow-up for long-term outcomes for patients with DSD including medical, surgical, and psychological. What is known is related mainly to surgical outcomes and sexual function. Early surgery, while successful in many cases, does run the risk of decreased sexual sensitivity, loss of clitoral tissue, and cosmetic

---

Box 1
Abbreviations of organizations

APEG-Australian Pediatric Endocrine Group

APPES-Asia Pacific Pediatric Endocrine Society

CPEG-Canadian Pediatric Endocrine Group

ESPCC-European Society for Pediatric Critical Care

ESPNIC-European Society of Pediatric and Neonatal Intensive Care

ESPE-European Society for Pediatric Endocrinology

GHRS-Growth Hormone Research Society

ISPAD-International Society

JDRF-Juvenile Diabetes Research Foundation International

JSPE-Japanese Society of Pediatric Endocrinology

LWPES-Lawson Wilkins Pediatric Endocrine Society

SLEP-Latin American Society of Pediatric Endocrinology

WFPICCS-World Federation of Pediatric Intensive and Critical Care Societies

---

concerns. The success of the surgery depends on the experience, skill, and technique of the surgeon. Scarring may need revision to insure proper sexual function. Surgery to construct a neovagina carries a risk of neoplasia. The degree of hypospadias and the amount of erectile tissue play a large role in the surgical result of undermasculinized males with a phallus. Feminizing genitoplasty requires less surgery to achieve an acceptable outcome compared to masculinizing genitoplasty and results in fewer urologic difficulties.

The highest tumor risk is found in TSPY (testis-specific protein Y-encoded) positive gonadal dysgenesis and PAIS with intra-abdominal gonads, whereas the lowest risk (<5%) is found in ovotestis and complete androgen insensitivity syndrome (CAIS). For a complete list please refer to the consensus statement (**Box 1**).

Addendum to Consensus Statement

Since publication of the consensus statement on management of intersex disorders, some have recommended the term atypical genitalia replace the previous term ambiguous genitalia.[17,18]

REFERENCES

1. Rycroft-Malone J. Formal consensus: the development of a national clinical guideline. Qual Health Care 2001;10:238–44.
2. Grimshaw JM, Russel IT. Achieving health gains through clinical guidelines: I. Developing scientifically valid guidelines. Qual Assur Health Care 1993;2:243–8.
3. Dunger DB, Sperling MA, Acerini CL, et al. European Society for Pediatric Endocrinology/Lawson Wilkins Pediatric Endocrine Society consensus statement on diabetic ketoacidosis in children and adolescents. Pediatrics 2004;113:e133–40.
4. Wolfsdorf J, Glaser N, Sperling MA. Diabetic ketoacidosis in infants, children, and adolescents. A consensus statement from the American Diabetes Association. Diabetes Care 2006;29(5):1150–9.

5. Wolfsdorf J, Craig ME, Daneman D, et al. ISPAD Clinical practice consensus guidelines 2006–2007. Diabetic ketoacidosis. Pediatr Diabetes 2007;8:28–43.
6. Dunger DB, Sperling MA, Acerni CL, et al. ESPE/LWPES consensus statement on diabetic ketoacidosis in children and adolescents. Arch Dis Child 2004;89: 188–94.
7. Cohen P, Rogol AD, Deal CL, et al. Consensus statement on the diagnosis and treatment of children with idiopathic short stature: a summary of the Growth Hormone Research Society, the Lawson Wilkins Pediatric Endocrine Society, and the European Society for Paediatric Endocrinology Workshop. J Clin Endocrinol Metab 2008;93(11):4210–7.
8. Lee M. Idiopathic short stature. N Engl J Med 2006;354:2576–82.
9. Wit J, Rekers-Mombarg L, Cutler G, et al. Growth hormone treatment to final height in children with idiopathic short stature: evidence for a dose effect. J Pediatr 2004;146:45–53.
10. Quigley C, Gill A, Crowe B, et al. Safety of growth hormone treatment in pediatric patients with idiopathic short stature. J Clin Endocrinol Metab 2005;90:5188–96.
11. Hero M, Norjavaara E, Dunkel L. Inhibition of estrogen biosíntesis with a potent aromatase inhibitor increases predicted adult height in boys with idiopathic short stature: a randomized controlled trial. J Clin Endocrinol Metab 2005;90: 6396–402.
12. Hero M, Wickman S, Dunkel L. Treatment with the aromastase inhibitor letrozole during adolescence increases near-final height in boys with constitutional delay of puberty. Clin Endocrinol 2006;64:510–3.
13. Clayton PE, Cianfarani S, Czernichow P, et al. Consensus statement: management of the child born small for gestational age through to adulthood: a consensus statement of the International Societies of Pediatric Endocrinology and the Growth Hormone Research Society. J Clin Endocrinol Metab 2007; 92(3):804–10.
14. Rapaport R, Saenger P, Wajnrajch MP, et al. Predictors of first-year growth response to a fixed-dose of growth hormone treatment in children born small for gestational age: results of an open-label, multicenter trial in the United States. J Pediatr Endocrinol Metab 2008;21:411–22.
15. Lee PA, Houk CP, Ahmed SF, et al. Consensus statement on Management of Intersex Disorders. International Consensus Conference on Intersex. Pediatrics 2006;118:e488–500.
16. Hughes I. Disorders of sex development: a new definition and classification. Best Pract Res Clin Endocrinol Metab 2008;22(1):119–34.
17. Rapaport R. Disorders of the gonads. In: Behrman RE, Kliegman RM, Jenson HB, editors. Nelson textbook of pediatrics. 17th edition. Philadelphia: Saunders; 2004. p. 1921–46.
18. Klein G, Rapaport R. Early diagnosis and management of atypical-appearing genitalia. In: Altchek A, Deligdisch L, editors. Pediatric, adolescent and young adult gynecology. West Sussex, UK: Wiley-Blackwell; 2009. p. 14–24.

Index

Note: Page numbers of article titles are in **boldface** type.

A

Accretropin (growth hormone), 1144
Acromegaly, genomics of, 1070
AD36 adenovirus infections, obesity in, 1224
Adiponectin, in metabolic syndrome, 1246
Adrenal gland
   congenital hyperplasia of. *See* Congenital adrenal hyperplasia.
   insufficiency of
      genomics of, 1068
      in newborns, 1088–1090
Adrenoleukodystrophy, 1068
AIRE gene, mutations of, hypogonadism in, 1191
Albright's hereditary osteodystrophy, obesity in, 1222
Alström syndrome, obesity in, 1223
Ambiguous genitalia, in congenital adrenal hyperplasia, 1290–1291
Amiloride, for diabetes insipidus, 1273
Anabolic steroids, for short stature, 1308
Anastrozole, for short stature, 1169–1176
Androgen insensitivity syndrome, 1068, 1187, 1189
Androgenization, in congenital adrenal hyperplasia, 1281–1284
Angelman syndrome, 1150
Anorexia nervosa, 1122
Anorexigenic agents, for obesity, 1228–1229
Anosmia, in Kollmann syndrome, 1182–1184
Anosmin-1 defects
   hypogonadism in, 1182–1184
   short stature in, 1066–1067
Antidiuretic hormone. *See* Vasopressin.
Antithyroid drugs
   for congenital hyperthyroidism, 1110–1112
   maternal, newborn thyroid dysfunction in, 1108
Aphallia, hypogonadism in, 1187–1188
Appetite suppressants, for obesity, 1228–1229
Aquaporin, deficiency of, 1069
Aromatase inhibitors, for short stature, 1169–1176, 1308
Asia Pacific Pediatric Endocrine Society, consensus statements endorsed by, 1301–1315
Athletic competition, aromatase inhibitors banned in, 1175
Australian Pediatric Endocrine Group, consensus statements endorsed by, 1301–1315
Autoimmune disorders
   gonadal failure, 1191
   polyglandular syndromes, 1068
   type 1 diabetes mellitus as, 1093–1094, **1257–1270**

Pediatr Clin N Am 58 (2011) 1317–1332
doi:10.1016/S0031-3955(11)00126-X
0031-3955/11/$ – see front matter © 2011 Elsevier Inc. All rights reserved.

pediatric.theclinics.com

United States Postal Service

Statement of Ownership, Management, and Circulation
(All Periodicals Publications Except Requester Publications)

1. Publication Title	2. Publication Number	3. Filing Date
Pediatric Clinics of North America	4 2 4 - 6 6 6 0	9/16/11

4. Issue Frequency	5. Number of Issues Published Annually	6. Annual Subscription Price
Feb, Apr, Jun, Aug, Oct, Dec	6	$179.00

7. Complete Mailing Address of Known Office of Publication (Not printer) (Street, city, county, state, and ZIP+4®)

Elsevier Inc.
360 Park Avenue South
New York, NY 10010-1710

Contact Person
Amy S. Beacham

Telephone (Include area code)
215-239-3687

8. Complete Mailing Address of Headquarters or General Business Office of Publisher (Not printer)

Elsevier Inc., 360 Park Avenue South, New York, NY 10010-1710

9. Full Names and Complete Mailing Addresses of Publisher, Editor, and Managing Editor (Do not leave blank)

Publisher (Name and complete mailing address)

Kim Murphy, Elsevier, Inc., 1600 John F. Kennedy Blvd. Suite 1800, Philadelphia, PA 19103-2899

Editor (Name and complete mailing address)

Kerry Holland, Elsevier, Inc., 1600 John F. Kennedy Blvd. Suite 1800, Philadelphia, PA 19103-2899

Managing Editor (Name and complete mailing address)

Sarah Barth, Elsevier, Inc., 1600 John F. Kennedy Blvd. Suite 1800, Philadelphia, PA 19103-2899

10. Owner (Do not leave blank. If the publication is owned by a corporation, give the name and address of the corporation immediately followed by the names and addresses of all stockholders owning or holding 1 percent or more of the total amount of stock. If not owned by a corporation, give the names and addresses of the individual owners. If owned by a partnership or other unincorporated firm, give its name and address as well as those of each individual owner. If the publication is published by a nonprofit organization, give its name and address.)

Full Name	Complete Mailing Address
Wholly owned subsidiary of	4520 East-West Highway
Reed/Elsevier, US holdings	Bethesda, MD 20814

11. Known Bondholders, Mortgagees, and Other Security Holders Owning or Holding 1 Percent or More of Total Amount of Bonds, Mortgages, or Other Securities. If none, check box. ☐ None

Full Name	Complete Mailing Address
N/A	

12. Tax Status (For completion by nonprofit organizations authorized to mail at nonprofit rates) (Check one)
The purpose, function, and nonprofit status of this organization and the exempt status for federal income tax purposes:
☐ Has Not Changed During Preceding 12 Months
☐ Has Changed During Preceding 12 Months (Publisher must submit explanation of change with this statement)

PS Form 3526, September 2007 (Page 1 of 3 (Instructions Page 3)) PSN 7530-01-000-9931 PRIVACY NOTICE: See our Privacy policy in www.usps.com

---

13. Publication Title	14. Issue Date for Circulation Data Below
Pediatric Clinics of North America	June 2011

15. Extent and Nature of Circulation		Average No. Copies Each Issue During Preceding 12 Months	No. Copies of Single Issue Published Nearest to Filing Date
a. Total Number of Copies (Net press run)		3935	3400
b. Paid Circulation (By Mail and Outside the Mail)	(1) Mailed Outside-County Paid Subscriptions Stated on PS Form 3541. (Include paid distribution above nominal rate, advertiser's proof copies, and exchange copies)	1665	1457
	(2) Mailed In-County Paid Subscriptions Stated on PS Form 3541 (Include paid distribution above nominal rate, advertiser's proof copies, and exchange copies)		
	(3) Paid Distribution Outside the Mails Including Sales Through Dealers and Carriers, Street Vendors, Counter Sales, and Other Paid Distribution Outside USPS®	1123	866
	(4) Paid Distribution by Other Classes Mailed Through the USPS (e.g. First-Class Mail®)		
c. Total Paid Distribution (Sum of 15b (1), (2), (3), and (4))	▶	2788	2323
d. Free or Nominal Rate Distribution (By Mail and Outside the Mail)	(1) Free or Nominal Rate Outside-County Copies Included on PS Form 3541	90	76
	(2) Free or Nominal Rate In-County Copies Included on PS Form 3541		
	(3) Free or Nominal Rate Copies Mailed at Other Classes Through the USPS (e.g. First-Class Mail)		
	(4) Free or Nominal Rate Distribution Outside the Mail (Carriers or other means)		
e. Total Free or Nominal Rate Distribution (Sum of 15d (1), (2), (3) and (4))	▶	90	76
f. Total Distribution (Sum of 15c and 15e)	▶	2878	2399
g. Copies not Distributed (See instructions to publishers #4 (page #3))	▶	1057	1001
h. Total (Sum of 15f and g)	▶	3935	3400
i. Percent Paid (15c divided by 15f times 100)		96.87%	96.83%

16. Publication of Statement of Ownership

☐ If the publication is a general publication, publication of this statement is required. Will be printed in the October 2011 issue of this publication.   ☐ Publication not required

17. Signature and Title of Editor, Publisher, Business Manager, or Owner

[signature] Date September 16, 2011

Amy S. Beacham, Senior Inventory Distribution Coordinator

I certify that all information furnished on this form is true and complete. I understand that anyone who furnishes false or misleading information on this form or who omits material or information requested on the form may be subject to criminal sanctions (including fines and imprisonment) and/or civil sanctions (including civil penalties).

PS Form 3526, September 2007 (Page 2 of 3)

Moving?

Make sure your subscription moves with you!

To notify us of your new address, find your **Clinics Account Number** (located on your mailing label above your name), and contact customer service at:

Email: journalscustomerservice-usa@elsevier.com

800-654-2452 (subscribers in the U.S. & Canada)
314-447-8871 (subscribers outside of the U.S. & Canada)

Fax number: 314-447-8029

Elsevier Health Sciences Division
Subscription Customer Service
3251 Riverport Lane
Maryland Heights, MO 63043

*To ensure uninterrupted delivery of your subscription, please notify us at least 4 weeks in advance of move.

Printed and bound by CPI Group (UK) Ltd, Croydon, CR0 4YY

03/10/2024

01040447-0008